A Nurse's Survival Guide to the Ward

To our families

For Churchill Livingstone:

Senior Commissioning Editor: Ninette Premdas
Project Development Manager: Katrina Mather
Design: Judith Wright

A Nurse's Survival Guide to the Ward

Ann Richards

RGN DIPN (LON) BA(HONS) MSC RNT
Senior Lecturer, Department of Nursing and Paramedic Studies,
University of Hertfordshire, Herts, UK

Sharon Edwards

MSC PGCEA RGN DIPN(LON)
Senior Lecturer, Department of Nursing and Paramedic Studies,
University of Hertfordshire, Herts, UK

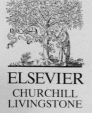

ELSEVIER
CHURCHILL
LIVINGSTONE

CHURCHILL LIVINGSTONE
An imprint of Elsevier Limited

First published 2003
Reprinted 2003, 2004 (twice), 2005

ISBN 0 443 05395 2

British Library Cataloguing in Publication Data
A catalogue record for this book is available from the British Library

Library of Congress Cataloguing in Publication Data
A catalogue record for this book is available from the Library of
Congress

Note
Medical knowledge is constantly changing. As new information
becomes available, changes in treatment, procedures, equipment and the
use of drugs become necessary. The authors and the publishers have
taken care to ensure that the information given in this text is accurate
and up to date. However, readers are strongly advised to confirm that
the information, especially with regard to drug usage, complies with the
latest legislation and standards of practice.

The Publisher

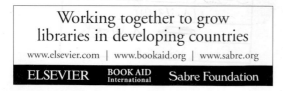

ELSEVIER   your source for books,
            journals and multimedia
            in the health sciences

www.elsevierhealth.com

Working together to grow
libraries in developing countries

www.elsevier.com | www.bookaid.org | www.sabre.org

ELSEVIER   BOOK AID   Sabre Foundation
            International

The
publisher's
policy is to use
paper manufactured
from sustainable forests

Printed in China

Contents

Preface   *vii*

SECTION 1 Your job and its organization   *1*
1.1 Organizing yourself   *2*
1.2 Emergency situations   *11*

SECTION 2 Assessing and investigating   *23*
2.1 Identification of patient problems   *24*
2.2 Assessment   *30*
2.3 Observations and measurements   *43*
2.4 Procedures and investigations   *56*
2.5 Nursing care issues   *81*

SECTION 3 Procedures   *101*
3.1 General principles and procedures   *102*
3.2 Infection and its control   *111*
3.3 Fluid and electrolyte balance   *117*
3.4 Nutritional support   *130*

SECTION 4 A systems approach   *137*
4.1 The cardiovascular system   *138*
4.2 The respiratory system   *159*
4.3 The blood   *172*
4.4 The gastrointestinal system   *189*
4.5 The renal system   *221*
4.6 The nervous system   *230*
4.7 The endocrine system   *249*
4.8 Diseases of bones and joints   *266*
4.9 The immune system   *283*
4.10 Cancer   *291*
4.11 Surgery   *305*

SECTION 5 Pharmacology   *307*
5.1 Drugs and the law   *308*
5.2 Administration of drugs   *309*
5.3 Nurse prescribing   *310*
5.4 Pharmacology in practice   *311*
5.5 Classification of drugs   *315*
5.6 Poisoning   *325*

References   *331*

Further reading   *333*

Appendix 1 Units of measurement   *335*
Appendix 2 Normal values   *339*
Appendix 3 Drug measurement and calculations   *343*

Glossary   *347*

Index   *351*

Preface

The ability to provide good evidence-based care for all patients on our ever busier hospital wards is what all practising nurses, both pre- and post-qualification, seek to achieve. This little book aims to be a survival guide and constant companion during those first early days in practice as a student and hopefully will also provide answers to some of the many questions you will continue to ask well beyond your qualification and early years as a staff nurse.

The book is a compact and pocket-sized companion that we hope will come to be regarded by its users as a friend in need. It is divided into five sections covering aspects of care and management on the ward today. Here, you will find not only information on clinical procedures, emergency situations and drugs but also common medical and surgical conditions briefly described using a body systems approach. The aim is to provide the factual information needed to assist in your provision of holistic care. Although the book is aimed primarily at nurses, we feel sure that its content will be relevant for all those working in healthcare today.

The idea for this book originally came from a student nurse at York who was, at the time, working in a frantically busy medical ward. His pleas for such a book were so heartfelt that Christopher Goodall, a lecturer at York, originally started to write the sort of text that the student felt was needed. Unfortunately, Christopher was unable to complete the book and we thank him for passing on to us the idea of his student, Jerome Whitfield, together with his enthusiasm for this text to be developed.

We hope you will enjoy using this little book and that it will provide some of the support and practical information needed for you to improve your patient care and to more than 'survive' in our hospital wards today! In writing this book it has been decided to use the terms she to refer to the nurse, and he to refer to the patient. The writers acknowledge that there are many male nurses and female patients, however, it was chosen to use these terms for brevity and clarity, and does not imply anything about the nature of nurses or patients.

We hope that this book will serve the reader well in the practice of patients in all areas of care. However, nursing practice is complex and includes many facets of care. Therefore, this book is not meant to replace all your nursing textbooks. It may detail areas of nursing care and the nursing process, drugs and their side effects, and pharmacological principles. The book sometimes explains nursing procedures but is not a complete procedure book. It sometimes outlines anatomy and physiological principles, and it occasionally describes pathophysiology but is not a complete text. This book is not meant to be all of these texts or a replacement of them, but contains material that nurses can refer to while working. You may need to refer to additional texts (see further reading section at the back of the book) either at home or from the ward, hospital or university library for more detailed information.

In addition, if you find areas missing or sections which you feel are not relevant or useful, please e-mail us your suggestions. You can e-mail either Ann Richards (A.C.1.Richards@herts.ac.uk), or Sharon Edwards (S.L.Edwards@herts.ac.uk). We will both be very glad to read and respond to your comments and incorporate your requests in any future editions of the book.

Ann Richards
Sharon Edwards

Hertfordshire 2002

YOUR JOB AND ITS ORGANIZATION

1.1 Organizing yourself 2

1.2 Emergency situations 11

1.1 ORGANIZING YOURSELF

The work of a nurse will vary from day to day and from hospital to hospital but the following factors should be considered in all cases.

- You should have a good working knowledge of all your patients: you should know who they are, where in the ward they are lodged and the principal diagnosis for each patient.
- If you are in charge of the ward, you should make a point of seeing all your patients each day.
- Do not be afraid to ask for advice from the sister, doctor or student. It is far better to ask too often than to struggle on not knowing if you are doing the right thing and feeling more and more inadequate.
- If you are not getting enough support from management, then your ward sister or equivalent person needs to be informed.
- Organize your off-duty time so that you get enough rest and sleep and ensure that you cook for yourself properly.
- Keep in contact with your friends; carry on with hobbies and interests, which will maintain your contact with the world outside nursing.

COMMUNICATING WITH OTHER TEAM MEMBERS (MULTIDISCIPLINARY)

Communication is recognized as an important aspect of healthcare with far-reaching effects. It is an essential and integral part of the care nurses provide. Communication needs to be clear and it involves verbal and non-verbal messages that convey feelings and information.

Do not be afraid of discussing patients' illnesses with them or their relatives in as much detail as is appropriate (remember that it is unethical to disclose sensitive information, such as a diagnosis of cancer, to the relatives without telling the patient). Effective communication makes a positive contribution to an individual's recovery by acting:

- as a buffer against fear and confusion
- as a relief of anxiety and stress
- to help decrease pain and reduce the number of complications and side-effects
- to improve compliance.
- as a way of improving coping ability
- to enhance convalescence.

When you go off duty do not forget you must tell the nurse responsible about any problems a particular patient may have or any care that you have been unable to achieve on your shift.

WORKING AS A TEAM

Teamwork is vital if care is to be carried out expertly and efficiently in any clinical area. The team consists of not only doctors and nurses but also many other personnel from both within and outside the hospital. These may include:

- the police
- security

- specialist hospitals
- laboratories, e.g. technicians, laboratory staff
- support staff, e.g. phlebotomists, ECG technicians
- theatres
- specialist nurses, e.g. diabetic, wound care, resuscitation
- other wards/departments, e.g. pharmacy, X-ray
- community carers
- helping agencies
- primary healthcare teams
- relatives and friends
- patients
- ambulance personnel.

Liaison and effective communication within the team are essential to ensure optimum patient care.

LEGAL AND SAFETY ISSUES

Property

In the rush and excitement of care, it is vital not to neglect or mislay any patient's property. Often the patient/family does not realize something is missing until discharge, which could be some weeks later, and difficulties can arise unless accurate records are kept. The following principles might help.

- It is always wise to keep a patient's property together and list it in detail as soon as possible in the property book on the ward (check hospital policy). Make a specific note of valuables such as money or jewellery.
- Note, too, if the patient is wearing or not wearing a watch or carrying any money so that there is a written record should any confusion arise.

- If the patient is unfit to make a decision, any valuables should be stored in a safe place in accordance with the hospital procedure (generally hospital property).
- If patients wish to remain in custody of their valuables they need to sign a disclaimer form that the trust cannot take responsibility for the loss of personal property and that it should be deposited in the hospital safe.
- A duplicate copy of the patient's belongings list sent to the property office should always be given to the patient.
- Property should not be handed to relatives other than at the patient's specific request and written documentation of this should be kept.
- When patients leave the department, all personal property should go with them, preferably in one large bag clearly labelled with name and destination. Receipts for any items taken into safe custody should be firmly attached to the notes or given to the patient if he or she is in a fit state.

Patient complaints

All patients have the right to make a complaint if they feel that their rights have been infringed and such complaints must be taken seriously. A formal complaint is usually made in the first instance to the hospital or community service involved, whether verbally or in writing, and is immediately reported to the senior manager who is responsible for investigating it. The patient and any staff involved are kept informed of any steps taken. Clinical complaints should be referred to the consultant in charge of the case who will discuss how it is to be handled with the senior manager.

Most complaints can be dealt with at a local level. When a complaint is likely to involve litigation, the health authority will seek legal advice and the staff concerned should be made aware of the help that is available to them through their professional association or trade union.

The complaints procedure usually involves the following steps.

1. The complaint will first be examined by the hospital or community services management before a decision is taken as to whether to refer the case to the nurse's national board.
2. The board decides whether the case should be referred to the Professional Conduct Committee of the UKCC, now the Nursing & Midwifery Council (NMC).
3. The health service ombudsman may be involved when a patient feels a case has not been dealt with satisfactorily by the health authority.
4. The health service commissioner publishes an annual report.

Informed consent

A person is regarded in law as able to give consent if he is able to understand what is being said and to make a decision based on that information. Sixteen years is generally regarded as the minimum age for consent to hospital treatment, though a 1985 House of Lords ruling established that a child could give consent to treatment if he fully understood the nature and purpose of the proposed treatment and the likely consequences.

Most procedures require written consent from the patient following detailed explanation by a doctor whose responsibility it is to ensure that written informed consent is obtained. For children under the age of 16, consent is generally obtained from an adult/parent who should be contacted and asked to come to the department as soon as possible.

In an emergency a doctor may decide to:

- treat a minor having received verbal consent over the telephone from a responsible adult
- accept the child's own consent
- assume consent for any treatment necessary to save life or limb or to alleviate great pain
- act despite refusal of consent from a patient's relative in some circumstances.

Failure to gain the consent of a mentally competent adult before touching him/her or even intending or threatening to touch may lead to legal action on charges of trespass, assault or battery. Consent may be implied, verbal or written, though the first two may be difficult to prove at a later date (see Autonomy p.8).

The patient who refuses treatment

Patients have a full legal right to refuse consent to treatment and to take their own discharge from hospital, unless they are deemed to be of such unsound mind that they cannot be allowed to do so. If patients wish to discharge themselves you should:

- try to persuade the patient to stay and explain to him why the investigation or treatment is necessary
- tell the patient that he is leaving against medical advice
- contact the doctor, who will get the patient to sign a self-discharge form (discharge against medical advice form).

Legally, patients are not obliged to sign a self-discharge form and some refuse to do so. In any case of self-discharge, and especially if the patient has refused to sign the form, you must write a full account of events in the nursing notes. In addition, you may be asked to sign the medical notes as witness to the truth of their account.

HEALTH AND SAFETY

Moving and handling

This may include lifting, putting down, pushing, pulling, carrying or moving. Any manual handling operation must meet two objectives.

1. The handler needs to employ minimal effort.
2. The patient experiences minimal discomfort.

These objectives can be achieved and the risk of injury reduced by undertaking a comprehensive assessment of the task's requirements. Risk assessment must be undertaken when manual

handling cannot be avoided and there is a risk of injury. When suitable equipment such as hoists, small handling aids and electronic profiling beds are provided these should be used, well maintained, serviced and in good working order.

Training and education in the use of manual handling equipment and practices should be an ongoing process with yearly updates for all staff. The aim is to have fewer nurses injured and to increase comfort and safety for patients. Factors that contribute to safer handling are:

- trained, fit staff
- adequate supervision
- ergonomic assessments
- planned maintenance
- repair and replacement of equipment
- control of purchasing
- suitable and sufficient handling aids
- influencing attitudes of patients and relatives
- reporting and investigation of incidents
- competent agency staff
- sufficient staff.

Many patients may be able to move themselves or assist nurses while being moved and should be encouraged to help in ways compatible with their capabilities or health status.

The principles of safer manual handling are as follows.

- Assess unavoidable handling tasks and update assessment regularly.
- Channel the effort through your legs to protect your back.

- Move your feet in turn, not your body. Turn feet successively in the direction of movement (rather than twist at the waist).
- Bend your knees when appropriate but avoid overbending.
- Keep close to the load (when safe to do so).
- Maintain the natural curves of your spine and avoid twisting.
- Wear a uniform that allows unrestricted movement at shoulders, waist and hip, with non-slip shoes that provide support.
- Try to vary your tasks (so that different muscle groups are used in turn).
- Relax and move smoothly; avoid sudden movements.
- Remember to look after yourself with enough rest, suitable exercise and a healthy diet.
- If in doubt, seek advice. **Do not risk it**.

Violence

Violence towards staff members is any incident in which a health professional experiences abuse, threat, fear or the application of force arising out of the course of their work, whether or not they are on duty. The management of violence is necessary when the person:

- shows a predisposition to violence
- makes a physical attack on another person or object
- becomes disturbed to the extent that his behaviour is considered a threat to his own safety and the safety of others.

The principles underlying the management of violent persons are as follows.

- Prevention of violent incidents is the foremost principle. This may not always be possible if physiological causes are the reason for the violence:
  —brain tumours
  —endocrine imbalance
  —hyperthyroidism
  —hyperglycaemia
  —convulsive disorders
  —HIV encephalopathy
  —dementia
  —neurological impairment
  —alcohol/substance abuse
  —pain
  —side-effects of medication.
- Restraint is always therapeutic, never corrective, and where a one-to-one violent confrontation arises the best method is to use a breakaway technique.
- The risk of physical injury should be minimized; any restraint should be appropriate to the actual danger or resistance shown by the person.
- In all situations of violence, the locally agreed procedure for the nursing management of care of violent patients should be adhered to. The policy for violence should include:
  —environmental and organizational factors
  —anticipation and prevention of violence
  —action following an incident.

Universal precautions

The problem with identifying infected patients has been

acknowledged and is incorporated into all areas of care to prevent the transmission of bloodborne pathogens. Universal precautions are employed to protect healthcare workers against infection by using appropriate protective clothing (plastic aprons, goggles, gloves) to prevent exposure of skin and mucous membranes to blood or body fluids.

These simple precautions should be included as part of the routine care of all patients. This level of precaution (e.g. gloves routinely worn for contact with excreta) could prevent the transmission of many pathogens and make a major contribution to the reduction of hospital-acquired infection (see Section 3.2, p. 111).

PROFESSIONAL ISSUES

Accountability

Accountability can be exercised in a number of different ways. The UKCC (1989) highlighted the following principles.

- The interests of the patient or client are paramount.
- Professional accountability must be exercised in such a manner as to ensure that the interests of the patients or clients are respected and are not overridden by those of the professions or their practitioners.
- The exercise of accountability requires the practitioner to seek to achieve and maintain high standards.
- Advocacy on behalf of patient or clients is an essential feature of the exercise of accountability by a professional practitioner.

- The role of other persons in the delivery of healthcare to patients or clients must be recognized and respected, provided that the first principle above is honoured.
- Public trust and confidence in the profession are dependent on its practitioners being seen to exercise their accountability responsibly.
- All registered nurses, midwives and health visitors must be able to justify any action or decision not to act in the course of their professional practice.

Responsibility

Responsibility takes three major forms.

- *Responsibility for self* is often captured in a professional practice code (UKCC 1992a). Wilful failure to adhere to these responsibilities usually results in action to exclude the individual from the right to practise.
- *Responsibility for others* is a much more complex issue which varies according to position, degree of authority delegated and the nature of accountability to be exercised. It includes:
  —concern for the safety of all in the shared work environment
  —the need to be explicit with all colleagues about authority and accountability issues as they affect both yourself and others
  —working only within your levels of knowledge and ability.
- *Professional responsibility* entails the legitimate freedom to choose one course of action or intervention over another, combined with the

responsibility for making correct choices in each clinical circumstance.

Professional responsibility is an important issue as all professionals can be required to provide service in areas in which they are not adequately prepared. This can occur because of pressure of work and because individual clients have a particular relationship with certain practitioners and seek help from someone they know and trust rather than a more appropriately prepared person. Being open about such limitations is not a sign of weakness but rather a key indicator of mature and caring practice.

Autonomy

Autonomy relates to independence of action, meaning that one can perform one's total professional function on the basis of one's own knowledge and judgement. It consists of making decisions and acting on them. To be autonomous, one must be accountable. Autonomy means:

- self-rule
- a patient is free to make up his own mind and act on his own decisions
- a patient has the right to be given all the information required to make an informed autonomous decision about care or treatment received
- ethical principles of self-determination and self-governance with concomitant responsibility for one's own actions.

The ethical principle is important as no one has the legal right to impose his will (however well intended) upon another and everyone has the right to determine his own actions and what is done to and for him. All surgical interventions and delivery of nursing care, in a legal or ethical sense, are possible solely because the client or patient has consented to them.

The principle of autonomy underlies concerns about informed consent for surgical, medical and nursing interventions. Patients have a right to be respected as autonomous beings capable of making decisions for themselves and responsible for their own actions. Therefore, they need to know their healthcare rights and responsibilities and what to expect when in hospital and even from individual nurses, doctors and other healthcare professionals whom they may encounter. Informed consent therefore consists of:

- the right to know
- the right to say no.

In addition, a patient has the fundamental right to give or withhold consent prior to examination or treatment. Sometimes it is difficult to give a patient all the facts needed to make an informed decision. The following must be borne in mind when giving information.

- Is something being withheld so the patient makes the decision as the doctor or nurse desires?
- If all the information were given, might the patient decide not to cooperate?

If information is withheld to persuade the patient to undertake a procedure, truth telling and honesty are compromised, trust is lost and individual autonomy cannot be exercised.

Most consent is implied, such as holding an arm out for a blood test or opening the mouth for an inspection or treatment. But such consent should not be taken for granted. It is not a signature which counts but respect for the other person. When consent is not sought, for whatever reason, that person's life is devalued (see Informed consent p. 4).

Confidentiality

The nurse is under legal obligation not to disclose confidential information without the patient's consent. Disclosure of information occurs in the following ways:

- with the consent of the patient/client
- without the consent of the patient/client when the disclosure is required by law or order of a court
- by accident
- without the consent of the patient/client when the disclosure is considered necessary in the public interest.

The UKCC published an advisory paper on confidentiality and a summary of the principles on which to base professional judgement in matters of confidentiality are as follows.

- A patient/client has a right to expect that information given in confidence will be used only for the purpose for which it was given and will not be released to others without his consent.
- Practitioners recognize the fundamental right of their patients/clients to have information about them held in secure and private storage.
- Where it is deemed appropriate to share information obtained in the course of professional practice with other health or social work practitioners, the practitioner who obtained the information must ensure, as far as is reasonable, before its release that it is being imparted to strict professional confidence and for a specific purpose.
- That the responsibility to either disclose or withhold confidential information in the public interest lies with individual practitioners, that they cannot delegate the decision and cannot be required by a superior to disclose or withhold information against their will.
- That a practitioner who chooses to breach the basic principle of confidentiality in the belief that it is necessary in the public interest must have considered the matter sufficiently to justify that decision.
- That deliberate breach of confidentiality other than with the consent of the patient/client should be exceptional.

Advocacy

Advocacy is defined as the act of pleading a cause for another. It is a process of acting for or on behalf of someone. The word *advocacy* is not specifically used in the UKCC Code (1992a) but it is implied in the first clause where nurses, midwives and health visitors exercising professional accountability must: 'Serve the interests of society and above all safeguard the interests of individual patients and clients'.

Advocacy is an important principle in nursing adult patients because it makes it clear that, generally, adults are rational. Adults are capable of making choices and making decisions; however, some illnesses and specific situations may mean they lose a certain amount of autonomy and need a person to speak for them. That person might be a nurse.

Codes of practice

The publication in 1983 of the first code of professional conduct for nurses, midwives and health visitors by the UKCC was a significant step forward for these professions in the UK. A code of practice is not a legal document but it gives direction and cohesion to the body for which it has been designed. The UKCC Code of Professional Conduct has become the basis for most major guidance documents (e.g. *The Scope of Professional Practice*, UKCC 1996; *Guidelines for Professional Practice*, UKCC 1996) and is the template against which misconduct is judged.

Hence it is important to be familiar with the code and to discuss cases and events at ward, departmental and community level, as well as in classrooms and study groups. In 1996 the UKCC published *Guidelines for Professional Practice*, to reflect on the challenges that face us

in day-to-day practice. As such it is achieving its aim and should be consulted widely.

Clinical supervision

Clinical supervision is an exchange between practising professionals to enable the development of professional skills. It is about exploring nursing practice and becoming more effective through helping nurses to think about and begin to reflect on their practice. Clinical supervision is a dynamic, interpersonally focused experience which promotes the development of therapeutic proficiency. One of the primary reasons for all supervision is to ensure that the quality of therapeutic work is of a consistently high standard in relation to the client's needs.

Clinical supervision is an important part of taking care of oneself and staying open to new learning, ongoing self-development, self-awareness and commitment to learning. It focuses on the essence of professional nursing practice and is linked to the process of guided reflection, which is necessary to increase effectiveness as a practitioner in today's healthcare climate.

Clinical supervision should be viewed as a way of increasing effectiveness through the provision of high challenge and high support, not as a means of monitoring and surveillance. The outcomes of using clinical supervision are suggested as:

- achieving therapeutic competence, professional skills and knowledge

- ensuring the quality and effectiveness of work with clients.

However, central to clinical supervision is guided structured reflection.

Reflective practice

Reflective practice involves practitioners paying attention to significant aspects of experience in order to make sense of them within the context of their work. By reflecting on and taking action to resolve the contradictions that occur in practice, practioners come to know themselves and, as a consequence, learn to become increasingly effective. There are many reflective practice tools available to assist nurses in their reflection, from simplistic models, e.g. Gibbs (1988) (Fig. 1.1), to the more complex, e.g. Johns (1994) (Box 1.1).

1.2 EMERGENCY SITUATIONS

CARDIAC ARREST

This is the cessation of cardiac mechanical activity with no clinical cardiac output. If immediate cardiopulmonary resuscitation (CPR) is not started, death or serious cerebral damage will result. Nursing staff should promote CPR training and be the driving force behind a hospital's resuscitation team.

Cardiac arrest may be primary or secondary.

Primary: sudden cessation of cardiac function

- Myocardial infarction
- Heart disease
- Electric shock
- Drugs, e.g. potassium

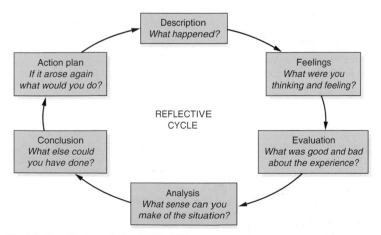

Fig. 1.1 The reflective cycle (from Gibbs 1988).

Box 1.1 Johns' (1994) model of structured reflection	
Cue questions	
Aesthetics	What was I trying to achieve?
	Why did I respond as I did?
	What were the consequences of that for:
	the patient?
	others?
	myself?
	How was this person(s) feeling?
	How did I know this?
Personal	How did I feel in this situation?
	What internal factors were influencing me?
Ethics	How did my actions match with my beliefs? What factors made me act in incongruent ways?
Empirics	What knowledge did or should have informed me?
Reflexivity	How does this connect with previous experience?
	Could I handle this better in similar situations?
	What would the consequences of alternative actions be for:
	the patient?
	others?
	myself?

Secondary: non-intrinsic cardiac causes

- Asphyxia, hypoxia, hypercarbia
- Exsanguination
- Central nervous system failure
- Metabolic/electrolyte disorders
- Temperature extremes
- Toxins
- Acute anaphylaxis

Cardiac arrest is usually associated with one of four rhythms:

- ventricular fibrillation (VF)
- pulseless ventricular tachycardia (VT)
- asystole
- electromechanical dissociation (EMD) – absent mechanical activity despite a coordinated ECG waveform; this is diagnosed infrequently.

Basic life support
The airway, breathing and circulation must be assessed before initiating active interventions. This can be achieved with the AABC of resuscitation.

- A – The initial assessment. Is the patient in any danger? Are you in any danger?
- A – Airway maintenance. Is the airway secure, free of vomit or debris? A Guedel's airway may be inserted.
- B – Breathing. Mouth-to-mouth breathing is started.
- C – Chest compression or external cardiac massage (ECM).

Basic life support implies that no equipment is used. The purpose is to maintain adequate ventilation and circulation until help arrives. Airway, breathing, circulation is always the priority order. The sequence of action is as follows.

1. Ensure the safety of yourself and the patient.

2. Check responsiveness of the patient. Ask 'are you all right?', give a verbal command and gently shake the shoulders.
3. If the patient responds by answering or moving, leave in position (if safe), assess condition and get help. If he does not respond, shout for help and then open the airway by tilting the head and lifting the chin.
4. Keeping the airway open, look, listen and feel for breathing for up to 10 seconds before deciding that breathing is absent.
5. If the patient is breathing, turn into the recovery position, check for continued breathing, get help. If he is not breathing, turn him on to his back and remove any visible obstruction from the mouth.
6. Give two effective rescue breaths, each of which makes the chest rise and fall. Mouth shields are recommended.
7. Assess casualty for signs of circulation. Check the carotid pulse for no more than 10 seconds.
8. If you are confident that you can detect signs of circulation, continue rescue breathing and every minute recheck for signs of circulation, again for no longer than 10 seconds each time.
9. If no signs of circulation, start compressions at the lower half of the sternum; depress 1.5–2 inches or 4–5 cm at a rate of 100 times per minute.
10. Combine rescue breathing and compression at a ratio of 2:15.
11. Continue resuscitation until the casualty shows signs of life and/or help arrives.

> ⚠ Adult tidal volume is 500 ml, dead space (air not involved in gaseous exchange) is up to 250 ml. Mouth-to-mouth resuscitation should reflect this and breaths given (adult) need to be greater than 250 ml to be effective.

Advanced life support

The European Resuscitation Council (ERC) recommends guidelines and protocols to manage VF (and pulseless VT), asystole and EMD. The protocol stresses early defibrillation and advanced care. Advanced life support involves:

- following the guidelines set out by the ERC
- giving 1 mg adrenaline and 10 sequences of 5:1 ECM/ventilation
- advanced airway care (intubation) after the first DC shock; once achieved, ventilation can proceed
- gaining venous access.

ENDOTRACHEAL INTUBATION

Advanced airway management involves endotracheal intubation which allows for spontaneous and positive pressure ventilation. Indications for intubation are:

- acute airway obstruction
- facilitation of tracheal suctioning
- protection of the airway in those without protective cough reflexes
- respiratory failure/arrest requiring ventilatory support and high inspired concentrations of oxygen.

Direct laryngoscopy is the most common method used in an

emergency, either in the mouth or through the nose. The tip of the tube may require direction with a Magill forceps to enter the glottis. Confirming correct tracheal tube placement is essential and therefore arterial blood gases need checking for expired carbon dioxide levels.

Complications of intubation include those that occur during intubation:

- trauma
- cardiovascular response to laryngoscopy and intubation
- hypoxaemia
- aspiration
- oesophageal intubation

and those that occur after the tube is in place:

- blockage
- dislodgement
- damage to larynx
- complications of mechanical ventilation.

SHOCK

Shock is a condition in which the cardiovascular system fails to perfuse the body tissues adequately, thereby causing widespread disruption of cellular metabolism, which results in functional disturbances at organ/tissue level. There are three stages of shock, each progressively worse.

1. Compensated (non-progressive) stage, where compensatory mechanisms stabilize the circulation.
2. Continuing hypoperfusion and deteriorating organ function mark the progressive stage.

3. Refractory (irreversible) stage, where severe cellular and therefore organ dysfunction leads to general decline and death.

There are many causes of shock, including any factor which affects blood volume, blood pressure or cardiac function. One classification of shock states that according to blood pressure, there are two forms:

- hypotensive shock – further subdivided into:
  —low cardiac output shock characterized clinically by cold skin
  —high cardiac output shock characterized by warm skin
- normotensive or hypertensive shock – blood pressure is compensated.

A more traditional classification categorizes shock according to the primary defect that produced it. With this system there are five forms of shock: anaphylactic, septic, neurogenic, cardiogenic and hypovolaemic.

Anaphylactic shock

Anaphylaxis occurs when a sensitized person is exposed to an antigen to which he is allergic. The antigen enters the body and combines with immunoglobulin E (IgE) antibodies on the surface of mast cells and basophils, primarily found in the lungs, small intestines, skin and connective tissue. An antigen–antibody reaction occurs which induces the release of histamine and prostaglandin into the blood, leading to:

- increased cell permeability, leading to oedema

- vasodilatation in some areas (beta-1 receptors and reduction in blood pressure
- vasoconstriction (beta-2 receptors) in others (breathlessness)
- third space fluid shifts, increased sodium in the intracellular and intravascular space; this fluid loss from the circulation causes circulatory collapse.

This results in reduced cardiac output and low arterial pressure. Cellular perfusion fails to meet the metabolic demands, resulting in acidosis, coagulopathies and capillary pooling.

Septic shock

The main organisms responsible are a Gram-negative enteric bacilli such as *Escherichia coli*, *Pseudomonas*, *Klebsiella*, *Proteus* and *Enterobacter* or Gram-positive organisms such as *staphylococci*, *streptococci* and *Clostridium*. These organisms enter the vascular system and release endotoxins, which cause an interstitial fluid leak, increased vascular permeability and vasodilatation, which leads to shock.

A great hazard for the development of sepsis is parenteral nutrition (PN).

- The PN solution is an ideal medium for bacterial growth if contaminated. All care of the feeding line must be aseptic.
- The feeding line may become infected (the catheter must be used for feeding only, not for taking bloods or drug administration). The most common infecting organisms are *Candida albicans* and *Staphylococcus epidermidis*, which are part of the skin flora.

- The practice of bypassing the gut and delivering nutrition directly into the blood can lead to problems, as the gut not only plays a major role in the digestion and absorption of nutrition but also acts as a protective barrier against the translocation of bacteria and endotoxins to the bloodstream (see p. 32).

The result of septic shock is:

- tachycardia;
- high cardiac output – maintained at a normal/high level by the increasing tachycardia
- the patient feels warm and has a high temperature
- a low circulating volume owing to venous pooling, increased capillary permeability and third space fluid shift.

If volume loss is not corrected, hypovolaemia will persist, cardiac output will decrease and the skin will become cool. As in all other types of shock, the primary problem is tissue hypoperfusion; consequently, nutrients and oxygen fail to be delivered to cells. Sepsis can be treated with antibiotics.

Neurogenic shock

Neurogenic shock causes changes to smooth muscle tension in the walls of the circulatory vessels through nervous system action, leading to an imbalance between parasympathetic and sympathetic stimulation. There is a loss of sympathetic tone, causing peripheral vasodilatation and resulting in severe hypotension. There is decreased vascular tone and systemic vascular resistance (SVR), inadequate cardiac output, reduced tissue perfusion and impaired cellular metabolism.

Neurogenic shock may be the result of:

- a severe brainstem injury at the level of the medulla
- an injury to the spinal cord
- spinal anaesthesia.

It may mask signs and symptoms of other types of shock.

If neurogenic shock is present, there should be a heightened suspicion for an undetected source of haemorrhage.

Cardiogenic shock

Cardiogenic shock occurs when the heart, due to impaired myocardial performance, cannot produce an adequate cardiac output to sustain the metabolic requirements of body tissues. Myocardial infarction is the most common cause of cardiogenic shock, as the area infarcted becomes dysfunctional and, depending on the size of the infarction, stroke volume and cardiac output may decrease with a concurrent increase in left ventricular end-diastolic pressure.

Compensatory mechanisms are stimulated by the decrease in blood pressure and catecholamines are released. This causes an increase in heart rate and contractility, blood pressure and SVR to maintain arterial pressure.

The compensatory mechanisms improve blood flow for a time but more oxygen is required by the already ischaemic cardiac muscle to pump blood into the constricted systemic circulation, consequently increasing cardiac workload. The heart becomes more ischaemic and

cardiac failure worsens, jeopardizing potentially viable tissue and increasing left ventricular function. As cardiac output continues to decline, blood pressure and tissue perfusion decrease, which results in cardiogenic shock and ends with the patient's death.

Hypovolaemic shock

Hypovolaemic shock is the most common type of shock and occurs due to a decrease in the circulating fluid volume so large that the body's metabolic needs cannot be met. The decline in blood volume is produced by:

- continued bleeding
- plasma loss
- bleeding disorders
- water or fluid shifts
- dehydration
- high temperature.

This decreases venous return and cardiac output, primarily affecting tissue perfusion.

The degree of shock depends on the amount of blood lost, the rate at which it was lost, the age and general physical condition of the patient and the patient's ability to activate compensatory mechanisms. Numerous compensatory mechanisms to increase venous tone are activated when the circulating volume and venous return are decreased. As a result, venous capacity is decreased to match the smaller blood volume and adequate transport of oxygen and nutrients is maintained.

If the fluid loss exceeds the ability of homeostatic mechanisms to compensate for the loss, the central venous pressure (CVP), diastolic filling pressure, stroke volume and systemic arterial blood pressure will fall. As the severity of shock increases, blood pools in the capillary and venous beds, with further impairment of the effective vascular volume available for oxygen transport and tissue perfusion.

Patients in shock will often have components of more than one of the forms of shock. For example, patients in cardiogenic shock may also be hypovolaemic due to loss of fluid into the tissues as a result of high venous pressures or increased capillary permeability. Hypovolaemia is also frequently a complication of septic shock and in the late stages of hypovolaemic shock patients usually have some degree of cardiac failure and vasomotor collapse complicating their shock picture.

FLUID OVERLOAD

An increase in circulating volume can occur for many reasons:

- circulation problems prior to admission
- fluid therapy given following surgery
- fluid therapy following hypovolaemia
- sluggish arterial and venous circulation caused by a stagnant flow of blood through the circulation due to continued bedrest or immobility.

Prior to problems being observed (cyanosis, pale skin) or measured (blood pressure, central venous pressure) in the patient's condition, these processes activate

compensatory mechanisms to maintain homeostasis e.g. ANF.

Factors that can precipitate fluid overload

There are many specific conditions which can precipitate fluid overload, by:

- reducing the body's ability to maintain homeostasis in the event of an increase in circulating volume
- stimulating control mechanisms that accelerate the symptoms of fluid overload
- causing the flow of blood to become turbulent, increasing SVR and blood pressure.

All these conditions may hasten fluid overload during or following an intravenous infusion. The most common of these are hypertension, heart failure and peripheral vascular disease.

In all cases of hypervolaemia there is an increase in circulatory volume. Cardiogenic shock is severe circulatory failure due to a primary defect in the pumping activity of the heart. The circulatory collapse becomes so profound that myocardial contractility is decreased and the body is unable to adequately compensate as cardiac output drops.

The principal aetiologies of fluid overload are as follows.

Blood transfusion
In this situation blood velocity reduces and blood flow becomes slow, leading to pooling of blood in the peripheries, lungs, liver, kidneys and possibly the brain. The heart can no longer pump the increasing amount of volume around the

circulation. As the signs of heart failure increase and the kidneys become swamped with fluid and start to receive a lower blood supply, renal failure ensues. The complications of pulmonary oedema, cardiac failure, renal failure, ascites, cerebral oedema and peripheral oedema can be very serious if not treated quickly.

In the majority of cases when a blood transfusion is being administered, a diuretic is generally given with each or every alternate unit. This is even more important in patients who have problems with maintaining an adequate circulation.

Salt/water overload
A fluid overload with normal saline and/or 5% dextrose can cause similar problems but for different reasons. When the body is functioning normally, it is almost impossible to produce an excess of total body water. However, this can occur during IV treatment with normal saline or 5% dextrose. The effects can be an overload of both salt and water (isotonic volume excess) or just salt (hypertonic volume excess) or a dilutional low sodium (hypotonic volume excesses).

TRAUMA

Patients with severe multiple trauma require care and attention to their primary injuries. This may include surgery, dressings, fluids, e.g. blood, crystalloid or colloid, oxygen, drugs and/or resuscitation. However, there is now a sophisticated understanding of the complex metabolic response of the human body to traumatic injury. Following trauma the initial

physiological responses that occur are neuroendocrine response; oxygen supply and demand; alterations in metabolism; inflammatory/immune response (IIR); and post-trauma capillary leak. These physiological responses are initiated to protect the body from cell/tissue/organ damage.

Neuroendocrine response to injury
One of the earliest responses to injury is neuroendocrine activation, which is intimately linked in the control of tissue function. Neuroendocrine activation occurs in response to cytokine release from the site of injury and stimulates the sympathetic nervous system, hypothalamus, pituitary and adrenal glands. The nervous system generates biochemical agents that act as hormones and the endocrine system produces substances that mediate activity within the central nervous system.

Following an insult, activation of the neuroendocrine system stimulates the release of numerous substances into the circulation, including:

- catecholamines (adrenaline and noradrenaline) via the sympathetic nervous system and adrenal cortex, causing tachycardia, increased cardiac output and blood pressure, rate and depth of respirations, blood flow redistribution, glycogenolysis, gluconeogenesis and lipolysis
- glucocorticoids via the hypothalamus releasing corticotrophin-releasing hormone (CRH) while the anterior pituitary gland secretes adrenocorticotrophic

hormone (ACTH). The adrenal cortex then releases cortisol, a glucocorticoid which causes gluconeogenesis, proteolysis and lipolysis, anti-inflammatory and cell-protective effects to prevent damage from excessive activation of the metabolic response.

The effect of catecholamines occurs almost immediately, effecting change in target organs with extreme rapidity and intensity. Heart rate can double in 3–5 seconds, cardiac output can increase fourfold, selective vasoconstriction and vasodilatation occurs to redistribute the circulating volume to vital organs (heart, brain).

The neuroendocrine response in injury protects the body from the effects of injury. However, it causes:

- an increase in oxygen consumption and myocardial work
- redistribution of blood flow away from the 'non-vital' gut which may result in translocation of bacteria and endotoxins into the circulation, resulting in septic shock
- high catecholamine levels which can lead to arrhythmias, causing cardiac arrest in a compromised heart.

Therefore, if this response is prolonged it is believed to contribute to shock and multiple system organ failure (MSOF).

Inflammatory/immune response (IIR)

The wound or injury site plays a role in the systemic response as the wound produces extensive inflammation by attracting nutrients,

fluids, clotting factors and large numbers of neutrophils and macrophages to the damaged site. These are activated to:

- protect the host from invading microorganisms
- limit the extent of blood loss and injury
- promote rapid healing of involved tissues.

This activation is known as the inflammatory/immune response (IIR) and represents a major physiological event in the body, which leads to an increased capillary permeability causing the swelling, redness, pain and oedema often observed in inflammation and stimulation of coagulation and fibrinolysis. The IIR is initiated to protect the host and to promote healing and is necessary for survival but it can lead to an uncontrolled intravascular inflammation that ultimately harms the host. This can be observed in such conditions as:

- adult respiratory distress syndrome (ARDS)
- systemic immune response syndrome (SIRS)
- disseminated intravascular coagulation (DIC)
- multiple system organ failure (MSOF).

Therefore, trauma requires immediate intervention as the process outlined above can lead to serious irreversible consequences and death. The nurse's immediate role is in:

- the administration of oxygen
- the instigation and administration of adequate nutrition

- maintenance of an adequate circulating volume.

FITTING/SEIZURES/ EPILEPSY

This is a common medical condition affecting at least five in every 1000 people. It is socially stigmatized and is defined as transient paroxysms of uncontrolled electrical discharges from nerve tissue in the brain which lead to epileptic attacks which can be recurring.

Normally in the brain there exists general stability between excitation and inhibition. In seizures the ability to suppress abnormal neural activity may be impaired or lost or there may be increased excitation within the neurons. This lowers the threshold and results in uncontrolled discharge of impulses in response to minimal stimuli which may occur in small groups of localized neurons or involve extensive areas.

Epilepsy is not an illness but rather a symptom of many diseases with different causes:

- raised intracranial pressure or brain damage
- systemic conditions, e.g. hypoglycaemia, hypocalcaemia (tetany), uraemia, fever, toxaemia, chemical poisoning, whereby the fits will disappear once the causative factor is corrected
- idiopathic, e.g. obscure cause such as inherited disposition.

The majority of patients develop recurring seizures before the age of 20. If they occur later an organic cause or previous tissue damage is considered.

Types of seizure

Characteristics of epilepsy vary in form and length, depending on the origin of abnormal neural activity and the extent and course of spread in the brain (Box 1.2). The manifestations may include:

- loss of consciousness
- changes in behaviour
- involuntary uncoordinated movements
- abnormal sensation.

Precipitating factors

May be unpredictable and random but may be linked to an identifiable trigger:

- external stimuli – noise, lights, TV, photosensitivity
- internal stimuli – stress, emotion, anger
- hormonal – menstruation
- precursory changes several days or hours before, e.g. irritability, headache, increased appetite.

Treatment is mainly drug therapy see p.236).

MANAGEMENT OF A TONIC-CLONIC SEIZURE

In a typical tonic-clonic seizure there is abrupt loss of consciousness and the person falls to the ground, sometimes calling out as they do so. Some will have a few seconds warning of a fit (an aura) and may be able to lie down before losing consciousness.

In the tonic phase (usually 10–30 seconds in length) there is sustained muscular contraction affecting all muscles including the respiratory ones. This means breathing may cease and

Box 1.2	Different types of seizures

Generalized seizures

Tonic-clonic — Used to be called grand mal and are the commonest of all types of seizures. Generally stop after a few minutes and followed by a deep sleep.

- The person is rigid
- Falls to the ground and jerks all over
- Breathing is laboured
- There is excessive salivation and cyanosis
- Incontinence may occur

Not all of these features may be observed.

Tonic — Sudden stiffness of muscles, person becomes rigid and falls (no jerking). Usually quick recovery, injuries often occur.

Atonic — Sudden loss of muscle tone, person collapses to the ground (sometimes called a drop attack). Quick recovery, injuries may occur.

Absences — There is a brief interruption of consciousness. Blank staring, fluttering of eyelids and nodding of the head may occur. Only lasts a few seconds and often goes unrecognized. Common in children. Sometimes known as petit mal.

Myoclonic — Abrupt, brief, shock-like jerks, may involve whole body, the arms or the head. Often happens shortly after waking up. The person may fall but recovery is immediate.

Partial seizures

Simple partial — There are a great variety of these and it is unusual for them to occur alone. They often develop into other forms of partial seizures.

- Consciousness and normal awareness are maintained
- Twitching of the limbs, pins and needles in a distinct part of the body
- A rising feeling in the stomach
- An unusual taste or some sensory disturbance
- Feelings of *déjà vu* or fear can also occur

Complex partial — Alterations in consciousness. The person may:

- pluck at clothing;
- fiddle with objects and act in a confused manner;
- make lipsmacking or chewing movements
- make grimacing, undressing, semi-purposeful movements
- walk around in a drunken fashion.

Secondary generalized — These are partial seizures, either simple or complex, in which the discharge spreads to the whole brain. This involvement of the whole brain leads to a clonic convulsive seizure with the same characteristics as a generalized tonic-clonic.

the patient becomes cyanosed. The nurse should not be unduly concerned, as when the patient starts breathing again, colour will return to normal. All muscles are contracted and the eyes are closed, the elbows flexed, the arms pronated and the legs extended. The teeth are clenched, the tongue may be bitten and the pupils are dilated. At the end of this phase bowel and/or bladder control may be lost resulting in incontinence, usually of urine.

After approximately 30 seconds the clonic phase supervenes and there are repeated violent jerking movements of the trunk and limbs. Self-inflicted injury is common during this phase. The clonic phase usually lasts between one and two minutes. The patient becomes tachycardic and breathing recommences at the end of the phase.

On cessation of the fit, consciousness is slowly regained. The patient sleeps with stertorous respiration and often cannot be roused. He/she may feel exhausted for hours or even days afterwards and muscles will ache as a result of the violent movements during the clonic phase.

It is most important that the patient is supported during the seizure by aiming to ensure an adequate airway and trying to protect them from injury whilst fitting. The progress of the seizure also needs to be recorded.

Wooden mouth gags, tongue forceps and physical restraint should not be used as they cause more harm than good.

1. Maintain an adequate airway

- Turn the patient onto their side and into the recovery position if possible.

- Never try and insert a mouth gag when the jaws are tightly clenched.
- When the patient becomes flaccid, turn this/her head to the side to enable any secretions to drain.
- Try and hold the jaw forward while the patient is flaccid.

2. Try to protect the patient from injury.

- Put a folded blanket under his head to prevent injury during the clonic stage.
- Loosen any constrictive clothing.
- Do not restrain the patient as this can lad to unnecessary injury.
- Stay with the person until they recover full consciousness.
- Ensure privacy for the patient.

3. Observe and record the progression of any seizure:-

- Note the time that the attack started if you were present.
- Observe where the movements or stiffness started.
- Note the type of movements and the parts of the body involved.
- Observe any changes in pupil diameter.
- Note incontinence of urine or faeces.
- Time the duration of each stage of the seizure if possible.
- Look for any weakness or paralysis following the fit.
- Note if the patient loses consciousness and for how long
- Is there any inability to speak following the seizure?

Most seizures are self-limiting events and it is important to stay calm and to reassure both the patient and those around that all is well (see also p. 237).

ASSESSING AND INVESTIGATING

2.1   Identification of patient
       problems   24

2.2   Assessment   30

2.3   Observations and
       measurements   43

2.4   Procedures and
       investigations   56

2.5   Nursing care issues   81

2.1 IDENTIFICATION OF PATIENT PROBLEMS

There are a number of elements and principles which help to identify values and beliefs concerning the nature of nursing. This section introduces nurses to how they can further articulate and understand the full potential of their practice.

HOLISTIC APPROACH TO CARE

It is important that nurses do not see patients in a reductionist way as just a collection of parts (brain, heart, lungs, kidneys, etc.) but try to understand their patients as a whole. Patients should be seen as members of communities and with a network of family roles and relationships. This view underscores the values and principles of holism. The core assumptions of holism are:

- the recognition that patients are whole people and cannot be viewed in reductionist terms
- the whole cannot be understood merely by isolating and examining its parts
- that nursing moves beyond disease management and requires that the nurse and patient collaborate to promote health
- the environment within which individuals live must be included
- that people live in cultural and social communities
- people have networks of relationships with others, most notably within the family
- that individuals have sexual needs as well as physical, psychological and social needs.

Each health experience is unique for both the person receiving care and for the caregiver. Holism is a concept centred around the needs of the patient and the nurse works with the patient from a basis of concern and mutual understanding.

NURSING PROCESS

The nursing process provides a framework for organizing individualized nursing care that focuses upon identifying and treating unique responses to actual or potential alterations in health. It consists of four steps: patient assessment, planning care, implementation of interventions and evaluation of the process and patient status.

- *Assessment* – all the patient information is gathered and examined to obtain all the facts necessary to determine the patient's health status and identify problems.
- *Planning* – once problems are identified those which need immediate attention are addressed. A plan of action is formulated which includes the following key activities:
  —setting priorities
  —establishing goals
  —determining nursing interventions
  —documenting nursing care plan.
- *Implementation* – putting the plan into action, which involves the following activities:
  —continuing to collect information about the patient

—performing the nursing interventions and activities

—recording the patient's health status and response to nursing interventions

● *Evaluation* – determining how well the plan has worked and whether any changes need to be made.

The purpose of the nursing process is to document information for other members of staff, to initiate support and continue observations and measurements to ensure the effectiveness of interventions.

GOAL SETTING

Goal setting takes place after patients have been assessed. Goals are sometimes referred to as aims of nursing, objectives, desired end results or expected outcomes of care.

To be useful, goals need to be stated in a clear and precise way. One way of achieving this is to state them in behavioural terms – what you would expect to observe, hear or see demonstrated if the goal is achieved. In other words, you set a measurable response which would be expected from the person for whom the goal is set and subsequently observe whether it has been achieved.

The five elements of a well-written goal statement are as follows.

1. Who, i.e. the patient.
2. Actual behaviour to demonstrate that the goal has been achieved: for example, reporting less anxiety, passing urine, touching, walking.

3. The relevant conditions under which the behaviour will be performed, such as the level of assistance needed from other people or aids (e.g. walks alone or with a stick) or where the behaviour will take place (e.g. on the level or on stairs).
4. The standard that will be needed to evaluate the behaviour. This entails specifying the criterion of success, which may relate to the frequency of the behaviour demonstrated (e.g. voids in the toilet *on each occasion*) or to a time limit (e.g. completes dressing *in 20 minutes*).
5. By what time it is expected that the behaviour will be achieved, e.g. immediately (those which have to be met first), over a number of days (short-term goals) or weeks/months (long-term goals).

Involvement of patients in goal setting can result in more-effective achievement and greater satisfaction for those providing healthcare. Using a goal-directed approach, which fully involves patients who are coherent and able to discuss their own goals and what they hope to achieve, produces better results for patients. However, not all patients are able to make decisions for themselves nor to be full partners in setting goals, such as those who are unconscious, confused or mentally handicapped. In these instances relatives or friends may become involved in establishing appropriate goals with nurses.

OBSERVATION OF THE PATIENT

Nurses may not realize it but they begin to 'assess' and 'make observations' about patients from the very moment they set eyes upon them.

- Are they on a trolley or in a wheelchair?
- Are they walking using a stick or do they have a limp or an unsteady gait?
- Facial colour, pallor, flushed or cyanosed
- Respiratory difficulty, rapid or shallow breathing
- Cool, moist or dehydrated skin
- Ischaemia of the eyelids, lips, gums and tongue
- Facial expression indicating pain, anxiety, fear, anger
- Oedema of the feet, legs or sacral area
- Increased or decreased body weight; loose-fitting clothing or false teeth
- Pulsating neck veins
- Poor posture
- Dry mucous membranes

Observations are made not only of the patient's physical condition but also of indicators of his psychological and emotional state too. An important point to stress is that observation depends not just on sight but also uses the senses of hearing, touch and smelling.

These observations will direct the nurse's subsequent, more systematic approach to data collection which includes further observation of specific factors.

INTERVIEWING THE PATIENT

The admission of a patient usually commences with an interview and it is from this structured discussion that a great deal of crucial information is obtained.

- Assess relevant health history, enquiring if there is any family history, any episodes of fatigue, restlessness, syncope or confusion.
- Ask patients to show you any medications that they are taking or take occasionally and check that the medications are taken as prescribed. If the patient does not have the medications on hand, ask a relative or friend to bring them in to you.
- Determine any risk factors for disease, such as diabetes, a high fat/cholesterol diet, does the patient smoke or take any exercise?
- Ask the patient about coping strategies which may help to determine how well the patient copes with stress.
- Determine any religious beliefs or preferences, sleeping and eating patterns.
- Ask about psychological status, e.g. recent bereavement, eating habits.
- Determine social status of the patient.
- Questions about diet, income, family concerns and job status are necessary as all can influence health and recovery.

A good nursing assessment relies heavily upon the nurse's skills in interviewing patients and nurses need to acquire a good interviewing technique. Observational skills also play a part in interviewing because information is forthcoming from patients' 'non-verbal communication', in addition to what they actually say. Whether the non-verbal cues appear to support or contradict the verbal communication may be of importance. For example, a patient in the postoperative ward might say to the staff nurse 'No, I do not have any pain' but at the same time be showing facial expressions which indicate anxiety, uncertainty and obvious pain.

Nurses should not underestimate the importance of skilled verbal communication in interviewing. The nurse needs to learn to ask the right questions, to know how to encourage the patient to give information and, perhaps most important, to recognize non-verbal cues given by the patient.

PATIENT COMMUNICATION

Communication can be verbal and/or non-verbal, conscious or unconscious. It is an essential activity of living, which is as important as physical support. Patients often express dissatisfaction with communication during their hospital stay, which relates to the quality and amount of information received and to insufficient, confusing and contradictory information being given by different healthcare professionals.

Nurses, by giving active information, can speed up recovery and reduce the number of complications and the need for pain relief. In the acute care setting, the development of verbal skills, the giving of information and the additional use of listening skills are insufficient on their own. The nurse needs to increase his/her proficiency at monitoring and interpreting non-verbal cues from physically dependent patients who are unable to communicate verbally, due to speech loss or factors affecting speech, such as breathlessness or pain.

Non-verbal communication is the term used to describe all forms of human communication not controlled by speech and it can be used therapeutically by nurses. The non-verbal component of communication is five times more influential than the verbal aspect.

Stress can be actively reduced using relaxation and soothing techniques and caring can be conveyed through touch. Touch is a means of giving and gathering information but consideration should be given to the fact that people are individuals, so interpretation of tactile communication will differ from person to person.

The communication process comprises five elements:

1. the sender or encoder of the message
2. the message itself
3. the receiver or decoder of the message
4. feedback that the receiver conveys to the sender
5. the environment in which the message is transmitted.

When planning to meet patients' communication needs there are six essential areas to include.

1. Orientation to the time, day, date, place, people, environment and procedures.
2. Specific patient teaching on any aspect of care.
3. Adopting methods to overcome patients' sensory deficits.
4. Comforting patients who are confused or hallucinating.
5. Communications which maintain the patient's personal identity.
6. Helping the communications of voiceless patients.

Resources, nursing actions and aids which can be used in connection with these six areas are suggested in Table 2.1.

Table 2.1 Communication aids to meet patient needs (Manley & Bellman 2000)

Essential areas of planning	Resource/aid/nursing action
Orientation to time, place, person, people, environment and procedures	• Information regarding: —treatment —care —progress —how patient can help himself • Visible clock and calendar • Daily newspapers • Day and night lighting • Positioning near windows • Use of glasses, hearing aids (if needed)
Communication which maintains patient identity	• Talking about normal life, home, family interests, preferences, concerns • Offering as many choices affecting the environment as possible • Enable the patient to maintain control of his own body – choices, decisions
Special patient teaching	• Rehabilitation programmes following myocardial infarction • Patient information booklets • Breathing / limb exercises
Overcoming sensory deficits	• Has aids he usually needs • Aids are functioning and effective • Verbal descriptions of environment if the patient cannot see • Tactile manipulation of equipment
Comforting patients who are confused or hallucinating	• Acknowledge and accept the patient's delusions or hallucinations while stating that you do not see or believe the same thing
Helping communication of voiceless patients	• Communication bells to attract attention • Communication cards • Pen and pad • Alphabet cards • Work out a system with patient and ensure continuity • Speaking appliances for tracheostomy tubes

It is important to remember that the information given through communication may not be remembered, especially by acutely ill patients whose drugs may interfere with information processing and storage; the patient may be unable to assign meaning to or organize the information at the time of exposure to it. This can lead to confusion and lack of memory with regard to the event.

Barriers to and interference with communication can occur at any point in the process. A summary of potential problems relating to the patient's reception of messages from the nurse in acute hospital settings is provided in Box 2.1.

CULTURAL ISSUES AND KNOWLEDGE OF CLIENTELE

Cultural issues

A patient's stay in hospital may be influenced by a number of factors,

---

Box 2.1   Potential problems relating to communicating in practice

Environment

Distortion of the message	• Noise
	• Poor/bright light
	• Vibration
	• Temperature
Distractions	• Other activity
	• Competing messages

Patient

Psychological	• Perception altered by drugs and/or pathology
	• Motivation/interest in message
	• Attitudes/values/beliefs
	• Anxiety/fear
	• Emotions/mood
	• Intelligence
	• Self-image
Physical	• Conscious level
	• Sensory deficits:
	—hearing (inpediments, tinnitis)
	—sight (short/long sighted, diplopia, hemianopia, blindness)
	—movement (paralysis/paresis)
	—sensation (loss)
	—speech (dysarthria/dysphasia/aphasia)
	• Constraints to movement (position, infusions, equipment)
	• Pain
Social	• Language
	• Culture/lifestyle
	• Isolation

e.g. religious beliefs or other strongly held principles, cultural background, ethnic origins and the availability of traditional foods. Whatever a person's ethnic and cultural background, food can play a role in maintaining good health but it will often have an important social or religious significance as well.

Some religious or cultural diets prohibit certain foods and have festivals which require strict fasting. Others require different activities following death. It is important for nurses to have knowledge and understanding of the diverse cultures currently resident in Britain and take their different practices into account.

Some religious beliefs may refuse specific treatments. Jehovah's Witnesses, Christian Scientists and members of other minority sects may refuse specific treatments such as blood transfusion. You should explain the nature of the treatment to such patients but if it is refused the doctor should be informed and the patient should sign a declaration to that effect. The patient's wishes must then dictate what treatment he then receives.

Knowledge of clientele

Psychological disturbances can influence recovery in many ways.

- Eating can be a way of finding comfort during periods of insecurity, depression, loneliness and boredom.
- Anorexia nervosa can be a way of coping with hate or anger

towards a parent or fear of maturity.
- Changes in roles within a family or society can cause psychological disturbances. Personal identity and functioning in a social setting can have an influence on recovery and might involve passive or active neglect of the patient's own needs.

Social and economic status can influence recovery due to the following.

- In low-income families food concerns are often of a low priority.
- Surviving in very poor housing.
- Families may have financial problems which compound the problem of maintaining health and recovery.

Elderly people can become anxious over issues concerning diet, become ill, confused or forgetful. Understanding the elderly clientele means:
- recognizing those in need of nutritional support in the community, e.g. meals on wheels or other services
- considering previous illness, e.g. physical disability, depression or loneliness, as this may affect recovery
- determining poverty, restricted access to food or shopping difficulties.

2.2 ASSESSMENT

A planned assessment often takes place when a patient is admitted and is an opportunity to collect detailed, specific information in order that the most effective interventions can be offered. It is essential that the focus is not on documentation but on the patient and the importance of communication skills as an essential part of the assessment process cannot be overstated.

A health assessment assists nurses in the identification of human responses and provides the basic data necessary to plan holistic care. It should cover areas such as:

- family history
- episodes of fatigue, restlessness, syncope or confusion
- current medications
- risk factors, such as diabetes, a high fat/cholesterol diet, smoking, exercise regime, coping strategies
- religious beliefs or preferences
- sleeping and eating patterns
- social status, to determine stress levels, diet, income, family concerns and job status.

AUTONOMIC NERVOUS SYSTEM (ANS)

To determine the mental state (both physiological and psychological), it is necessary to have knowledge of the autonomic nervous system. The ANS has two subdivisions: the sympathetic and the parasympathetic nervous systems. The sympathetic nervous system:

- is active in response to stressors

- is responsible for stimulating smooth muscle fibres to contract (i.e. excitation)
- stimulates the adrenal medulla to release the hormones adrenaline and noradrenaline.

The parasympathetic nervous system:

- is active in response to stressors
- causes relaxation (i.e. inhibition) and is most active during sleep and rest
- has a conserving effect on body resources.

These responses, under the control of the central nervous system, regulate other areas of the body to maintain homeostasis. An increase or decrease in either sympathetic or parasympathetic activity in the hospitalized person can often be reflected in other observations such as the blood pressure or heart rate. A general assessment of the patient's ANS may alert the nurse to impending neurological overstimulation or deterioration.

THE GLASGOW COMA SCALE (GCS)

The Glasgow Coma Scale (GCS) assesses the ANS via two aspects of consciousness: arousal, which involves being aware of the environment, and cognition, which demonstrates an understanding of what the observer has said through an ability to perform tasks.

The GCS was designed to:

- record conscious level and the activity of the ANS or mental state

- assess consciousness and standardize clinical observations of patients with impaired consciousness
- monitor the progress of head-injured patients and those undergoing intracranial surgery
- detect any other neurological disorder (cerebral vascular accident, encephalitis, meningitis)
- minimize variation and subjectivity in the clinical assessment of patients
- provide a neurological assessment that might indicate the level of patient dependency and subsequent need for nursing interventions.

It focuses on the evaluation of three parameters: eye opening, motor response and verbal response (Table 2.2). The patient's best achievement is recorded for each parameter. The scores are then added together to give an overall assessment of the patient's neurological status. A score of 15 represents the most responsive while a score of 3 is the least responsive.

Painful stimulus

If patients do not open their eyes or obey commands, the nurse must inflict a painful stimulus and view the response. The brain responds to central stimulation, the spine to peripheral stimulation.

- Central painful stimulation
  —The trapezium squeeze is the preferred method as supraorbital pressure and sternal rub can lead to bruising.
  —For best results the stimulus should last between 20 and 30 seconds.

—It should be carried out by the same member of nursing staff, using the same painful stimulus to assess the same patient's neurological status.
- Peripheral painful stimulation
  —Used to assess eye opening as central painful stimuli will often cause eye closure by inducing a grimacing effect.
  —It is applied directly to an unmoving arm or leg.
  —It will initiate a spinal reflex and the patient will pull the stimulated part away.
  —The best method of peripheral stimulus is to apply pressure on to the nail bed at the side of the finger so as to cause no damage to the structures under the nail bed.

Inflicting a painful stimulus may not always be needed, as the patient may find objects such as nasogastric tubes and oxygen masks irritating and may localize spontaneously to such sources.

It is important to remember that the nurse's goal is to assess the brain's best response to stimulation in order to catch early deterioration, not to cause pain for no reason.

Pupil size and reaction to light

Pupil size and reaction to light are tested by shining a torch onto the patient's eye. It is important to note whether the patient has any pre-existing pupil irregularities which are normal for them, e.g. previous eye injury, cataracts, blindness in one eye. Check the following factors.

Table 2.2 The three modes of behaviour used in the GCS (British Journal of Nursing)

Response	Description	Scale
Best eye opening response	Spontaneously: opens eyes spontaneously	4
	To speech: opens to verbal stimuli; not necessarily to command of 'open your eyes', a verbal stimulus may be normal, repeated or even loud	3
	To pain: does not open eyes to previous stimuli, opens eyes to central painful stimuli	2
	None: does not open eyes to any stimulus	1
Best verbal response	Orientated to time, place and person	5
	Disorientated and confused to any of the following: time, place or person; ability to hold a conversation but not accurately answering questions	4
	Inappropriate words: uses words or phrases making little or no sense, words may be said at random, shouting or swearing	3
	Incomprehensible sounds: makes unintelligible sounds (moans and groans)	2
	No response: makes no sounds or speech	1
	Other: if patient is intubated or has a tracheotomy, document ETT or trach; if dysphasia or aphasic document D or A	
Best motor response	Obeys verbal commands: follows commands, even if weakly	6
	Localizes to painful stimuli: attempts to locate or remove painful stimulus	5
	Withdraws from painful stimuli: moves away from painful stimulus or may bend or flex arm towards the source of pain but does not actually localize or remove source of pain	4
	Abnormal flexion and adduction of arms coupled with extensions of legs and plantar flexion of feet (decorticate posturing)	3
	Abnormal extension, adduction and internal rotation of upper and lower extremities (decerebrate posturing)	2
	No response, even to painful stimulus	1

- The pupil size (Fig. 2.1) – average pupil size is 2–5 mm
- The pupil reaction to light: brisk, sluggish or fixed
- The shape of the pupil – should be round
- If both pupils react equal to light and are equal in size

When undertaking the pupillary response the following should be observed.

- The light should be shone into the patient's eyes to see if they constrict.
- The light should not be shone directly into the patient's eyes; a

Pupil sizes in mm

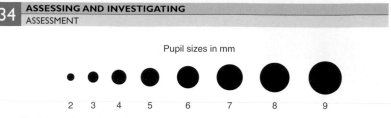

2   3   4   5   6   7   8   9

Fig. 2.1 Pupil size observed during the Glasgow Coma Scale (GCS) assessment.

torch should be shone from the side into the eye.

- It is best to carry this out in dim lighting as one sees the eyes constrict better when light is shone on them. Protocols should exist to eliminate any inconsistencies in the patient's score (e.g. discrepancies in dimming the light could occur during the night).
- Progressive dilatation and loss of pupil reaction on one side occur as a result of pressure on the third cranial nerve on that side, indicating an enlarged intracranial mass (haematoma).
- Progressive cerebral oedema eventually leads to compression of the third cranial nerve on the other side, so neither pupil then reacts to light (severe brain injury).
- Some drugs, e.g. atropine, dilate the pupil; opiates, e.g. morphine, constrict the pupil.

Observation of vital signs

The last section of the GCS is the observation of vital signs.

- A high temperature can be due to damage to the hypothalamus, which increases the cerebral metabolic oxygen requirement, an unwanted complication when oxygenation of the brain may already be depleted.
- Control centres for blood pressure, heart rate and respiration are all located in the brainstem so damage to this area of the brain can lead to:
  —changes in rate, depth and pattern of breathing, due to increases in carbon dioxide
  —other changes in heart rate and breathing, hypoxia, deterioration of brainstem function (Cheyne–Stokes respirations and/or central neurogenic hyperventilation)
  —increases in blood pressure: when there is an increase in intracranial pressure, cerebral resistance occurs and in order to maintain cerebral perfusion, blood pressure is raised.
- Neurological observations should be recorded at frequent intervals, one hour being the maximum time allowed.

The GCS provides a quick guide for evaluation of the acutely ill patient. The primary purpose of the GCS is to alert medical and nursing staff to deterioration in a patient's neurological status.

> ⚠ A continued rise in blood pressure and reduction in heart rate in patients with suspected increased intracranial pressure are indicative that their condition is worsening.

ANXIETY

A person's response to anxiety is due to activation of the sympathetic nervous system, potentiated by adrenaline and noradrenaline from the adrenal medulla. There are many factors in everyday life that provoke anxiety and hospitalization is one of them. Anxiety is difficult to define, mainly because it is often explained as a vague, uneasy feeling, the source of which is often non-specific or unknown to the individual.

Anxiety may be both positive and negative: positive in relation to learning ability, as a high anxiety level may have a motivating function, negative in relation to particular experiences, e.g. hospitalization.

Coping with the anxiety of hospitalization can sometimes lead to aggressive behaviour as a result of anger and frustration. Alternatively, coping may take the form of escape from the anxiety-provoking situation, resulting in withdrawal, due to the person's feelings of helplessness and the inability to gain control over events.

Anxiety is present in at least some hospitalized patients so there is a need for nurses to be able to make an accurate assessment. The assessment of anxiety relies on listening and talking to patients, questioning and discussion through interview, observation or the use of tools such as the:

- linear analogue scale (LAS)
- visual analogue scale (VAS)
- graphic anxiety scale
- Hospital Anxiety and Depression scale (HAD).

Nurses may already be familiar with their use.

STRESS

The concept of 'stress' is seen as an interaction process between the individual and his environment, rather than a single event or set of responses. Stressors make physical and psychological demands, which require individuals to assess and understand the situation and then to respond to it.

Situations where a person can understand and react to the circumstances in a satisfactory manner are less likely to be perceived as stressful by that individual. However, if the stressor demands new responses or ones which are undeveloped (e.g. illness) then it is likely that the experience will lead to stress.

Hence stress is taken to be the absence of or a deficiency in the individual's ability to cope with current environmental demands. The resulting illness caused by stress is linked to increased sympathetic nervous system arousal. The body's response to a stressor is reflected by a reaction which involves the whole body and generally consists of three distinct response phases.

1. *The alarm reaction* – widespread physiological response which includes a large outflow into the bloodstream of adrenal hormones in an attempt to defend the body from the stressor.
2. *Resistance or adaptation* – where an attempt is made by the body to reestablish equilibrium and to regain control to maintain

homeostasis. If the body is unable to re-establish homeostasis because of persistent exposure to the stressor then the third phase will result.

3. *Exhaustion* – ending in death.

The acutely ill individual in hospital is exposed to many stressors simultaneously. These act synergistically rather than cumulatively.

There are a number of events that make significant emotional demands upon the person while in hospital.

- Hearing the initial diagnosis may be a difficult and stressful process; the fear and anxiety generated by the news may be disruptive and debilitating, making it more difficult for the patient to absorb further information or to make informed choices.
- Perception of the situation itself is an intricate concept which may in turn be affected by past experiences, genetic predisposition, values and beliefs, self-concept and the level of anxiety at the time the stressor is perceived.
- Some treatments use powerful drugs, accompanied by side-effects which may include nausea and vomiting.
- Continued exposure to stressors can result in the development of stress ulcers, reduced wound healing and cardiac function and a reduced immune response to infection, amongst other physiological and psychological sequelae.
- Coping with specific life events – changes which occur through

choice (marriage or divorce) or may be totally unforeseen (bereavement, redundancy, accidental injury or long-term illness).

Therefore, the nurse caring for a patient in hospital needs to understand the relationship between the individual and his environment, life events and acute illness and as such take the following into consideration.

- Assessment of recent and current major life events and/or crises, as these may have precipitated the acute illness.
- Assessment of the individual's normal coping mechanisms and support networks, so that these can be enhanced or reinforced.
- Recognition that the present acute illness may cause stress in itself, particularly with regard to:
  —potential impact on employment
  —dependent family members
  —financial insecurity thus making the patient more vulnerable to infection, depression and slower recovery.
- The need to assist the patient's family members with positive coping mechanisms in a situation that may be perceived as stressful for them.

The ANS controls many other body functions and the physiological responses to stress can influence the measurements frequently undertaken by nurses during their daily work. The physiological responses to stress involve neuroendocrine activation and increased sympathetic activity, which stimulates the cardiovascular system and the adrenal medulla, resulting in the release of numerous substances into the circulation.

- *Catecholamines* – adrenaline increases heart rate, cardiac output, metabolic rate and blood glucose levels and causes dilatation of bronchioles; noradrenaline influences peripheral vasocontriction, increasing blood pressure.
- *Glucocorticoids* – cortisol from the adrenal cortex leads to gluconeogenesis, glycogenolysis, proteolysis and lipolysis and enhances adrenaline's vasoconstrictive effects.
- *Mineralocorticoids* – aldosterone increases sodium reabsorption in the renal tubules, resulting in the reduction of urine output and increase in intravascular volume, providing compensation for stress and fluid/ blood loss.
- *Antidiuretic hormone* (ADH) – targets kidney tubules and inhibits or prevents urine formation. Less urine is produced, blood volume increases and the thirst response will be aroused.

PAIN

Pain is one of the main symptoms that cause people to seek treatment. The presence of pain can interfere with obtaining accurate and reliable measurements, which can lead to false, inaccurate readings, and therefore it needs to be assessed early. Regular assessment of pain contributes to the quality of communication between nurse and patient and regular pain assessment can be a contributory factor in reducing pain.

Prior to effective treatment of pain, accurate assessment is essential. Because of its subjective nature, only patients can measure their own pain accurately and so nurses should provide simple pain assessment tools to help them assess and communicate their pain.

- *The visual analogue scale* – a straight line, usually 10 cm in length, with one extreme marked 'no pain at all' and the other end marked 'worst possible pain'. Descriptive words may be added.
- *Numerical rating scales* are marked 0–10, with 0 signifying 'no pain' and 10 meaning 'unbearable pain'.
- *Verbal rating scales* or verbal descriptors use 4–5 preset categories and consist of a list of adjectives that describe levels of pain intensity by extremes ('no pain', 'mild pain', 'discomfort', 'severe/distressing pain', 'excruciating/very severe pain').
- *The Bourbonnais pain assessment tool* – two pain assessment tools designed to complement each other, one for the patient and one for the nurse. The tool consists of two parts: a scale ranging from 0 (reflecting no pain) to 10 (reflecting excruciating pain) and a list of adjectives which describe different perceptions of pain. The person experiencing pain is then asked to match the word or words that describe his pain to the number, which corresponds to the intensity of the pain.

- *The London Pain Chart* – includes a body outline to record the site of pain, a verbal descriptor scale for intensity and measures to relieve pain.

It is important that the same tool is used throughout and that the tool chosen is the most appropriate for the patient's needs at that particular time. Also, when assessing patients' pain, it is vital to listen to what they are saying about their pain. Nurses persistently rate patients' pain as less than the patients do themselves.

Once assessed, it is imperative that the pain is treated as a failure to relieve pain is morally and ethically unacceptable (see Section 5 for pain relief). Pain can have a detrimental effect on patients' condition and can significantly slow recovery. The undertreatment of pain can lead to:

- decreased tidal volumes and alveolar ventilation, leading to decreased oxygen delivery to organs
- avoidance of coughing, resulting in an increase in secretions contributing to atelectasis and chest infections
- avoidance of movement, leading to an increased risk of deep vein thrombosis and pulmonary embolism
- increased stress response and sympathetic stimulation, resulting in vasoconstriction and tachycardia, raising blood pressure and increasing the workload of the heart
- stress, which interferes with intestinal smooth muscle and leads to an increase in metabolic rate, leading to difficulties in meeting nutritional needs and possible loss of weight.

Good pain relief can reduce these responses to pain and promote a safer and quicker recovery.

PRESSURE AREA RISK ASSESSMENT

Pressure sores are an avoidable complication of bedrest and decreased mobility. Patients at greater risk of developing pressure sores include:

- those who are in a poor state of health
- those who are malnourished
- those with some degree of immobility, particularly the elderly.

The pathogenesis of pressure sores is complex, since it is affected by so many predisposing factors. However, there are three major factors identified as significant.

- Pressure greater than 25 mmHg will occlude capillaries. The tissues are thus deprived of their blood supply and if the pressure is maintained for a sufficient length of time, the ischaemic tissues die.
- Friction is caused by dragging patients up the bed, which can seriously damage the microcirculation.
- Strain on structures so great that it tears the muscle and skin fibres from their bony attachments.

A patient suffering from a combination of predisposing factors is more susceptible to developing pressure sores. Predisposing factors can be subdivided into two main groups.

1. *Intrinsic factors* – aspects of the patient's condition, mental, physical and medical states, e.g. malnutrition, age, altered consciousness, immobility.
2. *Extrinsic factors* – external effects of drugs, treatment regimes, patient handling techniques, personal hygiene, weight distribution.

Those patients at greatest risk of developing pressure sores may be identified using a pressure sore prediction scale. The Waterlow Scale is the most widely used pressure sore risk calculator in the UK but the Braden Scale is often preferred because it is generally more reliable and valid, as the Waterlow Scale tends to overpredict risk. It is important to note that both scales are overcautious and potentially overpredict pressure sore risk. Yet it is better to overpredict than underpredict risk, as the cost of treating pressure sores is high, while the cost of preventing them is considerably less.

All patients admitted to hospital should be assessed for risk of pressure sore development within 2 hours of arrival. However, it is important to realize that a risk assessment score is not a definitive answer to the question of whether an individual will develop a pressure sore but rather an aid to professional and clinical judgement in determining what resources are needed. If used effectively, the calculator can justify a request for

resources, e.g. specialized beds and/or efficient moving and handling equipment.

WOUND ASSESSMENT

Wound assessment is a complex task that provides necessary information before deciding on a strategy for treatment. Using a measurement tool to assess wounds encourages consistent intervention irrespective of who assesses the wound at any time. A good wound assessment should include the following.

- A body diagram to record the patient's wound sites; in the case of multiple wounds these should be numbered individually.
- A separate assessment sheet should determine the site of each wound and/or the number identified from the initial body diagram.
- Consideration of the major areas in relation to the condition of any wound (Box 2.2).
- The maximum dimensions, traced and recorded, giving the length, width and depth of the wound in centimetres.

Charting wound healing facilitates accurate recording of observations and wound treatment. Which wound assessment documentation tool used is largely a matter of personal preference, so long as the user is aware of the tool's limitations. It is of paramount importance that the patient's wound(s) are assessed as soon as possible after admission and that the risk is reassessed whenever there is a significant change in his condition.

Box 2.2   Major areas that should be included in a wound assessment

Record of wound site	• Body diagram form different angles
	• Back
	• Front
	• Legs:
	—front
	—back
	—medial
	—lateral
Condition of wound	• Wound dimensions
	• Nature of wound bed
	• Exudate
	• Odour
	• Pain (site, frequency, severity)
	• Wound margin
	• Erythema of surrounding skin
	• Condition of surrounding skin infection
Dimensions/drawing	• Length
	• Width
	• Depth
	• Outside tracking
	• Healthy granulating tissue
	• Sloughy areas
Documentation	All these points need to be taken into consideration when documenting nursing observations and wound treatments in relation to wound care

---

NUTRITIONAL ASSESSMENT

Assessment of nutritional status is often omitted. However, most nurses are familiar with the use of assessment forms and protocols, including pressure sore management and risk assessment scales, which demonstrate how a simple tool employed at an early stage of patient contact can optimize care to produce the best outcome.

Nutritional assessment can be as simple or as complicated as desired but should be both subjective and objective. Information should be based on nurses' observations of the patient and on the collection of an essential core of material, e.g. patient history, psychological and social status, physical examination, diet history and appraisal of current nutritional intake, anthropometric measurements, biochemical and laboratory data.

Patient history, psychological and social status

A concise history provides the first clues about existing or potential malnutrition. The following patient factors are important.

• Recent bereavement
• Been ill at home for a long time
• Age
• Is he on income support?
• The type of accommodation he lives in

Observe the patient.

- Does he look thin?
- Assess the skin in terms of colour and condition.
- Are his clothes loose?
- Do his dentures fit properly?

These factors will all suggest that a problem with nutrition may exist and may also give information about any recent loss of weight.

Physical examination

A physical examination should include the following areas.

- The oral cavity.
- The presence of dysphagia, which may cause difficulty in chewing and swallowing, or any physical difficulties with feeding.
- Any nausea, vomiting, diarrhoea, which result in reduced absorption and appetite.
- Any constipation will affect nutritional intake and can lead to a feeling of fullness, discomfort, depression and confusion, thereby reducing food intake.
- Simple respiratory function tests can be recorded, such as vital capacity, maximum inspiration, maximum expiration, to determine respiratory muscle strength.

Diet history

A diet history should consist of questions about:

- likes and dislikes
- changes in weight
- type, quantity and texture of food eaten since the onset of illness, as disease often alters appetite

- any changes in taste and the ability to obtain and prepare food.

All these factors should be recorded in the patient's assessment and nursing care plan.

Anthropometric measurements

One of the most important anthropometric measurements in determining nutritional status is weight and changes in body weight can indicate the severity of malnutrition, a loss greater than 10% being indicative of malnutrition and a loss of 6–10% being potentially significant. It is important to note that weight is affected by certain disease processes, such as cancer, cachexia and oedema, which minimizes its usefulness as a measure of nutritional status. Ideal weight charts must be used with caution, as they do not take into account the effects of dehydration and fluid retention on weight. The charts are designed for the younger population and take no account of variations in weight due to illness or age.

Height can also be used to determine malnutrition but it is not always possible to measure height in hospitalized patients and it may not be an adequate guide in elderly patients. It is sometimes easier to ask the patient how tall he is – most people have a good idea and this is better than nothing.

Height and weight measurements can be used to determine body mass index (BMI) which is calculated by:

Weight (kg) divided by height (metres) squared.

The normal range is 20–25 and a BMI of less than 20 could be a serious risk to health.

More complicated anthropometric measurements can be used to gain more accurate information and can be useful in oedematous or dehydrated patients where body weight figures are meaningless. Body fat content is quickly and easily estimated from skinfold thickness measurements. Most commonly used is triceps skinfold thickness (TSF) which, in combination with mid upper arm circumference (MUAC), can be used to calculate mid-arm muscle circumference (MAMC) as an absolute index of muscle mass:

$$MAMC = MUAC - 0.3142 \times TSF$$

These measurements can be compared with standards and if performed serially, will reflect a change in body tissue. These measurements are only reliable if undertaken by a trained operator and are not always accurate or a true prediction of changes in body mass in overweight or elderly patients.

Biochemical measurements

Serum albumin
With a level of less than 35 g/l being indicative of protein energy malnutrition, it can be inaccurate as conditions such as stress, nephrosis and burns also exhibit hypoalbuminaemia. Thus the measurement is often misleading and not altogether reflective of nutritional deficiency in the short term. In the chronic situation, serum albumin remains a simple and reliable indicator of malnutrition.

Serum transferrin
Levels could be considered a better marker of acute nutritional depletion. Interpretation of serum levels is complicated by factors such as iron deficiency, which directly affects transferrin production, and so it may not be wholly appropriate as a predictor of malnutrition.

Serum haemoglobin
Measurements will highlight the presence of anaemia, which has been correlated with pressure sore development. Anaemia can occur for a variety of reasons but may be directly related to dietary inadequacy and questioning of dietary intake should always follow this up.

Undernutrition
Promising results have been demonstrated when nutritional assessment has resulted in initiation of preoperative feeding regimes. This method of identifying high-risk patients results in an optimization of their nutritional status and may help to ensure an uneventful recovery. The patient in hospital not only has an increased demand for energy but also, due to periods of reduction or cessation of nutritional intake, has a reduced supply of energy-containing nutrients. As a result, undernutrition or, in severe cases, malnutrition may occur.

Undernutrition reduces the body's ability to:

- heal wounds which increases the risk of pressure sores
- produce haemoglobin, which reduces the oxygen-carrying capacity of the blood
- produce white blood cells, causing suppression of the immune response and exposing the patient to the risk of infection
- maintain adequate respiratory drive due to reduction in pulmonary diaphragmatic muscle mass and strength, predisposing the patient to respiratory failure.

2.3 OBSERVATIONS AND MEASUREMENTS

Obvious examples of measurements are: heart rate, pulse rate, respiration, oxygen saturation and mental state, blood pressure, temperature, central venous pressure (CVP), urine output. These measurements may be carried out to substantiate information obtained from observing, interviewing or assessing the patient.

HEART RATE

The heartbeat originates in the sinoatrial node. The atria contract, followed by a short pause whilst the contraction wave moves down the bundle of His to the Purkinje fibres. Then the ventricles contract and blood is ejected from the right ventricle into the pulmonary artery and from the left ventricle into the aorta. The ventricular muscle relaxes and the heart returns to its initial position. There is then a longer pause, when all chambers are relaxed before the next beat occurs.

The heart beats continuously for the whole of a person's life. Each impact of the heart against the chest wall can be felt or heard with a stethoscope, in the fifth left intercostal space, generally under the left nipple.

PULSE RATE

The rhythmic contraction of the left ventricle transmits a pressure impulse through the arteries. This pulse is customarily palpated at the radial artery in the wrist. The important factors to consider in relation to the radial pulse rate are:

- rate
- rhythm
- pressure (volume)
- deficits with apex rate.

The pulse rate is an important component of cardiac output. Fluctuations of pulse rate in the well individual normally occur together with fluctuations in stroke volume to maintain optimum cardiac output for the activity being performed, for example rest or exercise.

In the resting adult, the pulse rate would normally be about 70 beats per minute. A rate greater than 100 beats per minute is termed a *tachycardia* and a rate less than 60 beats per minute is termed a *bradycardia*. The rhythm of the pulse may vary normally with respiration, especially in young adults, so that the pulse is irregular, speeding up at the peak of inspiration and slowing down with expiration. This is termed *sinus arrhythmia*. An irregular pulse is commonly categorized as regularly irregular or irregularly irregular. A regularly irregular pulse is most likely to be caused by ectopic beats (a beat originating from a site other than the sinoatrial node) which occur prematurely. Occasionally odd ectopic beats may occur in healthy individuals. If they are found to persist in an acutely ill person, the medical staff will require notification as they can be indicative of:

- increased cardiac irritability due to ischaemia or drugs (such as digoxin)
- increased sympathetic activity as a result of stressors (for example, hypoxia)
- potassium imbalance

all of which require further investigation. An irregularly irregular pulse usually indicates atrial fibrillation where atrial behaviour is chaotic and disorganized and the transmission of impulses to the ventricles is irregular.

The *pulse pressure* is a wave of pressure caused by a sequence of distension and elastic recoil in the wall of the aorta which forces blood rapidly down the systemic arterial system. It determines the strength of the pulse and can be defined as the difference between the systolic and diastolic blood pressures.

When the pulse pressure is low, the strength of the pulse may be feeble and thready. This may occur when hypovolaemia exists, because the stroke volume ejected by the left ventricle into the circulation is greatly reduced. When the pulse pressure is high, the pulse strength may be bounding and the person

experiencing this may feel palpitations or hear his heart pounding.

The *pulse deficit* is the difference between the heart rate counted at the apex of the heart using a stethoscope and the pulse rate counted simultaneously at the wrist. For the majority of patients the heart rate and pulse rate will be the same but for those who are in atrial fibrillation or who are having multiple ectopic beats, there will be a deficit which is important to monitor by recording both apex and radial rates.

There are many other pulses in the body and by measuring these, a nurse may help to determine the adequacy of circulation and where the problem may be. The main pulses in the body are:

- apical
- radial
- carotid
- femoral
- brachial
- aortic
- popliteal
- posterior tibial
- dorsalis pedis.

Peripheral pulses

As previously discussed, the pulse pressure is a wave of pressure which can be palpated near the body surface where large arteries are superficially located or where they pass over underlying bone. There are many pulses in the body (identified above) but the pulses of the lower limbs, the popliteal pulse located behind the knee and the dorsalis pedis and posterior tibial pulses in the feet, are important in determining adequacy of perfusion to the lower limbs.

RESPIRATION

Respiration is an essential body function necessary for the diffusion of gases between the alveoli and blood, as well as the maintenance of blood pH. Ventilation is the mechanical movement of gas or air in and out of the lungs. The respiratory rate is the ventilatory rate and is recorded in breaths per minute in order to:

- determine a baseline respiratory rate for compensation
- monitor fluctuations in respiration
- evaluate the patient's response to medications or treatments that affect the respiratory system.

Effective respiration is dependent on many factors, both nervous and chemical in nature, including the chemoreceptors and lung receptors, which control depth, quality and pattern of breathing.

Rate

The normal rate at rest is approximately 14–18 breaths per minute in adults and is faster in infants and children. Changes in the rate of breathing are defined as *tachypnoea*, an increase in respiratory rate, e.g. in fever, or *bradypnoea*, a decreased but regular respiratory rate, e.g. depression of the respiratory centre in the medulla by opiate narcotics.

Depth

This is the volume of air moving in and out with each respiration,

normally measured as the tidal volume of about 500 ml which is constant with each breath. Normal relaxed breathing is effortless, automatic, regular and almost silent. *Dyspnoea* is breathlessness and an awareness of discomfort with breathing.

Pattern

The pattern of breathing changes in disorders of the respiratory control centre. The respiratory pattern is normally regular and consists of inspiration, pause, longer expiration and another pause. In certain diseases the pattern changes.

- *Hyperventilation* – an increase in both the rate and depth of respiration to about 20–30 breaths per minute.
- *Apneustic* – a pattern of prolonged, gasping inspiration, followed by extremely short, inefficient expiration.
- *Cheyne–Stokes* – is periodic breathing characterized by a gradual increase in depth of respiration followed by a decrease in respiration, resulting in apnoea.

> ⚠ In hypovolaemic states haemodynamic measures, e.g. blood pressure, heart rate and respiration, may initially increase and then decrease as it becomes more difficult for the body to maintain adequate blood supply.

BLOOD PRESSURE (BP)

Taking the blood pressure (BP) remains one of the most important and widely used assessment tools in hospital, as from this one test much information can be gleaned about the patient's state of health. Nurses generally record blood pressure on admission to hospital to determine a baseline or as a determinant of risk factors for such diseases as cerebral vascular accident, ischaemic heart disease and renal disease, all of which can influence recovery.

The BP should be taken when a patient is admitted, postoperatively, when drugs that alter blood pressure are taken and when the patient's condition has deteriorated. It should also be taken when the patient is hypertensive, neutropenic, pregnant, critically ill, receiving an infusion or has an infection.

The BP is 'the force exerted by the blood on the walls of the arteries in which it is contained'. A number of factors determine it, most significantly cardiac output, peripheral resistance, elasticity of vessels and hormonal and chemical control mechanisms. Two components of blood pressure are evident.

- The *systolic pressure* – the amount of blood which is forced out into the arteries at ventricular contraction.
- The *diastolic pressure* – which is the fall in arterial pressure before the next ventricular contraction.

There are two methods of taking a blood pressure, direct and indirect.

- *Direct* monitoring of BP is accomplished by cannulating an artery and attaching the catheter to a fluid-filled tubing and transducer, which is connected to a voltage source.
- *Indirect* methods of BP monitoring are more commonly used and fall into two categories: the auscultatory (manual) method and computer-assisted automatic devices.

Two different sphygmomanometers are used for the manual method, the aneroid and mercury, but the use of the mercury sphygmomanometer is in decline. The reasons are:

- pressure from environmentalists to ban mercury as a toxic substance
- the failure to hear Korotkoff sounds in low-flow states
- there are more accurate automated devices to replace the conventional techniques, which may be inaccurate.

The traditional oscillatory technique uses a pneumatic cuff and stethoscope which monitors Korotkoff sounds (Box 2.3). Korotkoff sounds are generated by blood passing through the compressed artery under the cuff and meeting a static column of blood, resulting in turbulence and vibrations. To be detected by a stethoscope these

> ⚠ In low-flow states, such as those associated with hypotension, the auscultatory method has been demonstrated to fail, apparently because of the human ear's inability to appreciate low-frequency vibrations.

Box 2.3	Korotkoff sounds (Hinchliffe 1998)
Phase I	The pressure level at which the first clear tapping sounds are heard.
Phase II	The time during inflaction when a murmur and a swishing are heard.
Phase III	The point when the murmur disappears and the louder and more distinct sound is heard.
Phase IV	Muffling of sound.
Phase V	The sound disappears.

sounds must be at a frequency within an audible range.

The automatic cycling devices have gained increasing acceptance in an attempt to solve this problem. However, their reliability has been challenged as, like the auscultatory method, many of these devices are blood flow dependent.

Both methods of indirect BP monitoring are subject to error and may be unreliable in the very clinical situations where they are used the most (Box 2.4). This is mainly due to the fact that measuring and monitoring blood pressure are frequently carried out but often performed incorrectly. Recommendations on how to take an accurate blood pressure are given in Box 2.5.

> ⚠ Errors in measurement of blood pressure may mean wrong decisions being made in blood pressure management, thus compromising care.

OXYGEN SATURATION MEASUREMENT TO DETERMINE HYPOXIA

Adequate tissue oxygenation depends on a balance between oxygen supply and delivery and the tissue demand for oxygen. When oxygen demands exceed oxygen supply, hypoxia occurs. Alveolar hypoxia can cause pulmonary vasoconstriction, although hypoxia usually causes peripheral vasodilation.

Hypoxia may be due to:

- a blockage, whereby the tissues become hypoxic due to a reduced blood flow, as in arteriosclerosis
- the loss of red blood cells which carry oxygen to the cells, often observed in haemorrhage
- the inability to get oxygen into the circulation, seen in patients with impaired respiratory function.

The nurse is frequently the first to observe the presence of hypoxia and the one who can intervene to correct the problem with oxygenation.

Hypoxia may be observed in a number of ways. There may be changes in behaviour and level of consciousness. This is because the brain needs a continuous, steady supply of oxygenated blood and this is why the brain is a sensitive indicator of a patient's perfusion status. Very early signs of cerebral underperfusion are the inability to think abstractly or perform complex mental tasks, restlessness, apprehension, uncooperativeness and irritability.

Short-term memory may also be impaired. A family member may need to be called upon for

---

Box 2.4 Potential sources of error when taking a BP

The observer
- Observer bias – prior recording viewed by the nurse or a preference for a specific figure, known as digit preference.
- Cognitive deficits – education, inadequate training, no updating on the technique or principles.
- Lack of understanding of the correct procedure, e.g. incorrect positioning of the patient, sitting/standing, support of the arm, positioning of the cuff bladder over the centre of the brachial artery, the bladder / cuff not level with the heart
- Lack of concentration
- Hearing problems/deficit
- Sight problems

The equipment
- Cuff/bladder size
- Maintenance – BP machines should be calibrated and assessed every 6 – 12 months
- The level of mercury not at zero
- Defective control valves caused by leakage, making control of the pressure release difficult
- Leaks from cracked or perished rubber tubing
- The stethoscope should be in good condition and have clean and well-fitted earpieces

The patient
- The patient may be suffering from excessive heat or cold, be wearing constrictive clothing, have a full bladder, recently exercised, been smoking, just had a meal or there may be a distraction, all of which will serve to either increase or decrease the BP
- Older patients have calcified/rigid arteries or anaemia which can all influence the BP reading
- A patient suffering from a high temperature may have a low BP due to vasodilatation, causing the BP to fall
- In all patients the general consensus now is that disappearance of sounds (phase V) is the most accurate measurement of diastolic pressure with the stipulation that if sounds persist to zero (e.g. in pregnant women, children or patients suffering from anaemia), the muffling of sounds (phase IV) should be used
- In conditions where BP is low there may be distal vasoconstriction and it is common to underestimate the BP
- In some patients the white coat syndrome affects BP – this is caused when doctors appear at the bedside, giving an inaccurately high BP reading
- BP does vary during the day – higher systolic in the evening and a low recording in the morning
- Fear, anxiety, apprehension and pain can all raise the BP and these can be apparent on admission
- It is recommended in this instance to wait at least 1 hour following admission to take the BP

Box 2.5   Recommendations on how to take an accurate BP

- If possible the patient should not have eaten, exercised or smoked for at least 30 minutes prior to taking a BP.
- The patient should be sitting or lying down, in a quiet environment with his arm resting at heart level on a table or pillow (the antecubital fossa should be level with the fourth intercoastal space). An arm that is below this level results in a falsely high reading and vice versa.
- A rest period of at least 3 – 5 minutes should be allowed before the reading is taken.
- Measure the circumference of the arm and use the appropriate-sized bladder. However, it is possible with some cuffs to take an accurate BP even if the cuff is not an accurate size by placing the bladder centre over the brachial artery (an arrow on the actual cuff generally marks the spot) (Nolan & Nolan 1993).
- A gap of 2–3 cm should be left between the antecubital fossa and the bottom of the cuff.
- The sphygmomanometer should be placed near to the observer (no more than 3 feet away) on a flat surface with the mercury level at zero. If the mercury is not at zero it can produce false high or low readings.
- Locate the brachial artery by palpation.
- Assess the maximal inflation level of the cuff, to prevent causing pain to the patient. This is achieved by inflating the cuff and palpating the radial pulse at the same time; the maximal inflation level will be 20–30 mmHg higher than the level at which the pulse disappeared.
- The patient should not cross his legs as this will give a falsely high reading.
- Place the stethoscope over the brachial artery, being careful not to use too much pressure, as this lowers the diastolic pressure reading. Release the valve slowly and gently.
- The cuff should be rapidly inflated at 2 mmHg/s and deflated slowly. A slow inflation and a rapid deflation both result in inaccuracies.
- Note the systolic pressure at the onset of the first clear repetitive tapping sound of two beats or more.
- The diastolic pressure should be recorded at the cessation of sound (phase V) for all patients, unless the recording is zero, in which case the muffling of sound (phase IV) should be used. If phase IV is used it should be documented on the chart.
- The BP should be measured to the nearest 2 mmHg.
- The procedure should take no less than 5 minutes (Nolan & Nolan 1993).
- If the procedure is rushed, this will result in an underestimation of the systolic pressure and an overestimation of the diastolic pressure.
- The measurement should be recorded on the patient's chart. If it is not possible to achieve optimum conditions, this should also be noted with the blood pressure reading; for example, 'BP 145/95, L arm, phase V (patient very anxious)'.
- If the recording needs to be repeated, at least 1 – 2 minutes should have elapsed before reinflating the cuff.

information on the patient's normal personality and intellectual status. In addition, there may be changes in BP, pulse, and colour of mucous membranes. This may lead the nurse to extend the assessment for hypoxia by obtaining an oxygen saturation measurement (see p. 72) or by the doctor obtaining arterial blood for blood gas analysis (see p.67).

Oxygen saturation monitoring measures levels of haemoglobin and is widely used in many patient care settings. The normal percentage of oxygen saturated with haemoglobin is 98%. It is important for practitioners to note that the oxygen saturation monitor can give misleading information regarding the true nature of the patient's oxygen status.

The oxygen disassociation curve plots the relationship between the amount of oxygen bound to haemoglobin (oxygen saturation) and the partial pressure of oxygen (PaO_2) in the blood. The steep S-shaped curve highlights that at a normal PaO_2 of 13.3 kPa, oxygen saturation is 100%. If the PaO_2 drops by 5.3 kPa to 8 kPa the oxygen saturation will remain within acceptable limits at 90%. At a further drop of just 1.7 kPa, the oxygen saturation will drop from 90% to 70%. At this level breathing is difficult and respiratory arrest may occur, requiring emergency intubation.

An oxygen saturation of 90% may not indicate to the nurse that there is a low oxygen supply in the blood (determined by partial pressure of oxygen). An awareness of these principles will ensure that

oxygen saturation monitoring is safe and minimize the potential for unrecognized hypoxaemic episodes.

The oxygen saturation measurement is valuable as it allows nurses to evaluate the relative state of oxygenation and can help to improve the care the patient receives. However, when using pulse oximetry in practice, other observations should be undertaken in conjunction with it if hypoxia is suspected, e.g. colour, pulse rate, breathing pattern and rate, arterial blood gases (to give partial pressure of oxygen).

TEMPERATURE

The temperature can affect the circulation if it is abnormally low or high. If the temperature is high, as in infective states, the hypothalamus reflex initiates dilatation of arterioles and veins in the skin, causing a reduction in cardiac output and BP and an increase in heart rate. When the body's core temperature decreases below normal, surface blood vessels vasoconstrict to shunt the blood to the vital organs and prevent excess heat loss from skin surfaces, causing a decrease in oxygen consumption and heart rate and an increase in BP.

There are a number of ways to take the temperature:

- sublingually for 1 minute
- axilla for 2–3 minutes
- rectal temperature
- ear temperature.

Oral, axillary and ear temperatures are recommended as the most effective ways to take a temperature in the general wards. It should be noted that external variables affect oral temperature readings, including the ingestion of hot or cold substances, recent bathing, recent physical exertion and smoking. For the greatest accuracy, the bulb of the thermometer should be placed sublingually to the right or left and not the area in the middle of the tongue.

Different equipment is available to take the temperature and may influence the temperature reading.

- Glass thermometers containing mercury
- Electronic thermometer
- Single-use chemical thermometers – these use a chemical which changes colour with increasing temperature
- Electronic thermometers – a signal indicates when the maximum temperature has been reached, to prevent premature removal of the thermometer
- Tympanic membrane thermometer – uses an infrared light reflectance thermometer that detects heat radiated as infrared energy from the tympanic membrane.

The best time of day for temperature recording is important as there are diurnal variations in human body temperature owing to circadian rhythms and this will affect readings.

⚠ **Many standard thermometers do not record temperatures below 35°C, so for an accurate measurement of hypothermia, a low-reading thermometer is necessary.**

Temperature is most likely to be elevated at the peak of the circadian cycle, which is between 5pm and 7pm.

Infants and the elderly in relation to temperature control

Infants and the elderly require special attention to maintenance of body temperature.

- Infants produce sufficient body heat but are unable to conserve the heat produced.
- The poor heat conservation is caused by the infant's small body size and greater ratio of body surface to body weight, which gives the infant more surface area for heat loss.
- Infants also have a very thin layer of subcutaneous fat and thus are not as well insulated as adults.

The elderly have poor responses to environmental temperature extremes as a result of:

- slowed blood circulation
- structural and functional changes in the skin
- overall decrease in heat-producing activities
- decrease in shivering response (delayed onset and decreased effectiveness)
- slowed metabolic rate
- sedentary lifestyle
- decreased vasoconstrictor response
- diminished or absent sweating
- desynchronization of circadian rhythm
- undernutrition/dehydration
- decreased perception of heat and cold.

Toe temperature

When the main circulation is impaired there are changes to the peripheral circulation to the body's extremities. This will be reflected in the peripheral skin temperature, providing good indications of the presence and severity of a circulatory defect. The toe temperature gradient provides a valuable, inexpensive and non-invasive monitor of tissue perfusion.

Skin temperature

Skin temperature can be a useful guide to determining the severity of shock, as during hypovolaemia circulation to the major organs and central temperature need to be maintained. To do this the body under ANS control improves the circulation through baroreceptor activity, which will cause vasoconstriction and prevent heat loss from body surfaces. The end result is heat conservation, extremities that feel cool to touch, an increase in BP and improved circulation to the body's major organs.

CENTRAL VENOUS PRESSURE (CVP) MONITORING

The measurement of the central venous pressure (CVP) provides important haemodynamic information to guide therapy. The CVP reflects the volume of blood returning to the heart, which exerts pressure on the walls of the right ventricle. This blood will then be circulated through the heart and lungs and around the body.

CVP monitoring determines:

- the adequacy of the body's blood volume
- the pumping function of the right side of the heart
- vascular tone and pulmonary vascular resistance.

To determine an accurate CVP the patient should be placed in the supine position, with the backrest at an angle of up to 30°. It is essential that CVP measurement is made under identical conditions each time so that all possible variables (such as patient position) remain constant.

The most reliable external reference point used to take the CVP is the mid axilla, using a water manometer. Measuring a central venous pressure using a water manometer is demonstrated in Figure 2.2.

A fall in CVP may indicate:

- moderate hypovolaemic shock, in patients who are bleeding following surgery
- dehydration
- extreme vasodilatation, whereby the capacity of the circulation is increased but the circulating volume remains constant, as in patients with a pyrexia or from the excessive use of vasodilator drugs
- left ventricular failure.

An increase in CVP may represent:

- exposure to extreme cold, e.g. following surgery, causing severe vasoconstriction, which would return more blood to the heart as the veins are already filled
- fluid overload due to blood transfusion, colloid or crystalloid
- heart failure.

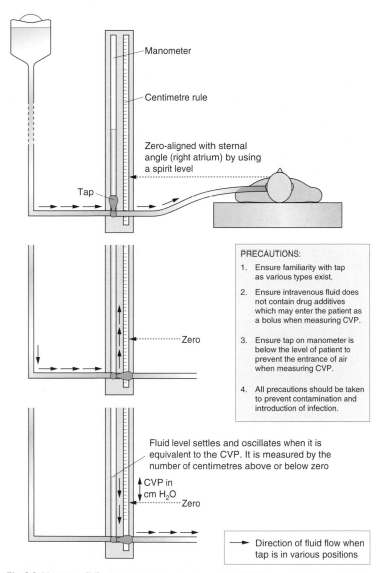

Manometer

Centimetre rule

Zero-aligned with sternal angle (right atrium) by using a spirit level

Tap

PRECAUTIONS:

1. Ensure familiarity with tap as various types exist.

2. Ensure intravenous fluid does not contain drug additives which may enter the patient as a bolus when measuring CVP.

3. Ensure tap on manometer is below the level of patient to prevent the entrance of air when measuring CVP.

4. All precautions should be taken to prevent contamination and introduction of infection.

Zero

Fluid level settles and oscillates when it is equivalent to the CVP. It is measured by the number of centimetres above or below zero

CVP in cm H_2O
Zero

Direction of fluid flow when tap is in various positions

Fig. 2.2 Measuring CVP via a water manometer. From Hinchliff S/Nursing Practice and Health Care 3e, reproduced with permission of Hodder/Arnold Limited.

Generally, the value of the CVP reading is overestimated. If a fall in CVP occurs this is proposed to indicate a moderate hypovolaemia while a consequent rise in CVP is proposed to suggest fluid overload. It is presumed by many that the CVP can be used as a guide to determine severity of fluid loss, measure when too much fluid has been administered and ascertain cardiac instability.

The suggestion is that a normal or reduced CVP will occur in hypovolaemia, during hypervolaemia and left-sided cardiac failure.

● In hypovolaemia due to the loss of fluid.
● In left-sided heart failure due to the left side of the heart generally failing first, causing severe systolic dysfunction of the left ventricle and a consequent reduction in stroke volume and cardiac output. As a result there is a decline in the amount of blood returning to the heart (venous return) and hence a reduction in CVP.
● In hypervolaemia, it may take nearly 24 hours for events occurring in the left side of the heart to reflect through the lungs into the right ventricle, atria and superior vena cava and be mirrored as an increased CVP reading.

This implies that CVP levels are not completely reliable in estimating circulatory function. Therefore, a more accurate measure would be that which could determine the pressure in the left side of the heart (see later) via pulmonary artery wedge pressure.

> ⚠ It is not the single CVP reading that is important but the trend demonstrated by a series of readings over time.

The CVP catheter can also be used for rapid infusion of fluids and blood or to withdraw blood for laboratory samples. The most common complications of a CVP line include pneumothorax, hydrothorax and ventricular arrhythmias, infection and air embolism, all of which should be observed for during the procedure.

PULMONARY ARTERY WEDGE PRESSURE (PAWP)

This indirectly measures the left ventricle's end-diastolic pressure and is an invaluable assessment. It is measured by a special catheter tip (Swan–Ganz or thermodilution pulmonary artery catheter) that sits at the distal port of the pulmonary artery and involves the threading of a catheter from a central vein through the right atrium and right ventricle and into the pulmonary artery. It is a highly invasive technique with a recognized risk of morbidity and mortality.

When the balloon is deflated the pressure reflected is the pulmonary artery pressure (PAP). The normal pressure is systolic 20–30 mmHg and diastolic 8–15 mmHg.

When the balloon is inflated the right pressures become blocked by the inflated balloon and the pulmonary artery wedge pressure (PAWP) recorded indirectly reflects left atrial pressure, left ventricular end-diastolic pressure (LVEDP) and left ventricular preload. Because of this the PAWP is a much more reliable measurement than the CVP in determining the circulating volume. The normal PAWP is 5–12 mmHg but many patients may require a much higher pressure, 15–20 mmHg, to achieve optimal preload and therapy often aims for a higher range.

The PAP catheter measures right atrial pressure, right ventricular pressure, PAWP, systemic vascular resistance (SVR) and cardiac output (CO).

The indications for haemodynamic evaluation are as follows:

- acute cardiac failure
- shock
- diagnosis of tamponade
- mitral regurgitation
- ruptured ventricular septum
- management of high-risk obstetrical patients
- intraoperative and postoperative management of high-risk patients.

If the PAWP is high and CO low, this may indicate hypervolaemia giving rise to left ventricular insufficiency and cardiac dysfunction. If hypovolaemia is present both PAWP and CO would be reduced. Hypervolaemia and hypovolaemia require different therapies to maintain adequate cardiac functioning.

INTRACRANIAL PRESSURE (ICP) MONITORING

The skull and meninges contain three major components.

- Brain tissue (80%)
- Cerebral spinal fluid (CSF) (10%)
- Cerebral blood flow (CBF) (10%)

The pressure these three components excert in the rigid skull is termed the intracranial pressure (ICP). The normal range of ICP is 0–15 mmHg. The brain maintains this normal pressure by compensation mechanisms known as *autoregulation*, which occurs following an insult or injury leading to increased brain, blood or CSF volume. To compensate the following occurs.

- Displacement of CSF from the cranial subarachnoid space, spinal and lumbar space. CSF production decreases and CSF absorption increases.
- Reduction in CBF as venous blood is shunted away from the affected areas. A widespread reduction in CBF to compensate can lead to further brain insult or ischaemia due to the reduced cerebral perfusion.

These compensatory mechanisms may become exhausted and an increase in ICP above 15 mmHg may occur as a result of:

- trauma
- hydrocephalus
- infection
- tumours
- metabolic disorders
- cerebrovascular accident
- encephalopathies.

In certain injuries monitoring techniques can be employed to measure the ICP. There are three types of ICP monitoring devices, all of which monitor but only one can drain the CSF.

- Ventriculostomy (intraventricular catheter; able to drain)
- Subdural bolt or catheter
- Epidural screw, bolt or sensor

Meticulous records of observations need to be kept, especially of mean arterial pressure (MAP). This is necessary to determine adequate CBF.

Cerebral perfusion pressure (CPP) is the pressure needed to perfuse the brain and the normal range is 80–90 mmHg. It is calculated by subtracting the ICP from the MAP.

CBF is compromised if the CPP is below 60 mmHg and reduced CPP may result in irreversible brain damage or death. It is thought that the threshold for mechanical brain injury is an ICP of 20–30 mmHg.

URINE OUTPUT

The kidney receives about 25% of the cardiac output. Glomerular filtration rate (GFR) is dependent on an adequate renal perfusion. When tissue perfusion is adequate the production of urine will exceed 0.5 ml/kg per hour. The average urinary output should be between 30 and 70 ml or more per hour. When blood flow to the kidneys is reduced an increase in vasoconstriction occurs. The overall net effect is that the GFR decreases, reducing urinary output. In contrast, when there is an increase in fluid administration causing hypervolaemia (fluid overload),

cardiac failure and pulmonary oedema may occur. In this instance kidney function may also become impaired, due to a reduction in the pumping action of the heart, a reduced cardiac output and blood flow to the kidneys.

In dehydrated or hypovolaemic states the kidneys play a complex role in restoring extracellular fluid volume and increasing systemic blood pressure. This system is stimulated principally when there is a decrease in blood pressure. This elaborate set of interlinked processes involves the renin-angiotensin-aldosterone system, osmoreceptors and baroreceptors.

If urine output falls below 25 ml per hour, fluid administration may be necessary. This is why urinary output should be measured, either at hourly intervals if a catheter is inserted or from a bedpan or bottle, and accurately recorded. Interpretation of urine output should also consider overall fluid balance (positive or negative over a 24-hour period), the quality and colour of urine.

2.4 PROCEDURES AND INVESTIGATIONS

COLLECTING AND SENDING SPECIMENS

The collection of a specimen involves obtaining a required amount of tissue or fluid for laboratory examinations. It is generally performed to:

- isolate and identify microorganisms that cause disease

- determine antibiotic sensitivity to guide the selection of appropriate antibiotic therapy
- measure levels of chemicals in blood and CSF to determine diagnosis and treatment.

In some instances nurses should be able to identify the need for microbiological investigation and, if appropriate, initiate the taking of a specimen. The types of specimens taken are:

- swabs of the eye, nose, throat, ear, wound, drain site, vagina, cervix, penis and rectum
- urine sample from a male or female
- faeces
- semen
- blood
- sputum
- cerebral spinal fluid.

When obtaining a sample for analysis the following should be considered.

- Explain and discuss the procedure with the patient and ensure privacy while the procedure is being carried out.
- Wash hands using bactericidal soap and water or bactericidal alcohol hand rub.
- Cleanse the area, if relevant, and collect the specimen, ensuring that no contamination of the specimen has occurred, as this will result in misleading information.
- Place specimen(s) and swabs in the appropriate correctly labelled containers. There are many types of specimen collection tools, e.g. swabs and pots. If you do not

know which is the correct container then seek advice from the microbiology department.
- The greater amount of material and information given to the laboratory, the greater the chance of isolating a causative organism. Therefore the request form must include the following information.
  —Patient name, ward and/or department
  —Hospital number
  —Date specimen collected
  —Time specimen collected
  —Provisional or diagnosis
  —Relevant signs and symptoms
  —Relevant history, e.g. recent foreign travel, recent toxic therapy
  —Any antimicrobial drugs being taken by the patient
  —Type of specimen
  —Risk of infection for staff
  —Consultant's name
  —Name of the doctor who ordered the investigation, as it may be necessary to telephone the result before the typed report is dispatched.
- The container should be leakproof and placed in a plastic bag before being sent to the laboratory.
- Dispatch specimens promptly to the laboratory with the completed request form.

URINE TESTING

This is a non-invasive technique to monitor the functioning of the kidney and in some instances other organs.

- Fluid balance, acid–base balance and kidney function may be evaluated.

- It can aid diagnosis in diabetes, weight loss, urinary tract infection, liver function, e.g. blockage of flow of bile, cancer of and trauma to the bladder.
- Circulatory status can be monitored.
- It provides valuable clues to the effectiveness of treatment.

The significance of the urine test strip results can be found in the specific gravity, pH or whether blood, protein, bilirubin and urobilinogen, nitrates, glucose and ketones are present.

The specific gravity (SG)

As urine is mostly water with a variable quantity of substances dissolved in it, the concentration of these substances will depend on the body's state of hydration and the amount of waste products to be excreted. Testing the urine for specific gravity(SG) can be one way to determine if hydration is adequate.

Dehydration is a common problem in hospital, especially in the elderly, so determining SG may give clues to the physiological status of the patient. Although inpatient monitoring of fluid balance with intake and output charts is essential, loss of water through the breath, sweat and faeces is not so easily measured. The SG of urine will give a good indication of the net fluid balance and is of particular value in patients where there is an unquantifiable loss, such as in burns cases, breathing difficulties, diarrhoea or fever.

In healthy adults, the SG varies between 1005 and 1035 (pure water

is the standard, with a SG of 1000). The SG depends on the state of hydration.

- The first specimen of the morning will tend to have a higher SG than one taken after the subject has had a drink.
- An isolated assessment of SG is of little value and the test should be repeated on samples taken at known times.
- Urine with a persistently low SG is suggestive of diabetes insipidus or renal damage. As the normal concentration power of the kidneys is lost, the urine passed will tend to be rather dilute.
- An increase in SG will indicate dehydration, perhaps due to bleeding, vomiting, diarrhoea, reduction in fluid intake or fever.

The method for measuring SG is the reagent strip, which measures the ionic strength of a urine sample and expresses this with a simple-to-read colour change. The colour changes on the reagent strips are easier to read than the gradations on the narrow stem of the hydrometer and thus the method is less prone to errors.

The pH

The pH of urine should reflect the acid–base balance of the body, as excess hydrogen or bicarbonate ions are excreted by the tubules to maintain the normal status. Under normal circumstances, the urine has a pH of around 6 but it can range from about 5 to 8.5. Metabolic acidosis arising from starvation, high protein diets or diabetic ketoacidosis will lead to an acid urine but diets including a lot of vegetables, mild or even bicarbonate-based antacids can cause an alkaline urine, when the pH will rise.

Urinary pH thus offers an opportunity to assess an aspect of the patient's metabolic state but it also has therapeutic implications. Renal calculi are formed from insoluble salts and other substances, such as uric acid, found in the urine which have precipitated out and aggregated into a discrete mass. In order to help dissolve the stones or prevent recurrence, the pH of the urine can be adjusted to create conditions where the constituents of the stone are more soluble or remain in solution. Knowing the urinary pH can be of use when attempting to diagnose a patient's symptoms. If a urinary tract infection is suspected, proteinuria combined with an alkaline pH is highly suggestive of bacterial infection but less likely if the urine is acid.

Blood

The presence of blood in the urine is a potentially serious sign and needs thorough and rapid investigation. Asymptomatic haematuria is usually the earliest sign of cancer of the bladder which can be treated if detected early enough. It can also be due to trauma, infection or stones. A reagent test strip is available which uses a colour change to blue or green if haemoglobin is present in the sample. Positive results must be followed up to determine where the blood is coming from and appropriate treatment instituted.

> **False-positive results** may occur from containers contaminated with bleach, skin preparation with povidone iodine or from the use of stale urine.

Protein

In early renal disease, the glomerulus and tubules may leak small amounts of protein into the urine. As renal disease progresses, detectable levels of protein will be found in the urine. There are a number of systemic diseases associated with proteinuria including:

- renal disease
- urinary tract infection
- hypertension
- preeclampsia
- congestive heart failure.

Transient positive tests are not always significant and normal urine contains small amounts of albumin and globulin, although generally not enough to give a positive result on a reagent strip. Thus, when testing for urinary protein, a morning specimen of urine is recommended to ensure sufficient concentration. Yet ultimately renal damage may be detected as an asymptomatic proteinuria before any other signs of disease are noticed.

> **Proteinuria is an early** sign as well as a means of monitoring the progress of disease or its response to therapy.

Bilirubin and urobilinogen

In normal health, bilirubin is not found in the urine but is excreted via the bile duct into the gut. However, when the liver is diseased or there is obstruction to the flow of bile into the gut, bilirubin or its metabolites are likely to be found in significant quantities in the urine.

> ⚠ Urobilinogen is normally present in urine but elevated levels may indicate liver abnormalities or excessive destruction of red blood cells, such as in haemolytic anaemia.

Nitrates

Urine normally contains nitrates from dietary metabolites and some of the common bacteria responsible for urinary infections will convert these nitrates to nitrites. Nitrites are not normally present in urine but are produced in increasing numbers when Gram-negative bacteria such as *E. coli* convert dietary nitrates (found in the preservatives in meat products, cheese and smoked food) to nitrites. As *E. coli* is responsible for 80% of urine infection the presence of nitrites is strongly suggestive of urinary tract infection. A reagent strip that will detect nitrites in urine can confirm a bacterial presence. The following should be considered.

● The specimen for testing should have been present in the bladder for 4 hours before voiding, to allow sufficient time for the nitrate/nitrite conversion.

● Visible signs may also be present (for example, is the specimen clear or cloudy?) and should be noted.
● If the specimen is clear and blood, protein, leucocytes and nitrites are not present, you can be sure there is no urinary tract infection.
● If the specimen is turbid and one or more of the four tests are positive, there is a 50% chance that the urine is infected.

It would be appropriate to send the specimen to the laboratory for culture and sensitivity and refer the patient to the doctor for treatment. A short course of low-dose antibiotics and increased fluid intake is recommended.

Glucose

Glucose is not normally found in urine. The presence of glucose may be due to raised blood glucose levels (hyperglycaemia). It can be associated with many medical conditions including:

● diabetes mellitus
● stress
● Cushing's syndrome
● acute pancreatitis.

There is a case for screening middle-aged and older people when admitted to hospital as they may, at an early stage, be relatively asymptomatic before more serious symptoms present. Once a diagnosis of diabetes is made, urinalysis for glucose can be a valuable method of monitoring the disease, particularly as diabetic retinopathy, kidney disease, peripheral vascular and cardiac disease are secondary to prolonged hyperglycaemia.

There are two categories of urine tests for glucose: the Clinitest and the impregnated test strips. The Clinitest is quite cumbersome but provides an accurate measure. Test strips do not measure the quantity of glucose in the urine so accurately and therefore are probably only adequate for screening purposes.

Ketones

When the body metabolizes fat, breakdown products include ketone bodies, which are excreted in the urine. In good health they are not detectable in urine. Usually ketones may be found in people who are fasting but can also be present in excessive amounts in people with uncontrolled diabetes. There are two tests available for ketones: Acetest, which is a tablet, and a strip test, which is available either as a single test, Ketostix, or incorporated into one of the combined multiple-strip sticks.

Ketones are acidic substances and when present in excess can lead to metabolic acidosis which, if untreated, can cause death. Early detection is therefore of value.

Appearance

The appearance of the urine should be noted for colour and clarity. Colour changes may be due to endogenous pigments such as haemoglobin (red or red/brown colour), bilirubin (yellow) or intact red cells (smoky red). Exogenous pigments may also cause colour changes:

- a red-coloured urine may be due to eating beetroot or to

contamination with menstrual blood
- orange discoloration may be due to the pigments found in some laxatives
- a blue/green colour may be caused by methylene blue in some proprietary medicines.

Odour

The odour of a urine specimen should be noted before further testing.

- Normal, freshly voided urine has very little smell but develops an ammonia-like smell on standing.
- Infected urine smells foul and may have a characteristic fishy smell which worsens on standing.
- Substances such as acetone excreted by diabetics with ketoacidosis or patients who have been starving or suffering from anorexia give urine a characteristic smell.
- Eating fish, curry or other strongly flavoured foodstuffs can also makes the urine smell.

The results of ward or clinic testing of urine should be recorded accurately in the patient's records, as soon as possible after testing. Remember, a negative test result may not only point to an alternative diagnosis but it is also a valuable baseline indicator to be referred to later in evaluating the progress of a patient during the course of an illness. A negative result should always be recorded even if at the time it appears unimportant or irrelevant.

BLOOD TESTS

Many early changes that occur in the body may be reflected in the results of a blood sample, well before they become clinically obvious. Blood tests can aid diagnosis, assist in monitoring circulatory status and help provide valuable clues to the effectiveness of treatment.

Blood cultures

Bacteraemia and fungaemia indicate failure of the host's immune system to localize infection and its primary focus. They are associated with significant morbidity and mortality and therefore, accurate and speedy microbiological detection of infection using blood cultures is essential. The timing of blood cultures is crucial, as most bacteraemias are intermittent. Blood cultures should be taken when the signs of infection are present, e.g. during fever, chills, rigors, changes in mental state and lethargy.

When taking blood cultures rigorous attention to aseptic technique is necessary as a failure to do so could result in a pseudo-bacteraemia, e.g. contamination of the culture from outside the bloodstream. A fresh sample of blood is preferred, as obtaining blood from an indwelling central venous catheter can increase the risk of contamination.

Haemaglobin(Hb) levels

The haemoglobin (Hb) level is the amount of red blood cells in the blood. Hb is contained in the erythrocyte's cytoplasm and is primarily responsible for carrying oxygen to and carbon dioxide from the body's tissues. Hb also plays a major role in blood viscosity.

The normal concentration of Hb in the blood is 12–15 g/100 ml of blood. A low Hb will indicate that red blood cells are being lost. When considering the Hb it is important to consider the patient's age, general state and the rate of fall of the Hb concentration. A Hb concentration that has fallen suddenly, such as in acute blood loss, is not well tolerated by the body and a transfusion is required to improve the delivery of oxygen to the tissues. A slow reduction in Hb is better tolerated as the body has time to adapt to the fall as it takes place gradually over weeks or months. This occurs in iron deficiency anaemia, megaloblastic anaemia, renal failure and anaemias associated with chronic disorders.

In addition to determining Hb levels, other signs may be present to confirm findings.

- In white skin the epidermis is nearly transparent and allows the colour of the Hb to show through as a pinkish tinge, as the blood circulates through the dermal capillaries. When Hb is poorly oxygenated, both the blood and the skin of white people appears blue (cyanosis).
- In black people, cyanosis of the skin can be observed in the mucous membranes and nail beds.
- By spending many hours in close contact with the patient,

undertaking careful monitoring and observation, the nurse may notice the more subtle changes that occur in the patient's condition (cyanosis) before the physiological parameter is actually measured (Hb).

> ⚠️ It is necessary to consider cyanosis in relation to the total clinical picture as it occurs in other clinical conditions such as respiratory diseases and heart failure.

Plasma osmolality

Osmolality is a measure of the number of milliosmoles per litre of solution or the concentration of molecules per volume of solution. When solute is added to water, the volume is expanded and includes the original amount of water plus the volume occupied by the solute particles (e.g. sodium, potassium, calcium, etc.). When there is an increase in osmolality there is a reduction of water in relation to the solutes contained within it, as the solute concentration has not changed.

The osmolality of intracellular and extracellular fluid tends to equalize and so provides a measure of body fluid concentration and thus the body's hydration status. The normal osmolality of body fluids is 280–294 mOsm/l. A serum osmolality of less than 280 mOsm/l will generally indicate an excess of fluids in the vessels, suggesting overhydration or hypovolaemia. An

increased serum osmolality greater than 295 mOsm/l indicates a loss of fluid and dehydration or hypovolaemia may be present.

> ⚠️ With an increase in osmolality, thirst and a dry mouth are often experienced. The nurse may then consider suggesting that the blood level be investigated.

Haematocrit levels

A factor which influences blood flow is the consistency of the blood. Flow varies inversely with the viscosity of the fluid. Thick fluids move more slowly and cause a greater resistance to flow than thin fluids. The viscosity of blood depends on its red cell content. The greater the percentage of red cells in the blood, the more viscous the blood. This relationship is expressed as the haematocrit, the ratio of volume of red blood cells to the volume of whole blood.

The haematocrit determination is the percentage of a given volume of blood that is occupied by erythrocytes. A high haematocrit reduces flow through the blood vessels, particularly the microcirculation (arterioles, capillaries and venules). Conditions in which the haematocrit is elevated, for example dehydration, haemorrhage, anaemias, leukaemias, cyanotic congenital heart disease and polycythaemia, can lead to an increase in cardiac work as a result of increased vascular resistance.

The viscosity of blood also increases if blood flow becomes very slow or stagnates. This condition is called *anomalous viscosity*. The haematocrit is a useful guide for determining if whole blood or some other intravenous fluid should be used for volume replacement in the haemorrhagic shock patient. Maximum oxygen-carrying capacity is achieved with a haematocrit between 35% and 45%.

Urea, creatinine and electrolytes

The doctor or phlebotomist often takes blood in the mornings. The results of these blood tests have a prime place in assisting the nurse to gain a full detailed assessment of the patient. For further details see Table 2.3.

Liver function tests

These determine how well the liver is functioning and can be obtained by sending a blood sample to the laboratory for liver biochemistry. They look at serum levels of the following substances.

Bilirubin

Normal range <17 μmol/l. Very high levels occur in biliary obstruction and serial measurements are useful in following the progress of some diseases, e.g. primary biliary cirrhosis, or response to treatment.

Aminotransferases

These enzymes are present in hepatocytes and leak into the blood with liver cell damage. Very high levels may occur with acute hepatitis (20–50 times normal). Aspartate aminotransferase (AST) (normal range 10–40 U/l) is also present in heart and skeletal muscle and seen in MI or skeletal damage. Alanine aminotransferase (ALT) (normal range 5–40 U/l) is more specific to the liver than AST.

Alkaline phosphatase

Normal range 25–115 U/l. Raised levels are seen in cholestasis from any cause. Alkaline phosphatase is derived from bone and is also raised in Paget's disease, osteomalacia, growing children, metastases and hyperthyroidism.

Gamma-glutamyl transpeptidase

Normal range, male <50 U/l, female <32 U/l. This is a liver microsomal enzyme which may be induced by alcohol and enzyme-inducing drugs, e.g. phenytoin. A raised serum concentration is a useful screen for alcohol abuse.

Serum proteins

Liver synthetic function is determined by measuring the serum albumin and the prothrombin time (clotting factors of the intrinsic pathway are synthesized by the liver).

Drug analysis

Therapeutic drug monitoring by blood analysis is available for a wide variety of antibiotics and some cardiac drugs. This is necessary for drugs that possess a narrow therapeutic range in serum. If the

Table 2.3 Normal blood values

	Values
Haematology	
Haemoglobin:	
● male	14.0–17.7 g/dl
● female	12.0–16.0 g/dl
White blood cell count	4–11 × 10^9/l
Platelet count	150–400 × 10^9/l
Serum B$_{12}$	160–925 ng/l
Serum folate	4–18 µg/l
Erythrocyte sedimentation rate (ESR)	<20 mm in 1 hour
Coagulation	
Partial thromboplastin time (PTTK)	35–50 seconds
Prothrombin time	12–16 seconds
Serum biochemistry	
Albumin	34–48 g/l
Amylase	<220 U/l
Bicarbonate	22–30 mmol/l
Bilirubin	<17 µmol/l(0.3–1.5 mg/dl)
Calcium	2.20–2.67 mmol/l(8.5–10.5 mg/dl)
Chloride	95–106 mmol/l
Creatinine	0.06–0.12 mmol/l(0.6–1.5 mg/dl)
Glucose	4.5–5.6 mmol/l(70–110 mg/dl)
Potassium	3.5–5.0 mmol/l
Sodium	135–146 mmol/l
Urea	2.5–6.7 mmol/l(8–25 mg/dl)

serum levels are too low the patient is jeopardized by the probable lack of efficacy; if they are too high, the patient may suffer serious toxicity.

The three most common drugs that require regular analysis are gentamicin, digoxin and phenytoin.

Drug monitoring is time consuming and costly but leads to improved drug administration by preventing toxicity and improving outcome.

Cardiac enzymes

When myocardial cells are damaged, they release a number of enzymes into the circulation known as cardiac enzymes (Table 2.4). It could be argued that interpretation of these specialist results is the domain of the doctor. However, holistic nursing involves the identification and understanding of all aspects of illness in order to provide effective and high-quality patient care.

Table 2.4 Cardiac enzymes

Enzyme release	Peak values	Normal values	Other situations
Creatinine kinase (CK) • released when cardiac muscle starts to die • is the first enzyme to increase after infarction	Values rise within the first 6 hours post MI. Reach a peak between 18–24 hours. Values may return to normal after about 72 hours as no more cells are dying. CK levels should be measured: • at the time of patient's admission • 24 hours later • at the end of the second and third day	Normal for men is 15–120 iu/l Women 10–80 iu/l CK values can rise 10-fold to thousands in severe cellular death	CK is not unique to cardiac muscle. Values can rise: • during trauma • in muscle disease • in cerebrovascular damage • after muscular exercise • with intramuscular injections
CK isoforms • MB is the one related to the heart • The presence of CK-MB in the plasma indicates myocardial necrosis	Measurement ensures levels are not confused with other muscle injury Helps to give an idea of the extent of muscle damage	If CK-MB levels are greater than 5% of the total CK level, the diagnosis of myocardial infarction is almost certain	It is only found in heart muscle
Lactic dehydrogenase (LDH)	LDH level is raised within 8–24 hours. Peaks in 3–6 days Returns to normal in 8–14 days	240–525 UI^{-1}	LDH release is also found in: • liver disease • renal disease • pulmonary embolism • shock • IM injection
LDH isoforms • Principally LD$_1$ • A rise in this isoform indicates myocardial necrosis	Has 5 isoforms denoted as LD$_1$ – LD$_5$ The pattern of LD$_1$ level greater than LD$_2$ occurs within 12–24 hours after the attack	If the LD$_1$ level is greater than the LD$_2$ level, a MI is indicated	Released by the myocardium
Aspartate aminotransferase (AST) • There are no cardiac-specific isoforms	AST concentrations rise in 8–12 hours. Approaching peak in 18–36 hours. Returning to normal in 3–4 days	10–40 UI^{-1}	AST is not specific to cardiac muscle and its use in the diagnosis of MI is limited

Table 2.4 Cardiac enzymes (Continued)

Enzyme release	Peak values	Normal values	Other situations
Troponins (Tn) ● Proteins present in striated muscle ● Function as regulators of muscle contraction	Has 3 isoforms: TnC, TnI, TnT TnI is cardiac specific and measured in MI. Rises within 4 hours and remains elevated for 10–14 days	Lower limit 0.4 ng/ml Upper limit 50 ng/ml Diagnostic level for MI 1.5 ng/ml	This test has improved sensitivity over CK-MB, allowing identification of patients that present 48 hours to 6 days after infarction

The estimation of myocardial enzymes is of great diagnostic importance in a myocardial infarction (MI). The enzymes most commonly measured are:

● aspartate aminotransferase (AST)
● lactate dehydrogenase (LDH)
● creatine kinase (CK)
● troponins.

These enzymes are normally present in low levels in the serum of healthy people, but their rise in concentration can be used to determine the diagnosis and severity of a MI. They cannot provide information about the location of the damage and CK and LDH only indicate muscle tissue injury. However, a precise investigation of MI can be made by analysing the concentrations of myocardial band (CK-MB) and isoforms of these enzymes, e.g. LD_1, LD_2.

Arterial blood gases

Blood can be taken from an artery and analysed to determine partial pressure of oxygen and carbon dioxide to understand the patient's acid–base balance. The movement of oxygen from the alveoli in the lungs to the pulmonary blood occurs due to the pressure gradient that exists. The partial pressure of oxygen in the alveoli is 13.7 kPa as compared to 5.3 kPa in the pulmonary capillaries, which allows exchange of oxygen through diffusion. Similarly, oxygen is easily exchanged between the capillaries to the tissues, because of a steep partial pressure gradient.

Measuring these partial pressure and other values in arterial blood can determine:

● whether the patient is acidotic or alkalotic
● the cause of the condition (respiratory or metabolic)
● whether the condition is being compensated.

When attempting to analyse a person's acid–base balance, scrutinize the blood values in the following order.

1. Note the pH. This tells whether the person is in acidosis (pH <7.35) or alkalosis (pH >7.45) but it does not tell you the cause.

2. Check the PCO_2 to see if this is the cause of the acid–base imbalance. The respiratory system acts fast and an excessively high or low PCO_2 may indicate either that the condition is respiratory or metabolic or if the patient is compensating.
   —The PCO_2 is over 5.7 kPa (40 mmHg): the respiratory system is the cause of the problem and the condition is a respiratory acidosis.
   —The PCO_2 is below normal limits (5.2 kPa, 35 mmHg): the respiratory system is not the cause but is compensating.
3. Check the bicarbonate level. If step 2 indicates that the respiratory system is not responsible then the condition is metabolic and should be reflected in increased or decreased bicarbonate levels.

   —Metabolic acidosis is indicated by HCO_3^- values below 22 mmol/l.
   —Metabolic alkalosis by values over 26 mmol/l.

Notice that PCO_2 levels vary inversely with blood pH (PCO_2 rises as blood pH falls) while HCO_3^- levels vary directly with blood pH (increased HCO_3^- results in increased pH).

If any changes occur in the partial pressures of oxygen or carbon dioxide, e.g. due to respiratory disease (asthma, COPD, ARDS) or metabolic disease (diabetes, renal failure, vomiting, diarrhoea) disruptions in the acid–base balance of the body may result.

Metabolic acidosis (HCO_3^- <22 mmol/l; pH <7.40)
Occurs in conditions such as:

- severe diarrhoea
- renal disease
- untreated diabetes mellitus
- starvation
- excess alcohol ingestion
- high ECF potassium concentrations.

Metabolic alkalosis (HCO_3^- >26 mmol/l; pH >7.40)
Occurs in conditions such as:

- vomiting or gastric suctioning of hydrogen chloride-containing gastric contents
- selected diuretics
- ingestion of excessive amounts of sodium bicarbonate
- constipation
- excess aldosterone (e.g. tumours).

Respiratory acidosis (PCO_2 >5.7 kPa; pH <7.4)
Occurs in conditions such as:

- any condition that impairs gas exchange or lung ventilation (chronic bronchitis, cystic fibrosis, emphysema)
- rapid, shallow breathing
- narcotic or barbiturate overdose or injury to brainstem.

Respiratory alkalosis (PCO_2 <5.7 kPa; pH >7.4)
- Direct cause is always hyperventilation.
- Brain tumour or injury.

END-TIDAL CARBON DIOXIDE ($P_{ET}CO_2$) MONITORING

The end-tidal carbon dioxide ($P_{ET}CO_2$) monitors exhaled carbon dioxide on both intubated and non-intubated patients. The normal range for expired $P_{ET}CO_2$ is generally 4.5–5.7 kPa. This method of expiratory gas analysis can be undertaken through a nasal cannula which simultaneously delivers supplemental oxygen. In lungs where ventilation is uniformly distributed and evenly matched to perfusion, $P_{ET}CO_2$ reasonably reflects partial pressure of arterial CO_2.

- Pulmonary embolism or decreased cardiac output is associated with a decrease in $P_{ET}CO_2$, because of decreased alveolar blood flow.
- An increase in $P_{ET}CO_2$ reflects the presence of airway narrowing or other lung disease associated with respiratory changes in the mechanical properties of the lungs.

This method of expiratory gas analysis is not commonly used in all clinical practice areas but studies are showing its benefits and value in respiratory management. In the future it may become as normal as attaching an oxygen saturation monitor.

ELECTROCARDIOGRAM (ECG) RHYTHM STRIP

The electrocardiogram (ECG) rhythm strip records the electrical activity of the heart in one particular lead, generally lead II. Cardiac cells are specialized and are unlike any other cells in the body, as each individual cell can initiate its own electrical impulse. The ECG can give information about:

- the heart rate and rhythm
- the effects of electrolytes on the heart
- the effect of drugs on the heart
- electrical orientation of the cardiac muscle.

In a normal heart the sinoatrial (SA) node, situated in the right atrium, initiates the cardiac electrical impulse. The SA node is often called the *cardiac pacemaker* as it beats the fastest, between 60 and 100 beats per minute (bpm). Following discharge of the SA node, waves pass through specialized conducting pathways in the atria, each cell acting as stimulus to the next. This process causes atrial depolarization (contraction) and is represented on the ECG as the P wave.

The impulse then reaches the atrial ventricular (AV) node, then passes through the bundle of His and down the right and left bundle branches to finally arrive at the Purkinje fibres. The time it takes an impulse from the SA node to reach the Purkinje fibres is represented as the P–R interval (significant in some heart blocks). The Purkinje fibres give rise to ventricular depolarization (contraction), represented on the ECG as the QRS complex. The T wave soon follows which depicts repolarization (the heart going back to the resting phase) of the ventricles (Fig. 2.3).

The whole sequence of the PQRST portrays the systolic phase of the heart (heart contraction). The space between each beat is known as the repolarization or diastolic phase (resting phase) of the heart, whereby the arteries of the body are perfused with nutrients and oxygen is exchanged for carbon dioxide at cellular level.

The rate of discharge of the SA node can increase (*tachycardia* – over 100 beats per minute) due to:

- disease of the heart, e.g. heart failure, hypertension, myocardial infarction (MI)

- blood loss
- pain
- stress or anxiety
- haemorrhage, dehydration.

The SA node may reduce its rate of discharge (*bradycardia* – less than 60 beats per minute) due to:

- over administration of certain drugs (digoxin)
- a lack of oxygen supply
- myocardial infarction (MI).

Abnormal rhythms can occur from:

- heart failure
- coronary artery disease
- myocardial infarction
- arteriosclerosis

Waveform	Time	Voltage	
P interval	Not longer than 0.11 seconds or 3–4 small squares	2.5 mm–3.0 mm in any lead	
PR interval	0.12 seconds or 3–5 small squares	Not significant	
Q wave	0.03 seconds	Less than 25% of the R wave	
QRS	0.04–0.11 seconds or 2–3 small squares	Not significant	
R wave	See QRS	The total QRS (above or below the isoelectric line) must be 5.0 mm or greater in leads I, II, III to be considered normal	
ST segment	Not significant	Normally isoelectric but may be elevated 2.0 mm above isoelectric line or depressed 0.5 mm below the isoelectric line	
T wave	Not significant	No more than 5.0 mm in standard leads, 10.0 mm in chest leads	
U wave	Should be in the same direction as the proceeding T wave	Less than 1 mm	

Fig. 2.3 The PQRST waveform of an ECG. Edwards 2002. In: British Journal of Nursing II 454–468, reproduced with permission.

- fluid overload
- fluid and electrolyte imbalance.

Changes to an ECG rhythm strip can be determined by interpreting changes that occur in time and voltage to the PQRST waveforms and by using a standardized approach to the diagnosis of arrhythmias. An ECG rhythm strip can identify abnormal rhythms, such as:

- sinus bradycardia
- sinus tachycardia
- sinus arrhythmias
- atrial fibrillation
- atrial flutter
- atrial ectopics
- ventricular ectopics (unifocal, multifocal)
- ventricular tachycardia (SVT)
- ventricular fibrillation
- asystole.

THE 12-LEAD ECG

A 12-lead ECG, which gives 12 readings, will be undertaken to confirm diagnosis and determine any other cardiac damage present. It is more useful when diagnosing a MI or other cardiac problems, e.g. heart block. It can be performed simply and quickly and views the heart electrically in a three-dimensional manner. The limb leads are attached to the forearms and calves, with a small amount of conduction gel, and three bipolar leads (I, II, III) and three augmented unipolar leads (AVR, AVL, and AVF) can be recorded. Chest precordial unipolar lead placements are secured again by applying a small

amount of conduction gel over the six V lead positions (V_1, V_2, V_3, V_4, V_5 and V_6) and allow the heart to be viewed in the horizontal axis from the chest wall.

The 12-lead ECG produces a representation of what is happening directly underneath the electrode so that a practitioner can determine if the conduction pathway of the heart is normal or damaged. During a MI, changes on a 12-lead ECG over a period of days can be detected. These changes occur if cardiac muscle is damaged, so that the electrical waves within the heart have to travel via an alternative route, and this will alter the pattern of the ECG and identify the affected area.

RESPIRATORY INVESTIGATIONS

The gas inspired and expired per minute can be measured as lung volumes and capacities.

- Tidal volume (TV) is the amount of gas inspired and expired during normal breathing.
- Inspiratory reserve volume (IRV) is the amount of gas that can be inspired in addition to tidal volume.
- Expiratory reserve volume (ERV) is the amount of gas that can be expired after a passive (relaxed) expiration.
- Residual volume (RV) is the volume of gas that cannot be expired and is always present in the lungs.
- Total lung capacity (TLC) is the total gas volume in the lung when

it is maximally inflated. It is made up of RV, ERV, TV and IRV.

The lung capacities are always the sum of two or more volumes.

- Vital capacity (VC) is the maximum amount of gas that can be displaced (expired) from the lung and includes IRV, TV and ERV.
- Functional residual capacity (FRC) is the amount of gas remaining in the lung at the end of a passive expiration (RV and ERV). The lungs are at rest or in a state of mechanical equilibrium.
- Inspiratory capacity (IC) is the amount of gas that can be inspired after a passive expiration (from FRC) and includes TV and IRV.

Norms for volumes and capacities are based on age, sex and height and are referred to as predicted values. Changes from predicted or baseline values are taken into account in diagnosing and assessing respiratory disorders.

The volume of air exhaled in a minute of resting breathing is known as the *total minute volume* (MV) and is equal to tidal volume (millilitres per breath) multiplied by the frequency of breathing (breathing per minute). Only about two-thirds of this volume actually reaches the alveoli (this is known as the *alveolar minute volume*). Not all the air entering the airways and lungs participates in gas exchange. The remaining one-third stays within the trachea, bronchus and bronchioles of the lungs. This volume of wasted ventilation is called *dead space ventilation* (VD).

Chronic pulmonary disorders include:

- *obstructive* disorders of the bronchioles (emphysema, bronchitis and asthma), whereby the patient has difficulty moving air rapidly into and out of the lungs
- *restrictive* disorders of the lungs (fibrosis, adult respiratory distress syndrome).

The measure that is most commonly used in practice is the forced expiratory volume in 1 second (FEV_1) or peak expiratory flow (PEF) rate, which is a useful indicator of a worsening condition.

PULSE OXIMETRY

This non-invasive technique is used to measure the saturation of blood in the arterial capillaries. It is a spectrophotometric measurement of the proportion of oxygenated haemoglobin in the arteries. The absorption of light by desaturated and fully saturated haemoglobin is different. This light absorption is measured by a special light detector and appears as the percentage oxygen saturation of the haemoglobin in the arteries.

The light detector of the oximeter is attached to a tissue that is reasonably transparent to these wavelengths of light. This may be the finger, the toe or the ear lobe. As such, it is very useful in following changes in arterial oxygenation. There must be:

- a good flow of blood to the area (not effective if severe vasoconstriction is present)
- no mechanical movement of the probe, which will cause interference
- no nail varnish, which will affect the normal haemoglobin saturation measured.

If the oxygen saturation falls below 85% the pulse oximeter may become progressively less accurate. Pulse oximetry cannot be used in any form of carbon monoxide inhalation because the carboxyhaemoglobin will cause the oximeter to over-read the saturation level. Pulse oximetry is used:

- to estimate arterial oxygen saturation (SpO_2)
- to monitor changes in arterial oxygen saturation
- alongside blood gas analysis to monitor the adequacy of ventilation.

LUMBAR PUNCTURE

In this procedure cerebrospinal fluid (CSF) is withdrawn following the insertion of a hollow needle into the lumbar subarachnoid space. The needle is usually inserted between the second and third or third and fourth lumbar vertebrae (L2 and L3 or L3 and L4). This is below the level of the spinal cord, which extends to L1 or L2, and is in the region of the cauda equina.

The fluid obtained is examined for diagnostic purposes and may be required:

- to record the pressure of the CSF using a manometer
- in suspected meningitis or encephalitis to look for bacteria in the CSF
- in suspected malignant tumours to look for cancer cells (cytology)
- to aid diagnosis in subarachnoid haemorrhage when there would be blood in the CSF
- to introduce intrathecal medication such as antibiotics or cytotoxic drugs
- to introduce contrast media for radiological examination.

A lumbar puncture is contraindicated in the following circumstances.

- In patients with papilloedema or deteriorating neurological symptoms, where raised intracranial pressure is suspected.
- In the presence of infection, as this may lead to meningitis or abscess formation:
  —localized skin infection around the insertion site
  —the presence of frontal sinusitis
  —middle ear discharge
  —congenital heart disease or prosthetic heart valves.
- In patients who are unable to cooperate or who are too drowsy to give a history.
- In patients who have severe degenerative spinal joint disease.

- In those patients undergoing anticoagulant therapy or who have coagulopathies or thrombocytopenia.

A doctor carries out the procedure using an aseptic technique. The position of the patient is vitally important and the nurse may be responsible for helping the patient to maintain this position during the procedure.

- The patient should be in the left lateral position, with maximum flexion of the spine and as near the edge of the bed as possible.
- There should be one pillow under the patient's head.
- To gain maximum stretching of the lumbar vertebrae the client should flex his head to the chest and draw his knees to the abdomen, holding them with his hands.
- The nurse can help by supporting the client behind the knees and neck, thus ensuring the widening of the intervertebral space.

Careful positioning is necessary so that the doctor can feel the lumbar spine more easily and so insert the needle accurately. It is imperative that the lumbar puncture is performed below the first lumbar vertebra where the cord terminates.

When the needle is in position the stylette is removed and a manometer attached to record the pressure of the CSF. The normal pressure of the CSF is 60–180 mmH$_2$0. For laboratory analysis

> ⚠ If the lumbar puncture is difficult, for example in an obese client, the doctor may request that the patient sits straddled on a straight-backed chair with their arms folded round the back of the chair and their head resting on their hands. The patient will need support and reassurance throughout.

approximately 5–10 ml of CSF is withdrawn.

The nurse should note:

- the colour of the CSF – it should be colourless
- the presence of blood in the CSF – the first few millilitres may be bloodstained due to trauma following insertion of the needle but after this the fluid should run clear
- the consistency of the CSF – it should be like water
- the opacity of the CSF – it should be clear; cloudy CSF is typical in bacterial meningitis.

A Queckenstedt's test is done when an obstruction to the flow of CSF in the spinal pathway is suspected. Pressure is recorded using the manometer whilst jugular compression is applied. Normally the pressure of the CSF would rapidly rise when jugular compression is applied and just as rapidly fall when the pressure is released. If an obstruction such as a spinal tumour or dislocated vertebra is present the rise and fall of pressure will occur much more slowly. Pressure is applied for a maximum of 10 seconds and recordings taken via the manometer. Further recordings are then taken for 10 seconds when the pressure is released. When pressure recordings are complete, the specimens of CSF will be collected in culture bottles.

Following the completion of the procedure:

- the needle is withdrawn and the wound sealed with a plastic sealant dressing
- the patient is asked to lie down flat in bed for 6 12 hours. This should prevent the development of a headache
- observations for leakage from the puncture site together with neurological observations should be continued for up to 24 hours.

RADIOGRAPHY (X-RAYS)

Radiography enables film views of the internal structures of the body to be taken by the passage of X-rays (gamma rays) through the body onto a specially sensitized film.

Very high-energy X-rays or radioactive substances are also used in the radiotherapy department to treat some forms of cancer. This is radiation therapy. Protection from this radiation is necessary in both the above cases. The radiographer is qualified to take X-rays for interpretation by a radiologist, who is a physician who has specialized in the use of radiography to diagnose and treat disease.

X-rays are electromagnetic vibrations of short wavelength produced by passing a high voltage through a cathode ray tube. The beam crosses the patient and is partially absorbed in the process. Those energy waves (photons) that leave the patient are captured by an image receptor. The energies of the photons are decreased by differing amounts as they pass through different tissues in the body. The remnant radiation that leaves the patient produces the photographic image on the radiographic film.

- *Radiolucent* materials allow X-rays to pass through them easily. Air is radiolucent.
- *Radiopaque* materials do not easily allow light to pass. Bone is a relatively radiopaque material.
- On a plain radiograph, gas and fat absorb few X-rays and appear dark.
- Bone and other calcified regions absorb most of the X-rays and appear white.
- Some foreign bodies such as metal and some glass are radiopaque but wood and plastic cannot be seen.

Protection from ionizing radiation

Exposure to radiation always involves the risk of biological changes within the body. The benefits of better diagnosis outweigh the risk to the patient but great care has to be taken to protect both the patient and the staff involved with taking X-rays. The patient should always be exposed to the lowest amount of radiation possible and all individuals coming into contact with radiation should be protected.

Protection occurs by:

- minimizing the time the patient is in the path of the X-ray beam
- maximizing the distance between the radiation source and the patient
- shielding the reproductive organs of the patient if they are within 4–5 cm of the beam. This is extremely important in children and young adults. The shields are made of lead which absorbs X-rays
- improvement of X-ray machines so that there is less scatter of the radiation.

Time, distance and shielding are also used to protect staff.

- The time spent in the room where the radiation source is active should be as short as possible. The risk is only there when exposures are being made.
- Increasing the distance from the source of the beam greatly reduces the quantity of radiation that will reach the radiographer or nurse. This means that if the nurse has to hold the patient while he is X-rayed there will be much greater exposure.
- If the nurse does have to support the patient, a shield should be worn. Lead aprons or gloves are used where a fixed shield is not in place.
- Any worker regularly exposed to ionizing radiation must be

monitored, usually by the use of a film badge. The film inside gets darker in response to the amount of radiation exposure and it is analysed, usually monthly.
- Contact with X-rays should be *avoided in pregnancy* as exposure can lead to malformations of the fetus. There is a safe limit of 0.5 rem for a declared pregnant woman.

Contrast media

These are diagnostic agents introduced into the body by injection or via an orifice to enhance the X-ray picture in areas of the body where there is insufficient natural contrast.

- Air may be used to study the ventricles of the brain and to aid localization of tumours in the brain.
- Barium sulphate is used to study the digestive tract. It is an inert and insoluble compound that is non-toxic, cheap and readily available.
- Iodine contrast media are used to study the renal tract and vascular system.

Preparation for barium studies
- For upper gastrointestinal studies the patient should be fasted overnight, except for water.
- Smoking should be avoided to minimize bowel gas.
- For small bowel studies, laxatives are sometimes taken the day before to empty the colon.
- For a barium enema laxatives are given and sometimes rectal washouts so that any defects in the mucosa can be seen.

Care with contrast agents
- Barium sulphate is not used if a perforation is suspected. The body cannot remove it if it enters the peritoneum and peritonitis follows.
- Care should be taken in the elderly, especially those on steroid drugs, as there may be a danger of perforation.
- Barium sulphate should not be taken by mouth in bowel obstruction as it will solidify and can turn a partial obstruction into a complete one.
- Plenty of fluids should be taken orally following barium, as it is very constipating and can dry in the bowel, forming an obstruction.
- Any iodine-containing contrast medium may provoke an anaphylactoid action (see p. 285). It may be minor, resulting in urticaria (hives), or there may be wheezing and laryngeal oedema. Sometimes steroids and antihistamines are given as premedication to reduce these effects.
- Resuscitation equipment will always be at hand.
- Non-ionic iodine contrast media with less risk of side-effects have now been introduced, e.g. ioxaglate and iodixanol.
- In sickle cell trait the injection of contrast media can cause sickling to occur.

Biliary contrast radiology

Cholecystography
- Contrast that is excreted in the bile is given orally and it weakly opacifies the gall bladder and bile ducts.
- The gall bladder concentrates the contrast and the films are taken 12 hours after its administration.
- A fatty meal is then given and this causes contraction of a healthy gall bladder that can be seen on the X-ray.
- If there is no contraction, this suggests damage to the gall bladder by inflammation.

Intravenous cholangiography
This is done less frequently now as the contrast material is relatively toxic. It has been replaced by percutaneous transhepatic cholangiography (PTC or 'perc'). This is used to diagnose the cause of obstructive jaundice (see p. 213).

Angiography
- This is the opacification of the veins or arteries by the injection of appropriate contrast media.
- The femoral vessels in the groin are the favourite entry points for the catheter through which water-soluble contrast is injected and images recorded on a video recorder.
- Obstructions due to thrombosis, atheroma or embolism can be seen.
- Clotting studies should be done first to ensure there is no bleeding tendency.
- Following cannulation there is a risk of trauma to the vessel causing bleeding or thrombosis and occasionally part of the catheter has been lost into the lumen of the vessel.

- There is also a risk of allergic response to the contrast media.

Ultrasound

High-frequency sound waves are used in diagnostic medical sonography to visualize structures in the body by recording the reflections of high-frequency pulses directed into the tissue.

- Non-invasive.
- Painless and almost certainly safe.
- Uses a transducer, which both emits and receives the ultrasound.
- Based on the emission of sound waves and the reflection of ultrasound echoes.
- The ultrasound probe containing a transducer is applied to the skin over the area of interest and the image is displayed on a screen.
- Jelly is used to exclude air and ensure a good connection to the skin.
- The probe is moved at different angles and in different directions to display any abnormalities. 'Spot' films are also taken to record any images.
- Minimal patient preparation is needed.
- The bladder needs to be full of urine to examine the pelvis and the patient should be fasted to minimize gas shadows in gall bladder studies.

Ultrasound is used to examine virtually all areas of the body. It:

- distinguishes solid from cystic lesions
- assesses abdominal masses (difficult to see on X-ray)

- detects abnormal material in an organ, such as metastases
- detects movement, as in the pulsation of an aneurysm
- can measure physical dimensions, such as the diameter of the aorta
- detects stones in the urinary bladder or the gall bladder
- guides intervention procedures such as aspiration or biopsy.

Limiting factors of ultrasound
- Bone completely reflects ultrasound and obscures any tissues beyond it. This means it cannot be used to examine the brain or the spinal cord.
- Bowel gas partly reflects the ultrasound and here starving the patient or using laxatives may help.
- A thick layer of fat scatters ultrasound and so it may be better to investigate the gall bladder by other means in the very obese.

Doppler-shift ultrasound
This method is used to study blood flow. The beam is directed towards the artery and is reflected from the red cells. It can be used to generate an audible signal for detecting blood flow or may be processed to give information on the nature of the flow. Other uses include:

- measuring systolic blood pressure when low. A portable Doppler is used to detect flow beyond a sphygmomanometer cuff placed around the arm or ankle
- detecting the fetal heart
- studying flow dynamics, for example in carotid artery disease.

Computed tomography (CT)

Computer tomography (CT) allows the visualization of the anatomy from various sectional planes by X-raying a series of thin transverse 'slices' of the patient's head or body that are then analysed by a computer. Very specialized equipment is needed and the radiographer needs extra training in this field. CT uses computerized digital imaging, as does ultrasonography and magnetic resonance imaging. Eventually digital imaging will be used more and more in the X-ray department, reducing the use of film.

- Pathological anatomy can be studied in great detail. Can reveal as much as an explorative operation, especially following injury to the brain. The management of serious head injuries has been transformed by the use of CT scanning. It enables appropriate surgical intervention only when necessary.
- Good images can be obtained in the obese this time! This is because fat separates the organs.
- Water-soluble contrast can be given before the scan to enhance the image.
- Very useful for areas where radiography is unsuitable:
  —the pancreas (deep inside the body)
  —the lungs and mediastinum
  —the brain and spinal cord.
- Planning radiotherapy or chemotherapy and staging
- tumours, e.g. lymphomas.
- Planning surgery, e.g. establishing the extent of invasion of oesophageal cancer.

- Assessing damage in abdominal or thoracic trauma.
- Guiding needles in biopsy, drainage of fluid or aspiration.

Radioisotope scanning

This is the diagnostic application of nuclear medicine to identify sites of abnormal pathology, e.g. presence of pus, extensive bone turnover, but it gives poor anatomical detail. A radioactive label is combined with a substance taken up readily by the tissue – this combination is called a tracer agent. The tracer is concentrated in a specific tissue type, e.g. the thyroid gland, and detected by a gamma camera that collects and counts the level of radioactivity across the area of interest. It is used for:

- liver and spleen scans to investigate unexplained abnormalities in liver function tests or suspected liver metastases
- bone scanning – areas of increased bone deposition and reabsorption take up the tracer. This includes secondary tumours
- renal scans, giving information not available from any other source
- labelling the patient's white blood cells
- lung scanning, to detect pulmonary emboli.

Magnetic resonance imaging (MRI)

Strong magnetic fields and radio waves are used along with a computer in magnetic resonance imaging (MRI) to generate sectional images of the anatomy. It is a rapidly expanding diagnostic field and involves applying a powerful magnetic field to the body, which causes all the protons of all the hydrogen nuclei to become aligned. Pulses of radio waves, which emit signals that are recorded electronically, then excite these. Images are produced using sophisticated equipment that can be viewed in any plane.

- Lipids have a high hydrogen content and so are clearly seen on MRI.
- Very useful for examining the brain and spinal cord.
- Atheroma can also be demonstrated.
- Can be used to investigate blood flow and cardiac function without the use of contrast media.

ENDOSCOPY

Any method of looking into the body uses an instrument. This can either be via an orifice, such as the nose or mouth, or via an artificial opening such as an arthroscopy. Endoscopes are now illuminated by the use of fibreoptics enabling accurate diagnosis to be made.

- Gastroscopy, oesophago-gastroduodenoscopy (OGD) – enables the whole area to be viewed and peptic ulcers to be seen. The source of haemorrhage can often be identified.
- Duodenoscopy – allows the injection of contrast into the common bile duct.
- Colonoscopy, large bowel endoscopy – can be used to

remove polyps and to biopsy suspicious lesions.
- Bronchoscopy – inspecting the bronchi with a narrow fibreoptic endoscope.
- Cystoscopy, cystourethroscopy – inspection of the bladder and urethra is very important in both diagnosis and treatment of diseases of the prostate, urethra and bladder.
- Ureteroscopy – can now be used to remove stones from the lower half of the ureter.
- Laparoscopy is used by gynaecologists to diagnose pelvic disorders. The abdomen is inflated with carbon dioxide and a scope passed into the peritoneal cavity. Can also be used to obtain liver biopsies.

BIOPSY

This is the removal of a small amount of tissue for diagnostic purposes. The lesions are usually removed under local anaesthetic or at operation, e.g. lymph nodes.

CYTOLOGY

This is the study of cells by the application of special staining techniques for malignancy. A negative result may be due to sampling error. Uses include:

- early detection of cancer as in cervical cytology
- examining fluid as in a needle biopsy of the breast
- examining ascitic fluid obtained via paracentesis or pleural effusions from chest aspiration

- examining cells from solid masses such as the pancreas, the breast or the thyroid.

2.5 NURSING CARE ISSUES

TRACHEOSTOMY CARE

A tracheostomy is an opening into the anterior wall of the trachea to facilitate ventilation. It comprises:

- a curved tracheostomy tube which conforms to the neck anatomy and is available in many different sizes
- an inner cannula which should be removed and cleaned frequently to ensure patency of the tube
- a high-volume, low-pressure cuff that helps to prevent occlusion of capillary blood flow in the trachea.

There are three major factors in effective pulmonary hygiene for the tracheostomy patient, as it bypasses the normal protective processes of the upper respiratory tract and inhibits the cough reflex: humidity, mobilization of secretions and suctioning.

Humidity

When a patient breathes through a tracheostomy, air is not warmed, moisturized or filtered. Therefore, additional humidity is required to keep the patient's secretions thin and mobilized as thick, crusty secretions can result in infection.

Mobilizing secretions

Regular physiotherapy aids the mobilization of secretions. Also important is frequent turning of the patient as well as encouraging deep breathing to prevent pulmonary complications. Depending on the activity level of the patient, sitting in a chair should also be encouraged.

Suctioning

Suctioning is needed when the cough becomes ineffective or secretions too thick for the patient to cough out easily. An inability to expectorate secretions is a common problem for patients with a tracheostomy and suctioning forms a significant part in maintaining a patient's airway. If the clinical signs of the patient indicate suctioning, the correct catheter size must be at the bedside and used to minimize trauma to the tracheal mucosa. The size of the catheter should be approximately one half the internal diameter of the tracheostomy tube.

The pressure used for suctioning is important. If the pressure is too low, suctioning will be ineffective, if too high it can cause:

- atelectasis
- hypoxaemia
- airway collapse
- ulceration.

A higher negative pressure does not directly relate to the quantity of mucus extracted. Therefore, suctioning pressure of between 80 and 120 mmHg should be used.

In some patients it may be necessary to preoxygenate with 100% oxygen using a ventilation bag prior to suctioning. This procedure compensates for the oxygen removed from the trachea and bronchi during suctioning and prevents hypoxaemia. The procedure should be explained to the patient since suctioning can have a frightening effect. A clear explanation with reassurance decreases the patient's fears.

The procedure is as follows.

- A sterile or non-touch technique is followed throughout using a clean or sterile glove, protective goggles and mask.
- Normal saline instillation is not recommended as good humidification, in the form of nebulizers and a cold-water humidifier, eliminates the need for this practice.
- The catheter is inserted about 6 inches into the trachea. Suction is not applied during insertion but rather as the catheter is being withdrawn.
- Gently rotating the catheter as it is being withdrawn will facilitate the removal of secretions, but when using a multiple-eyed catheter this may not be necessary.
- Suctioning should be no longer than 10–15 seconds.
- Catheter tubing may require:
  —sending to CSSD
  —effective disposal
  —cleaning with special attention to aseptic technique.
- The patient should rest between suctioning attempts to allow for adequate reoxygenation.
- Some patients may require manual ventilation with the ventilatory bag between attempts and after suctioning has been completed.

Suctioning of the upper airway may also be indicated if secretions or vomit are evident or suspected. Patients with a tracheostomy might find it difficult to swallow their saliva adequately or at all. Suctioning in this instance must be applied with care to avoid damage to mucosal surfaces.

Preventing complications

Complications of a tracheostomy can be prevented or minimized through meticulous nursing care and assessment.

Wound care

Attention to the tracheostomy wound can lessen the severity of infection and so it should be treated as a surgical wound. The wound may be cleaned and covered with a precut tracheostomy dressing to absorb drainage and to keep the neck plate from injuring the neck tissue. This dressing should be changed whenever it becomes soiled.

Accidental extubation

This complication can be a life-threatening situation. To lessen the chance of such an occurrence, it is essential that tracheostomy ties be secured in a knot, not a bow, at a tension allowing one finger to slip between the ties and the neck. It is recommended that a replacement tube of the same size and type and a pair of trachydilators be kept at the patient's bedside at all times, in case of extubation. The tracheal opening should be held open with the dilators until the replacement tube can be inserted.

Mucous plug formation

This complication can be avoided if adequate humidification is provided.

A mucous plug that obstructs the airway occurs largely as a result of:

- retained secretions
- inadequate humidification
- inadequate mobilization of secretions
- lack of a properly fitted inner cannula.

Special care considerations

Probably the greatest fear of the tracheostomy patient is the inability to speak or call for help when necessary so everything must be done to facilitate communication. Writing boards and cards should be available for the patient at the bedside and placed within easy reach. The following suggestions may be useful when communicating with tracheostomy patients.

- Allow ample time for the patient to respond since writing takes longer than speaking
- Speak in a normal tone. Although the patient cannot talk, he can hear (often there is a tendency to speak too loudly)
- Avoid asking two questions at once. Again, allow extra time to respond in writing.
- Encourage use of the paper, writing pad or slate to ensure privacy of the communication. What is written should be destroyed or erased.

WOUND CARE

Caring for patients with wounds can be very challenging and complex, as wounds occur in people of all ages.

The structure of the skin

The skin is one of the largest organs of the body and it occupies a surface area of approximately 2 square metres. It can be divided into two main parts.

- The epidermis – composed mainly of stratified squamous epithelial tissue and four major cell types:
  —keratinocytes
  —melanocytes
  —Langerhans cells
  —Granstein cells.
- The dermis – composed primarily of connective tissue containing collagenous and elastic fibres. Other structures found in this region include:
  —blood supply
  —lymph vessels
  —sensory nerve endings
  —sweat glands and ducts
  —hair, roots and follicles
  —sebaceous glands
  —arrectores pilorum (involuntary muscle attached to hair follicles).

Functions of the skin

When intact, the skin essentially forms a barrier between the external and internal environments of the body. Its principal functions are as follows.

- *Protection* – against invasion by bacteria and foreign matter.
- *Perception of stimuli* – enables constant monitoring of the external environment.
- *Absorption* – allows certain topical compounds such as drugs to be absorbed.
- *Synthesis of vitamin D* – synthesized by the body as a

result of direct exposure to ultraviolet radiation.

- *Maintenance of body temperature* – through metabolic processes the body is continuously producing heat. This is primarily dissipated through the skin, facilitated by three processes:
  —*radiation*: the ability of the body to give off its heat to another object of a lower temperature
  —*conduction*: the transfer of heat from the body to a cooler object in contact with it
  —*convection*: the movement of warm air molecules away from the body.
- *Water balance* – a small amount of fluid is lost each day (approximately 500 ml) through evaporation. This is termed *insensible loss*.

The healing process

The healing process includes three classifications of healing.

1. Healing by *primary intention* – the skin edges are brought together with the aid of sutures or clips (surgical wounds), butterfly plasters or Steristrips (minor trauma).
2. Healing by *secondary intention* – the skin edges are deliberately not brought together (pressure ulcer). The wound is encouraged to fill with granulation tissue from its base. Common in chronic wounds.
3. Healing by *tertiary intention* – a wound has been sutured but has broken down and been resutured later.

Phases of healing

There are three phases of wound healing which are continuous, overlapping and merging with the next.

1. *The inflammatory phase* – the formation of a blood clot, loosely uniting the wound edges and stimulating the inflammatory response and leading to the characteristic appearance of a wound, e.g. swelling, heat, redness, pain, facilitating healing and repair (0–3 days).
2. *The regenerative phase* – the tissue starts to fill and granulation tissue starts the process of wound contraction. The signs of inflammation start to subside but the wound may be raised in relation to surrounding tissues (0–24 days).
3. *The maturation phase* – the process of re-epithelialization begins. The scab should now slough off, as the epidermis is restored to its natural thickness (21 days–2 years).

Wound drainage

This is an abnormal opening in the skin that produces exudate or drainage, which may be caused by disease, trauma or surgery (as a method of treatment, e.g. therapeutic, or to prevent complications, e.g. prophylactic). All drainage should be accurately measured and recorded on either a wound assessment or fluid balance chart. The common types of wound/ surgical drainage are as follows.

- Corrugated strips of rubber or plastic – used to drain fat layers and the subcutaneous tissues and occasionally the peritoneal cavity. They guide exudate onto the surface absorbent dressing, can be messy and affect normal skin.

- Tubes and catheter-type drains – most efficient type of drain and can be connected to closed drainage bags. These drains include:
  —Portex drains (paediatric surgery)
  —Shirley drains (liver transplants to assess/contain bleeding)
  —Sterimed drains (minor orthopaedic surgery)
  —silicone drains (laparotomy or bowel resection procedures)
  —Yate's drain (hysterectomy).
- Suction drainage systems – these may involve a closed suction system, ideal for removal of blood and serous fluid. Examples include:
  —Dre-vac drain (laparotomy, cholecystectomy)
  —Porto-vac drains (plastic surgery)
  —Redivac drains (hip surgery).

Wound dressing materials
To undertake appropriate and effective management of wound, drainage and intravenous line sites, knowledge of the structure of the skin and the natural healing process is essential. In addition, the nurse should be able to recognize the various stages of wound healing and assess the wound using an assessment tool.

The best dressing
The ideal dressing product should ensure that the wound remains:

- moist with exudate but not macerated
- free from clinical infection and excessive slough
- free from toxic chemical particles or fibres released from the dressing
- at an optimum temperature for healing to take place
- undisturbed by frequent or unnecessary dressing changes
- at an optimum pH value.

Classification of wound dressing types
Nurses are often restricted to using what is available. However, with so many similar dressings, an appropriate alternative should be available. Wound dressings are classified by their primary functions.

- Film membranes (Opsite, Tegaderm, Cutifilm, BioClusive, Opraflex) – these:
  —are permeable to water vapour and oxygen
  —are impermeable to water and microorganisms
  —provide a warm, moist environment
  —are comfortable and convenient and permit constant observation.
- Alginates (Kaltostat, Sorbsan, Tegagel) – used to fill cavities and sinuses. They are useful around drainage sites as they absorb exudate and serous fluid and are easily removed by irrigation techniques.
- Foams (Allevyn, Cavi-Care, Lyofoam, Dermasorb, Tielle) – absorb exudate which then evaporates into the cells of the dressing and is lost as water vapour. They are non-adherent.

- Hydrogels (Gelliperm, Granugel, second Skin, Intrasite gel) – they swell when wet and can retain significant proportions of water within their structure. Therefore they:
  —rehydrate wounds
  —debride and clean
  —are painless to apply and remove
  —are soothing.
- Hydrocolloids (Comfeel, Cutinova, Granuflex, Tegasorb) – take up wound fluid to form a gel that produces a moist environment on the wound surface in order to facilitate healing.

Additional therapies

Not all wound dressing materials are suited to all wound types, in particular, to the treatment of non-healing or copiously draining wounds. However, an alternative method is beneficial in such situations – the vacuum-assisted wound closure (VAC) system.

- A closed, non-invasive, active therapy system.
- It uses negative pressure, which increases the effectiveness of the local circulation in the wounded area.
- Actively removes excessive exudate, reducing oedema and haematoma formation.
- Assists with the control of wound leakage.
- Promotes angiogenesis (growth of new blood capillaries).

This method of treatment is often considered when other conventional methods of wound management have failed.

MOUTH CARE

Mouth care (oral hygiene) is the scientific care of the teeth and mouth. The aim of oral care is to:

- keep the mucosa clean, soft, moist and intact and prevent infection
- keep the lips clean, soft, moist and intact
- remove food debris as well as dental plaque without damaging the gingiva
- alleviate pain and discomfort and enhance oral intake
- prevent halitosis and freshen the mouth.

The oral cavity harbours many varieties of bacteria, which do not normally pose any problems. Immunosuppression and systemic treatment such as cytotoxic, antifungal or radiation therapy and steroids may increase the pathogenicity of these organisms, leading to local infection. Oral complications can lead to pain, ulcers, infection, bone and dentition changes and bleeding and functional disorders affecting verbal and non-verbal communication, chewing and swallowing, taste and respiration. Therefore, mouth care is an important part of nursing practice.
   Mouth care involves:

- cleaning the teeth with toothpaste and toothbrush after meals
- chlorhexidine gluconate 0.2% 5 ml, four times a day, diluted in 100 ml of water which should be retained in the mouth for at least 1 minute before discarding.

> ⚠ A comfortable mouth will not only assist with appetite and food intake but will help the patient feel more sociable and confident.

ABDOMINAL PARACENTESIS

Abdominal paracentesis is the puncture of the abdominal wall with an abdominal trochar and cannula inserted into the peritoneal cavity. It is usually performed:

- to obtain a specimen of fluid for analysis
- for the management/relief of symptoms, e.g. associated with ascites
- for the administration of solutions into the peritoneal cavity, e.g. radioactive gold colloid or cytotoxic drugs (bleomycin, cisplatin).

Abdominal ascites is an accumulation of serous fluid within the peritoneal cavity. It can be caused by:

- non-malignant conditions such as advanced congestive heart failure, chronic pericarditis, cirrhosis of the liver
- malignant conditions such as metastatic cancer of the ovary, stomach, colon or breast.

Abdominal ascites is accompanied by symptoms of:

- breathlessness (due to pressure on the diaphragm)
- indigestion
- alteration in bowel habits
- fatigue

- ankle oedema (due to reduced serum albumin)
- reduced mobility
- nausea and vomiting, loss of appetite (leading to weight loss or anorexia)
- abdominal swelling (can cause bowel obstruction, decreased bladder capacity)
- pain (due to the increase in intra-abdominal pressure and pressure on internal organs)
- change of body image.

It makes sense therefore to relieve the pressure but abdominal paracentesis is not undertaken lightly due to the risks of hypovolaemia, hypokalaemia, hyponatraemia or protein depletion.

Special care considerations

Abdominal paracentesis is an invasive procedure performed by the doctor assisted by the nurse at the patient's bedside.

- The patient should be informed about the procedure, the results that might be obtained/expected, information regarding quality of life and full knowledge of the course of the disease.
- The area of skin is prepared and draped with sterile towels and a local anaesthetic is administered.
- A specimen of 20–100 ml is obtained, then a closed drainage system is attached, a dressing applied and taped in position.
- A drainage pattern of 1 l every 4 hours is recommended. If fluid is draining too fast a clamp should be applied to reduce the flow.
- Fluid drained and any other input and output should be measured

and volumes recorded. A high protein and calorie diet may be ordered.

- Regular observations must be carried out to detect early signs of shock and infection.
- Patients may require assistance to move and gain a comfortable position.
- Appropriate pain assessment and analgesia.

INTRAPLEURAL DRAINAGE

Intrapleural drainage is a method used to remove a collection of, air, fluid, pus or blood from the pleural space in order to restore normal lung expansion and function. The tubing used is clear, fairly rigid and may have a radiopaque strip, which enables X-ray detection.

Conditions which require intrapleural drainage include:

- pneumothorax
- pleural effusion
- haemothorax
- haemopneumothorax
- empyema.

In any of these conditions the pleural fluid seal is broken (e.g. by a spontaneous intrapulmonary air leak, during chest surgery or by a stab wound) and air, pus, blood or fluid will be drawn into the intrapleural space. The lung in the affected area collapses, the chest wall is no longer effective in expanding the lung and gas exchange is seriously impaired. Rapid diagnosis is essential.

- Decreased chest movement and breath sounds on the affected side of the chest on inspiration.
- Difficulty in breathing (dyspnoea).
- Increased respiratory rate.
- Cardiovascular changes, e.g. increasing heart rate, decreasing blood pressure.
- Sudden deterioration in condition.
- Cyanosis and pleuritic chest pain.
- Confirmed by chest X-ray.

Treatment is aimed at restoring the lung to its original size, usually achieved by the insertion of a wide-bore intercostal catheter under sterile conditions. The positioning of the drain depends on whether it is being inserted to remove air or fluid.

- In the case of air – the drain should be placed in the second, third or fourth intercostal space in the mid-clavicular line, which is in the anterior and apical part of the chest.
- In the case of fluid – the drain should be placed in the fifth or sixth intercostal space in the mid-axillary line, which is in the posterior and basal part of the chest. This uses the principle of gravity for drainage, as fluid and blood are heavier.

Once this has been accomplished, a chest tube should be inserted and underwater seal drainage attached to draw air, fluid, pus or blood from the pleural space to prevent any further fluid build-up.

The basic principle is always to allow air and excess fluid to escape from the pleural cavity. The drainage tube from the patient is connected to a long catheter, the end of which is submerged below a few centimetres of sterile water in a calibrated drainage bottle. The decrease in pressure inside the pleural cavity during inspiration causes air to be sucked up the tube, usually to a height of about 10–20 cm (a *swing*).

It is important that:

- drainage bottles are kept below the level of the patient's chest, preferably on the floor, to prevent water being sucked into the chest
- drains should not be clamped during movement of the patient or routinely stripped or milked
- if suctioning is applied, it is of low pressure, e.g. 10–25 cmH$_2$o
- regular observation of the drain takes place, e.g. drainage, swing, suction
- regular observation of the patient should take place and if any complaints of chest pain or difficulty in breathing or a rise in pulse rate occur immediate investigation is warranted
- deep breathing and coughing are encouraged to promote drainage
- the volume of fluid drained is recorded
- precautions are in place to ensure that drainage bottles are not accidentally moved or knocked over and a spare set of equipment is available in case of emergency
- the drainage tubes are secured or supported so that they do not pull on the chest wall or become dislodged.

> ⚠ Drains should only be clamped in the case of tube disconnection, bottle/system breakage, check X-ray or when the bottle and tubing needs to be changed, and then the clamp should be in place for the least time possible.

> ⚠ A chest drain attached to a suction unit which is turned off is considered to be a clamped drain. Turned off suction must be disconnected from the suction pump.

URINARY CATHETERIZATION

This is the passage of a catheter into the bladder using aseptic technique. It is indicated:

- for retention of urine – especially common in men with prostatic enlargement
- for accurate measurement of urine output in the very ill client, especially if he is unconscious
- for the relief of incontinence of urine if all other measures have failed
- to empty the bladder before surgery or certain investigations
- occasionally to empty the bladder before childbirth
- to bypass an obstruction and thus provide a channel for micturition
- to allow irrigation of the bladder or the administration of certain drugs.

There are several types of urinary catheter available and the reason for the catheterization will determine the type to be used. If a catheter is required for medium or long-term insertion, a latex catheter should not be used as this material is likely to irritate. A Silastic or silicone catheter is less irritable to the lining of the urinary tract. A catheter that stays in the bladder is called a retention catheter and has a balloon which is inflated following insertion.

A 5–10 ml balloon is used for adults and 3–5 ml for children.

The smallest catheter necessary for drainage should be chosen. If the urine is clear this is likely to be a 12–14 for men and women. If there is sediment or blood present, a larger size may be needed. There are different lengths of catheter available for men and women.

Procedure for a female catheterization

(Male catheterization is usually carried out by a medical practitioner or a male nurse.) The procedure is invasive and aseptic technique is essential throughout the procedure (washing of hands and sterile gloves) as bacteria may be introduced into the urinary tract.

- The procedure should be explained to the patient and their cooperation and privacy ensured.
- Prepare the trolley. A good light might be needed to view the genitalia.
- Place a waterproof protection underneath the patient (an incontinence pad would suffice). The patient needs to be in the supine position with knees bent, hips flexed and feet resting 60–70 cm apart.
- Clean the urethral orifice with normal saline or an antiseptic solution. Downward strokes should always be used (i.e. away from the urethra towards the anus).
- Lubricate the catheter with jelly to prevent urethral trauma.
- The catheter is inserted for 5–6 cm in an upward and backward direction following the natural route of the urethra. Urine should now flow. If the catheter is to remain in situ it should be advanced about 6 cm and the balloon inflated according to the manufacturer's instructions.
- Never inflate the balloon until some urine has drained and you are absolutely sure the catheter is in the bladder.
- A specimen of urine for the laboratory analysis may be needed and a drainage bag may then be attached to the catheter which is secured in position.
- Ensure the patient is comfortable following the procedure.

If the bladder is very full, as in retention of urine, rapid emptying may result in haemorrhage from the bladder mucosa so 200–300 ml should be released about every 30 minutes. Never leave the catheter clamped for long periods as this encourages the growth of micro-organisms.

Bladder lavage is the washing out of the bladder using sterile fluid to aid removal of blood clots or sediment from the bladder or to relieve an obstructed catheter. Normal saline may be used and it should be at body temperature. The procedure is aseptic and the fluid is introduced into the bladder slowly using a 50 ml syringe. The fluids are then allowed to drain from the bladder into a sterile receiver and the procedure is repeated until the prescribed amount of fluid has been used.

> ⚠ It is important to note that the bladder is normally a sterile environment and the introduction of a catheter for urinary drainage is a potential source of micro-organisms and infection. Great care is needed at all times to reduce this risk.

OXYGEN THERAPY

Increased oxygen content in the air used for breathing is needed when the patient is suffering from hypoxia. Hypoxia is oxygen deficiency in the body cells and may be caused by:

- deficient oxygenation of the blood – due to respiratory disease or chest injuries
- inadequate transport of oxygen by haemoglobin – as in anaemia or haemorrhage
- circulatory inadequacy – as in heart disease or emergency situations, e.g. cardiac arrest
- inability of cells to use oxygen – rare; an example is cyanide poisoning.

Oxygen therapy is a specific medical treatment and is given as prescribed by the medical staff who will write the percentage of oxygen and the method of administration on the prescription sheet. The concentration given depends upon the condition being treated and an inappropriate concentration may have lethal effects.

Low concentrations of oxygen (24–28%) are used to treat patients with chronic obstructive airways disease. A higher concentration in these patients can occasionally be dangerous and is therefore not given unless prescribed.

Higher concentrations of oxygen are often prescribed in a severe asthma attack and in pneumonia but may also be used in shock or haemorrhage.

Oxygen toxicity may follow prolonged periods (over 24 hours) of administration of high (over 50%) concentrations of oxygen. The end result of this may be fibrosis.

The equipment used varies and oxygen may be given by:

- mask
- nasal cannulae
- oxygen tent
- ventilator
- endotracheal tube
- Ambu-bag in an emergency.

There are many kinds of oxygen mask and the flow rate needed to achieve a certain percentage of oxygen will always be stated in the instructions that come with each mask. Some types have specific attachments that can be used to give certain percentages of oxygen and may be colour coded.

Nasal cannulae are not suitable for all patients because they are not accurate when giving lower percentages of oxygen and if a higher percentage is needed there is inadequate humidification. They are useful when the patient finds the conventional mask claustrophobic, as often happens in pulmonary oedema associated, for example, with acute left ventricular failure.

If high concentrations of oxygen are used, some form of humidification will be needed or the oxygen will have a very drying effect on the mucosa. If the patient's own airways have been bypassed, as when oxygen is given via an endotracheal tube, humidification is essential.

The effects of oxygen can be monitored with pulse oximetry, which records the oxygen saturation using a non-invasive procedure (see p. 72). The aim is to keep the saturation above 90% if possible.

> ⚠ **Oxygen is an inflammable gas so great care must always be taken because of this. Most hospitals are 'no smoking' zones now but smoking must never be allowed near the oxygen.**

THE UNCONSCIOUS PATIENT

Consciousness is an awareness of oneself and the surrounding environment. There are three properties of consciousness, which are affected by the disease process.

1. Arousal or wakefulness (eyes open to command)
2. Alertness and awareness (orientation and communication)
3. Appropriate voluntary motor activity (obeying commands)

The causes of unconsciousness are numerous and may indicate the length of time required for recovery. The nurse should be aware of the cause of the coma and be observant for indications of deterioration in the patient's condition. The following is a list of the common causes for unsciousiouness which is, of course, not exhaustive.

- Poisons and drugs, e.g. alcohol, overdose, gases, lead
- Vascular causes, e.g. post cardiac arrest, ischaemia, haemorrhage, hypovolaemia
- Infections, e.g. septicaemia, encephalitis, HIV, meningitis
- Seizures
- Metabolic disorders, e.g. hyperglycaemia, hypoxia, renal failure, hepatic failure
- Other causes, e.g. neoplasm, trauma, cardiac failure, tetany, degenerative disorders

Complete care of the unconscious patient demands all the expert skills of the nurse, as the patient is totally dependent for his comfort and essential needs.

Special care considerations

The care of the unconscious patient is geared to the preservation of life and the avoidance of further disabilities. In addition to physiological effects, consideration should be given to the psychological effects of coma, e.g. isolation, sleep deprivation, sensory deprivation and overload.

The main factors of caring for the unconscious patient are:

- establish and maintain a clear airway, remove any vomit from the mouth and position in the

unconscious position to prevent aspiration
- oxygen, suction, airway, Ambu-bag and mask, intubation by the bed or close by are essential
- assess the level of consciousness (use the Glasgow Coma Scale; see p. 31) and record it on the appropriate chart
- record and evaluate vital signs
- administer oxygen, prescribed drugs, IV fluids and nutrition
- maintain fluid and electrolyte balance
- carry out essential nursing care as appropriate to the patient's condition, e.g. mouth care, eye care, catheter care, turning, bed bathing, shaving, hair washing and communication
- positioning in the unconscious position may be required to enhance pulmonary function
- passive physiotherapy exercises of the limbs
- observe colour, temperature and pulses.

POSITIONING

Positioning is a fundamental and essential care element that nurses undertake on a daily basis. It is important to stress the need to correctly position and reposition patients frequently in order to decrease the risk of pressure sores and respiratory complications.

The semi-sitting or sitting position well supported with pillows, to prevent pressure sores or nerve damage, is recommended for optimizing and matching ventilation and perfusion following or during:

- thoracic surgery
- asthma
- acute exacerbation of COPD
- pneumonia/chest infection.

This will reduce the risk of increased breathlessness; it also reduces abdominal pressure on the diaphragm and minimizes the risk of aspiration.

The patient should be turned from side to side in the lateral or semi-prone position at least every 2 hours (unless contraindicated, e.g. lobectomy, pneumonectomy, chronic lung pathology) to change the distribution of ventilation and blood flow through the lungs and mobilize secretions. This has positive cardiopulmonary effects in enhancing oxygen transport by changing ventilation/perfusion of the lungs through gravitational effects.

The log role should be used when patients have to lie in the prone position and they are in danger due to their injury of further damage occurring during ordinary turning. This is a labour-intensive process and requires seven individuals: one for the head (the leader) and three either side of the bed.

Procedure

- The nurse at the head of the bed should be a qualified nurse experienced in log-rolling procedure.
- The head is maintained in position by the nurse holding the shoulders while her lower arms secure the head on either side.
- The other six nurses:

- no. 1 holds the patient from shoulder to middle waist
- no. 2 places arms over the middle and the upper thigh
- no. 3 places arms over upper thigh and knee
- no. 4 places arms at the thigh and knee
- no. 5 holds the feet
- no. 6 will carry out any other care required.
- When everyone is in position, the leader will decide how to indicate that all participants turn together.
- Once the signal is decided, all roll the patient with the spine in line and another nurse performs the change of sheet or necessary essential care.

MOBILIZATION

Early and progressive mobilization is an important aspect of caring for patients. It is an extension of the physiological principles of turning and repositioning the bedbound patient. Ambulation:

- encourages ventilation
- increases perfusion
- promotes secretion clearance
- promotes oxygenation
- decreases venous pooling, which reduces the risk of thrombus formation and pulmonary embolism
- improves functional residual capacity (FRC)
- reduces muscle wasting
- decreases the potential for psychological distress, e.g. feelings of helplessness, depression and lack of control.

When and how the patient should be mobilized is decided on an individual basis in conjunction with the patient, nurse, surgeon and physiotherapist. For effective mobilization it is paramount that the nurse monitors, observes and provides optimal pain and comfort strategies and interventions during this period.

PYREXIA AND HYPERPYREXIA

A pyrexia is a body temperature between 37.6° and 40°C and hyperpyrexia is a temperature >40°C. They are conditions in which the thermoregulatory mechanisms are intact but the body temperature is high. Infection is the most common cause of pyrexia and sepsis of hyperpyrexia but there are other causes. A number of drugs have been associated with pyrexia, e.g. diuretics, antiseizure therapy, analgesics, antiarrhythmics and antibiotics. Other causes of pyrexia include neoplasm, surgery, acute myocardial infarctions, heart failure, haemolysis (seen in reactions to blood transfusions) and hyperthyroidism.

There are four stages associated with pyrexia.

1. The *chill stage* is the cold stage when the hypothalamic thermostat is reset to a higher level – the patient feels chilly, has goosebumps, is cool to touch and pale.
2. The *plateau* is the hot stage when the body temperature has been raised to a level equal to the

hypothalamic set point – the patient feels hot, warm to touch, is flushed and has raised heart and respiratory rates.

3. In the *difervescence stage* the temperature returns to normal, heat is dissipated through heat loss mechanisms, the skin remains warm to touch and flushed and eventually there is a drop in body temperature to a normal level.

4. The *crisis stage* occurs if the temperature fails to respond to treatment, the micro-organism responsible cannot be eradicated and thermoregulation mechanisms can no longer control heat loss. Death may ensue.

These stages account for the discomfort experienced by patients with high temperatures. They also explain why a patient with a high temperature may initially feel cold and want to wrap up rather than be uncovered.

There are also different patterns of a pyrexia, which exhibit recognizable changes in temperature over time. These patterns vary according to the time of day, which may influence decisions regarding when to monitor body temperature.

Beneficial effects of a pyrexia

Pyrexia can be beneficial and is an important host defence mechanism.

- A body temperature of 40.9°C will kill some Pneumococcal and Gonococcal organisms.
- The high temperature causes a reduction in serum levels of iron, zinc and copper, which inhibits the replication of certain micro-organisms.

- Pyrexia as a result of viral infection increases interferon production by the infected cells, which then enters non-infected cells to inhibit infiltration by the invading virus.
- The activity of phagocytes and leucocytes is increased at temperatures between 38°C and 40°C, thus improving the infection-fighting ability of the immune system.
- A high temperature causes the breakdown of lysosomes (involved in the intracellular digestive system, which allows cells to digest and remove unwanted substances such as bacteria) in infected cells, thereby destroying cells and preventing them from initiating viral replication.

Detrimental effects of a pyrexia

A pyrexia can also be detrimental to the patient.

- Basal metabolic rate will be increased, eventually leading to exhaustion.
- Glycogen stores in the liver become reduced and lead to nitrogen wastage (as protein is used for energy) and, if prolonged, may result in debility, impaired healing and delirium.
- In patients who have compromised cardiopulmonary function, the effects of increased metabolic, heart and respiratory rates can be quite dangerous. These effects can lead to an increase in carbon dioxide

production and oxygen consumption.

- Dehydration may result from fluid loss during sweating and from the lungs due to increased respiratory rate, leading to hypovolaemia and electrolyte imbalance, which can be life threatening.
- The patient feels uncomfortably hot and sweaty, with a loss of appetite, weakness and malaise, apathy and confusion.

HYPERTHERMIA

A hyperthermia is defined as an increase in body temperature, with increased cellular metabolism, oxygen consumption and carbon dioxide production but where the body fails to activate compensatory cooling mechanisms (Morgan 1990). This condition is caused by problems of the central nervous system and does not respond to antipyretic therapy.

A hyperthermia causes cerebral metabolism to increase and the brain has great difficulty keeping up with the increase in carbon dioxide production. Cerebral vasodilatation occurs which may increase intracranial pressure and is thus dangerous in neurologically compromised patients. A temperature between 41°C and 43°C produces nerve damage, coagulation, convulsions and death. Unless effective cooling measures are initiated, irreversible brain damage and death will occur (Holtzclaw 1993).

A hyperthermia also presents in five other conditions:

1. heat cramps
2. heat exhaustion
3. heat stroke
4. malignant hyperthermia
5. neuroleptic malignant syndrome (NMS).

Heat cramps and exhaustion, even though they can be severe, do not generally warrant admission to hospital and those at risk can be taught ways to avoid it. However, heat stroke, malignant hyperthermia and NMS must be recognized quickly as, untreated, they may be fatal.

Tepid sponging/fanning

During a high temperature due to an infection
Treatment by cooling methods such as tepid sponging or fanning has been criticized. Cooling methods are of no use, as they result in:

- a compensatory response by the hypothalamus, which will activate heat-generating activities like chills and shivering
- compromising an unstable patient by depleting his metabolic reserve and can create a new temperature spike, which is as high or higher than the original one and may even increase the patient's temperature
- the patient feeling weak, especially during the early stages when the temperature is still rising.

Treating a high temperature by cooling and tepid sponging can only serve to increase the temperature further and cause the patient discomfort and possible harm. The best way to treat a high temperature is by the use of antipyrexial drug therapy, in preference to cooling methods.

> ⚠ Treating a high temperature by cooling and tepid sponging will increase the temperature further and cause the patient discomfort and possible harm.

During a hyperpyrexia due to damage of the hypothalamus
In this situation the body fails to activate compensatory cooling mechanisms. This tends to increase cellular metabolism, oxygen consumption and carbon dioxide production. As cerebral metabolism increases, the brain has great difficulty keeping up with the increase in carbon dioxide production and can potentially increase intracranial pressure in already neurologically compromised patients. Unless the temperature is monitored carefully and cooling methods are instituted, irreversible brain damage and death occur.

Artificial cooling methods like tepid sponging and fanning are valuable in hyperthermia, heat stroke and malignant hyperthermias, as these generally do not respond well to antipyretic therapy. Aggressive cooling should be commenced early, as temperatures of above 41°C cause coagulation, nerve damage, convulsions, cell, tissue and organ damage and eventually death.

HYPOTHERMIA

A hypothermia is defined as a core temperature of less than 35°C and affects virtually all metabolic processes in the body (Fritsch 1995).

In acute hypothermia, peripheral vasoconstriction shunts blood away from the cooler skin to the core in an effort to decrease heat loss. This peripheral vasoconstriction leads to peripheral tissue ischaemia, which causes the hypothalamus to stimulate shivering in an effort to increase heat production. At 34°C, thinking becomes sluggish and coordination is impaired. Degrees of hypothermia are classified as follows.

- In a mild hypothermia with a body temperature of 32–35°C, severe shivering occurs at core temperatures below 35°C and will continue until the core temperature rises or drops further to 30–32°C.
- A moderate hypothermia is between 28 and 31.9°C. At 31°C the individual becomes lethargic, heart and respiratory rates decline, cardiac output is diminished and there is confusion, hyperactivity and exaggerated tendon reflexes. Cerebral blood flow is decreased. Metabolic rate declines, further decreasing core temperature. This has an effect on drug metabolism as the drug half-life is increased. Sinus node depression occurs with slowing of conduction through the atrioventricular node and premature ventricular contractions (ectopics) are

common. There is also an increased risk of atrial fibrillation and other dysrhythmias.
- In severe hypothermia, pulse and respiration may be undetectable and the blood coagulates more easily. Dehydration is common after a lengthy exposure to the cold. Loss of consciousness and the absence of neurological reflexes follow.
- As the temperature falls below 20°C, the profoundly hypothermic patient becomes unable to regulate his body heat and the thermoregulatory mechanisms fail. Ice crystals form inside cells, causing them to rupture and die.

The degree and length of exposure of the patient are important. Thus, the length of time hypothermia has taken to occur is significant in that it can influence outcomes. After 12 hours there will be significant fluid loss from the blood, due to shifts of fluid from extracellular to other fluid spaces and from cold-induced diuresis. In addition, there is a marked increase in mortality. It is also significant when rewarming patients as the timespan of hypothermia will determine the best method of achieving this.

Accidental hypothermia
Accidental hypothermia is defined as a core body temperature below 35°C that results from sudden immersion in cold water or prolonged exposure to cold environments. It may occur in accidents involving immersion in cold water or near drowning. Older adults are at risk of accidental

hypothermia, as they have poor responses to extremes of environmental temperature as a result of slowed blood circulation, structural and functional changes in the skin and overall decrease in heat-producing activities.

Therapeutic hypothermia
The term *therapeutic hypothermia* generally refers to a deliberately induced state of hypothermia, which is used to slow a patient's metabolism and thus preserve ischaemic tissue during some types of major surgery. However, hypothermia that occurs inadvertently during surgery is also termed therapeutic hypothermia because it presents during a therapeutic procedure. Both types of hypothermia can sometimes extend into the postoperative period. Therapeutic hypothermia is therefore classified into the following three categories.

Induced hypothermia
This is the intentional lowering of a patient's body temperature. It is generally used in neurosurgery and to treat hyperthermia and during cardiac surgery to decrease metabolic rate and tissue oxygen demands, protect the brain, decrease the risk of ischaemic tissue damage to the heart and thereby protect other vital organs from hypoxia.

Inadvertent, intraoperative or unintentional hypothermia
Major surgery often induces significant hypothermia (termed *inadvertent hypothermia*) because of the exposure of body cavities to the

relatively cool operating room environment. In addition, procedures often involve irrigation of body cavities with room temperature solutions, infusion of room temperature intravenous solutions, inhalation of unwarmed anaesthetic agents and the use of drugs that impair thermoregulatory mechanisms. Older adults are at greater risk of suffering from this type of hypothermia.

This type of hypothermia occurs because:

- patients undergoing surgery do not adapt quickly enough to cool intraoperative environments
- patients are transported along cold draughty corridors before being exposed to operating theatres that have an ambient temperature of 21°C
- skin preparation may include the use of volatile fluids or fluids that must be allowed to dry on the skin, which leads to an increase in heat loss by evaporation
- medications such as muscle relaxants, narcotics and inhaled anaesthetics also contribute to decreasing body temperature as they affect the temperature regulation mechanisms and prevent body movement
- the ability of patients to produce heat is blocked and they become dependent on the temperature of the environment.
- once surgery begins, the use of intravenous solutions and blood at temperatures below that of the patient's body can compound the problem.

Postanaesthesia or postoperative hypothermia
This has been recognized to be an extension of induced or inadvertent hypothermia.

Rewarming methods

Passive external rewarming
Remove any wet clothing, gently dry the patient if needed and then insulate him with blankets. The patient may then be allowed to rewarm using only normal metabolic heat production. Recommended for both mild (32.2–35°C) and moderate (28–32°C) hypothermias that have an onset of less than 12 hours. Movement will contribute to heat loss through convection and may reduce temperature further if not closely monitored.

If the patient's temperature fails to rise and he becomes persistently hypotensive, active external rewarming should be commenced.

Active external rewarming
The patient's skin is warmed using hot baths, hot air blowers or radiant heat. This method can also be used as an adjunct to internal active rewarming, using connective warming. It uses the principles of convection, forcing heated air directly onto the patient's skin through a disposable blanket. Used when the hypothermia has occurred slowly, e.g. over a 12-hour period, and is mild or moderate in nature. However, the patient's vital signs and peripheral temperature must be closely monitored, as rewarming shock may occur in the severely hypothermic patient as a

consequence of rewarming the peripheries before the core.

Active internal rewarming
These are invasive procedures, whereby the deep tissues of the body are warmed. They allow the lungs and heart to be rewarmed first. Methods include:

- warm fluid for gastric and peritoneal lavage
- mediastinal and pleural irrigation
- continuous arteriovenous or venovenous rewarming
- extracorporeal rewarming
- cardiopulmonary bypass – the fastest method.

These are not readily available in all hospitals and require critical care input so are not methods of choice for use in general wards. The easiest methods are:

- warmed gases to the respiratory tract – gases should be humidified as well as warmed
- warmed intravenous (IV) fluids – observe CVP and urine output.

If this method is used the nurse needs to be vigilant to observe for afterdrop, which occurs after internal active rewarming is discontinued. A decrease in temperature of as much as 2°C may occur as blood circulates to the peripheries, recools and returns to the core. When invasive active internal rewarming methods are

discontinued, attention is directed to the need for passive and active external rewarming, to prevent afterdrop in temperature.

This method is best used when the hypothermia has occurred very quickly, e.g. in less than 12 hours, and is moderate or severe in nature. The treatment reduces the risk of cardiac arrest, by reducing the time the patient's core temperature is below 32.2°C.

Special care considerations
The whole process of rewarming should proceed no faster than a few degrees per hour. If a patient is rapidly rewarmed oxygen consumption, myocardial demand and vasodilatation increase faster than the heart's ability to compensate and death can occur. Hypothermia in the elderly need not be treated any differently to that in younger patients.

Heat warming processes are not the only aspects to be considered in the care of hypothermic patients. The nurse has a broader role in managing and caring for these patients and should:

- be vigilant during fluid administration
- observe blood results and the ECG
- document urine output
- ensure that any drugs administered during rewarming are not toxic.

PROCEDURES

3.1 General principles and procedures 102

3.2 Infection and its control 111

3.3 Fluid and electrolyte balance 117

3.4 Nutritional support 130

3.1 GENERAL PRINCIPLES AND PROCEDURES

This section discusses how nurses can further broaden and expand their knowledge of the person as an individual.

PROMOTING REST AND SLEEP

Sleep can be defined as an altered state of consciousness from which a person can be aroused by stimuli of sufficient magnitude. The function of sleep is far from clear. It is considered as restorative and energy conserving, as protein synthesis and cell division for the renewal of tissues take place predominantly during the time devoted to rest and sleep. Sleep is needed to avoid the psychological problems resulting from inadequate sleep which might hinder recovery and if the function of sleep is correctly assumed, then sleep deprivation could be considered as a stressor, over and above those physical and emotional traumas already suffered.

During an average night's sleep individuals pass through four or five sleep cycles, each cycle lasting about 90–100 minutes. Within the sleep cycle, five successive stages have been defined by their distinctive characteristics. The first four stages of sleep are called collectively *non-rapid eye movement* (NREM) sleep and demonstrate a progressive increase in the depth of sleep. Stage five is called rapid eye movement (REM) sleep, or paradoxical sleep,

and is associated with dreaming, learning and memory.

Perpetual awakening and sleep interruption have been associated with increased anxiety, irritability and disorientation, which may have a negative influence on recovery. Total sleep deprivation for 48 hours can result in changes such as:

- behavioural irritability
- suspiciousness
- speech slurring
- minor visual misperceptions
- reduction in motivation and willingness to perform tasks which could include mobilization and other aspects of self-care
- lethargy, irritability and disorientation and confusion
- later, delusions and paranoia.

Recommendations for minimizing sleep interruption in patients are listed in Box 3.1.

ADMISSION TO HOSPITAL

Prior to admission to hospital the patient may have come into contact with the ambulance service or paramedic team (prehospital care), his GP, the primary healthcare team or the police. He may have referred himself to the local A&E department or the minor injuries unit or be a booked admission from home.

In the A&E department the first impressions of the hospital are formed. An A&E nurse may undertake the initial assessment and a decision may be made as to the urgency/priority of the case.

The transfer to the ward may have been a lengthy process and the patient may have been in A&E for a

---

Box 3.1   Minimizing sleep interruptions in patients

- Turn off maximum number of lights, especially at night.
- Keep noise to a minimum (switch off suction equipment, reduce talking and whispering).
- Offer cotton wool balls for patients' ears.
- Continually reassess the need to interrupt patients' sleep to perform observations.
- Perform as many nursing observations as possible together.
- Chart amount of uninterrupted sleep per shift and evidence of sleep stages
- Communicate the patients' need to sleep to other professionals.
- Use knowledge of patients' normal sleeping patterns and supportive family relationships to optimize environment for sleep.
- Administer analgesics and sedatives according to the patients' felt need and monitor events.

---

number of hours before being admitted. In addition, the patient may have been waiting a long time before being admitted from home. On admission to the ward, a welcoming approach, good communication, effective use of assessment tools, observation, measurement, interviewing and documentation (nursing process) skills are paramount (see Section 2).

The often-neglected psychological and social factors need to be included. These identify the close interrelated concepts of physical, psychological and social well-being, as disruption in any one of these aspects will have implications for the others.

DISCHARGE PLANNING/ TRANSFER

This is a process of developing a plan of care for a patient who is transferred from one environment to another. The significance of early discharge planning cannot be overestimated. The average length of hospital admission has been reduced

dramatically owing to advances in technology, financial considerations and contracting requirements of purchasers. Discharge planning should be initiated prior to admission and should include the following.

- Patients and their families/ partners to be informed of the requirements on discharge.
- It should be designed to promote self-care or to assist with care needs when necessary.
- Involvement of the multidisciplinary team.
- The patient's physical, psychological, social, cultural and economic needs.
- The degree of support needed at home after discharge, which should be to a safe and adequate environment.
- Planning on who will look after the patient.
- Consideration for those patients who may have specific care needs.
  —Live alone, frail and/or elderly
  —Have a limited prognosis

—Have serious illnesses, who may be returning to hospital for further treatments
—Have a continuing disability, learning difficulties, mental illness or dementia
—dependants
—Have limited financial resources
—Are homeless or living in poor housing
—Do not have English as a first language
—Require aids/equipment at home
—Have spent an extended time in hospital

- Consideration of the need for external agencies to be involved. Assessment of needs at home may involve the:
  —occupational therapist
  —social services.

Discharge should not be a matter of chance. There is the potential for patients to occupy beds unnecessarily due to late decisions regarding discharge.

Occasionally the discharge process may not proceed as planned or may be delayed. Patients may take their own discharge against medical advice and this should be documented accordingly. Some patients receiving a bad prognosis may prefer to go home and plans may need to be set up at short notice.

PREOPERATIVE CARE

The nurse needs to provide safe, effective and consistent care for patients prior to surgery. This includes ensuring a positive experience and outcome for the pre-operative patient and their carers. As part of preoperative care the nurse needs to consider patient participation and partnership.

- Shared decision making, inclusion of the patient.
- Information giving (verbal or written) including education about the forthcoming operation (preferably 10–14 days preoperatively), explanations of any drugs and pain management preferences, specific postoperative equipment or techniques that may be employed.
- Good communication skills; preoperative communication/ visiting, identifying the barriers to good communication, e.g. anxiety and stress.
- Identify culture differences in interpretation and understanding. Spiritual requirements should be explored.
- Develop an effective nurse–patient relationship. Assessment of the patient's understanding and explanation of words and phrases used during information giving should be undertaken.
- The opportunity to ask questions.
- Informed consent (see p. 4). The nurse needs to ensure that the patient comprehends what is likely to happen to him. The nurse must act in the patient's best interests.

Screening prior to surgery

Screening prior to anaesthetic and surgery is an essential part of patient preparation. There are many specific investigations and preparations that are required for different types of surgery, e.g. of the bowel; these are detailed in Section 5. There are also standard test results that will enhance the surgeon's understanding of the patient's general condition prior to surgery.

- Baseline clinical observations: blood pressure, temperature, pulse, respiratory rate and urine analysis.
- Laboratory tests: full blood count (FBC), to ensure normal haemoglobin to enhance postoperative recovery, blood crossmatched for transfusion, blood urea, creatinine and electrolyte (U&E) levels to check renal function.
- Further investigations, if necessary, may involve chest/abdominal X-ray, ECG, lung function tests and a CT scan.

PERIOPERATIVE CARE

Care in the period before going to theatre may include the following.

- Ongoing physical and psychological care.
- Skin or bowel preparations (may need to commence 48 hours preoperatively).
- Nil by mouth for 4–6 hours is safest since the stomach and small intestine should be empty of the last meal by this time.
- IV cannulation and infusion if relevant.
- Personal hygiene.
- Preoperative checks and premedication: this is to ensure patient safety so name bands are mandatory. A premedication may

not be required and this is generally considered on an individual basis.
- Consider the removal of wigs, hairpieces, jewellery (can cause burns if diathermy is used; wedding rings can be covered with tape), dentures, glasses, contact lenses and prostheses. Removal should be delayed as long as possible to maintain body image.
- The removal of make-up and nail varnish is essential as these prevent the observation of true skin colour and the recording of oxygen saturation monitoring is affected by nail varnish
- Preparation of the bed area for return of the patient (see below).
- Escorting patient to the operating theatre: ideally this should be done by the named nurse.
- Transportation to the operating theatre: the patient should be allowed to sit up whether travelling on a bed or trolley.
- Reception in the operating theatre complex: the patient is generally received from the ward nurse in a reception area and 'handed over' to the theatre nurse, then taken to the anaesthetic room when the anaesthetist is ready.

It is important to highlight that having to undergo surgery is one of the most stressful events in a person's life. The significance of the nurse's knowledge and skill in providing a safe and meaningful preoperative experience for the surgical patient can never be overestimated.

POSTOPERATIVE CARE

There is a range of activities that nurses need to undertake when caring for postoperative patients. There are also specialist areas of surgery, e.g. bowel and thoracic surgery, which require more specific care and these are covered in Section 5.

- The patient is placed in the recovery room attached to theatre. The patients' condition is assessed and he is nursed in the lateral recovery position to minimize risks of aspiration until fully conscious, when he can be transferred back to the ward.
- The bed area has been prepared and includes:
  —airways, various sizes
  —oxygen supply, disposable mask and tubing
  —suction equipment, selection of catheters
  —disposable gloves, gauze swabs, bowl of water and receiver
  —oxygen saturation monitor
  —emergency cardiopulmonary resuscitation equipment.
- A significant aspect of a surgical nurse's role is to reduce the risk of postoperative complications for patients. Surgical complications carry a potential risk to a person's recovery, as well as incurring significant financial costs. Some of the more common postoperative complications are:
  —wound infection
  —deep vein thrombosis (DVT)
  —bleeding (hypovolaemia, hypovolaemic shock)
  —chest infection
  —urinary retention
  —urinary tract infection (UTI)
  —paralytic ileus
  —nausea and vomiting
  —joint stiffness
  —pressure sores
  —shock
  —hypothermia
  —restlessness/confusion/hypoxia.
- It is necessary for the nurse to undertake regular monitoring of the patient and ensure the correct postoperative instructions are adhered to.

Special nursing considerations

These may include an assessment of the patient's risk of DVT formation and instigating preventive measures such as:

- ensuring patient cooperation through education
- encouraging deep breathing and coughing at regular intervals, movement around the bed
- early mobilization
- antiembolic stockings
- administration of postoperative heparin/warfarin
- effective observation and monitoring of peripheral circulation.

Other considerations during the postoperative period can be found elsewhere in the book and include:

- dignity
- urinary catheterization
- nasogastric tube
- intravenous infusion
- nutrition
- wound care
- rest and sleep
- pain assessment and management
- discharge planning

- patient discharge education and health promotion.

PALLIATIVE CARE

Palliative care is the active total care of patients whose disease is not responsive to curative treatment, encompassing both the patient and their family/carers. Issues of death and dying are often not discussed with ease. It is important that health professionals develop skills and strategies for caring for the dying patient and his family.

The principles of palliative care originally focused on patients with advanced cancer but the scope has broadened and it is now offered to patients with a wide range of life-threatening illnesses such as multiple sclerosis, motor neuron disease, AIDS, chronic circulatory or respiratory disease.

Kinghorn and Gamlin (2001) state that palliative care:

- affirms life and regards death as a normal process
- neither hastens nor postpones death
- provides relief from pain and other distressing symptoms
- integrates the psychological and spiritual aspects of patient care
- offers a support system to help patients live as actively as possible until death.

This care takes place in hospitals and is an integral part of all clinical practice. The quality of palliative care in the hospital setting is of crucial importance despite the rapid growth of hospices and home care schemes.

The key principles underpinning palliative care comprise:

- whole-person approach
- care which encompasses both the patient and those who matter to them
- emphasis on open and sensitive communication, including adequate information about diagnosis and treatment options
- respect for patient autonomy and choice
- focus on quality of life which includes good symptom control and nursing care.

The role of the nurse is central to the care of the dying patient and family. It requires the utmost sensitivity and attention to detail. Many dying patients wish to remain independent for as long as possible. The nurse is in a position to offer:

- skilled, supportive care to patients and families
- sensitive nursing care enabling the patient to remain independent for as long as possible
- reporting of presenting symptoms and monitoring of symptom control
- coordination of care between the multiprofessional team.

Nursing intervention in common symptoms

There are some aspects of symptom control that will be directly helped by skilled nursing.

- *Anorexia* – providing extra nutrition will not prolong life; liaise with the dietitian for ideas on presentation and supplements.

- *Mouth care* – assess the oral cavity; can be helped with ice cubes, boiled lemon sweets or fresh pineapple chunks.
- *Constipation* – a high-fibre diet is inappropriate; appropriate use of laxatives, privacy for defaecation and mobilization for as long as possible.
- *Dyspnoea* – involves relaxation and a range of pharmacological interventions.
- *Fungating wounds* – sight and smell; need to eradicate smell and use a dressing that is cosmetically acceptable to the patient.

Emotional care

Emotional care relies on openness and sharing the truth about the illness. The patient will feel loss and grief for the lack of:

- independence (holidays, trips out)
- self-esteem (body image, appetite)
- status, job and income
- role and relationships
- a future.

Spiritual care

Spiritual care gives the patient and family an opportunity to examine the impact of the illness on their belief systems. They need to be given the opportunity to ask questions.

- Why me?
- Why now?
- What have I done to deserve this?

Staying with this sort of spiritual pain and not being afraid of the questions is a helpful response. Offering the support of a relevant religious figure may not be appropriate for all but listening and being present will be appreciated.

Cultural diversity

Making nursing practice relevant to people of many cultures is a constant challenge to the nurse. Cultures differ with regard to:

- the meaning of illness
- attitude to pain and symptoms and to medication
- ways of coping with illness
- attitude to place of care, physical and emotional care
- the roles of the family
- rituals around death, the funeral and bereavement.

Social needs

The nurse needs to ensure that patients and families have adequate information regarding the benefits to which they may be entitled. This includes:

- Disability Living Allowance (DLA)
- attendance allowance
- free prescriptions
- housing benefits
- income support
- council tax
- Macmillan cancer relief grants
- power of attorney (the legal right to act on someone's behalf)
- drawing up of a will.

DEATH/DYING

The majority of people would prefer to die at home but this is not always feasible and only about 25% of people in the UK do so. Maintaining comfort is paramount and the last few days of life are likely to be spent in bed.

- Some people fear terrible pain or dying in a dramatic fashion and the nurse can do much to reassure and comfort the patient.
- A few patients find the last days intolerable and it is compassionate for the medical and nursing team to offer medication that will help relieve this.
- The majority of patients become sleepy and this merges into drowsiness and unconsciousness.
- Cheyne–Stokes breathing may occur (periods of apnoea followed by more respirations, a cycle which continues until breathing stops).

Complementary therapies

These are becoming increasingly popular for people who are dying and include:

- acupuncture
- aromatherapy
- massage
- reflexology.

These are generally safe and free from the side-effects of orthodox anticancer treatments.

Potential organ donation

Many patients in the UK die or suffer prolonged dependency because of a lack of organs for transplantation. Therefore, if a young or middle-aged patient with a fatal condition has healthy kidneys, liver, heart or corneas, it might be relevant to discuss organ donation with the medical team. Suitable organ donors include:

- victims of severe head injury
- severe subarachnoid or intracerebral haemorrhage
- in the case of corneal donation, any young patient with healthy eyes or a rapidly fatal illness.

Patients who are unsuitable organ donors:

- where brain death is uncertain
- those over 60
- where there has been significant hypotension or hypoxia during a fatal illness
- where there is a history of previous disease affecting the potential donor organ (e.g. hypertension, diabetes, hepatitis B, alcohol abuse)
- where the patient has received drugs or other treatment which might have affected the organs to be transplanted
- in the case of the kidneys, where there is persistent oliguria.

What to do after the patient has died

- The family should be able to spend as much time with the dead person as they want.
- The doctor or GP will be called to certify the death.
- Date and time of death are recorded.
- There is no need for children to be excluded from this time.
- Inform surrounding patients of the death.
- If a doctor has not seen the patient within 14 days before the death, a postmortem examination may be needed.

Last offices

This is the care given to a deceased patient, which is focused on fulfilling religious and cultural beliefs as well as health and safety and legal requirements. It should be remembered that this is the final demonstration of respectful, sensitive care given to the patient.

- It is important that the nurse knows in advance the cultural values and religious beliefs of the family, as there are considerable cultural variations between people of different faiths, ethnic backgrounds and national origins in their approach to death and dying.
- Individual preferences should be determined and patients should be encouraged to talk about how they may wish to be treated upon dying. If in doubt, consult the family members.
- Catheters and other appliances should be removed (except in a coroner's case – a medical enquiry into the cause of death) and any dentures replaced.
- Orifices that are leaking fluid should be packed with gauze.
- Relatives should be asked whether jewellery should be left on or taken off.
- Wash the patient, unless requested not to do so for religious/cultural reasons. It may not be acceptable for the nurse to undertake this task or sometimes, a relative may want to help.
- The body is dressed in nightwear, a shroud or other garments selected by the family.

- The body needs to be labelled (if in an institution) on one wrist, one ankle and on the outside of the shroud, with an identification bracelet and the property identified and stored.
- Wrap the body in a mortuary sheet and secure the sheet with tape.
- Tape a notification of death card on the outside of the sheet (refer to hospital policy for details).
- Request the portering staff to remove the body.
- Screen off appropriate areas from view of other patients when the body is being removed.
- Update nursing records, transfer property and patient records to the appropriate administrative department.

A death certificate will be issued the next day from the hospital and needs to be registered within 5 days at the registrar's office in the district in which the death took place.

Bereavement

A nurse working with dying patients needs to have an understanding of bereavement and how to recognize abnormal grief and to refer to specialist help. Most of the country is now covered by local bereavement services.

Grief is not an illness, it is a pattern of reactions that take place while the person adjusts to the death of his loved one. The nurse is not expected to be a bereavement counsellor but to be there for the relative before the patient has died. A well-managed death will help with the emotional health of a family. Listening and understanding imply concern and care while acknowledgement of their pain and sorrow may help relatives to move forward.

Recognizing abnormal grief

- Are grief reactions prolonged, excessive and seeming incapable of resolution?
- Are grief reactions absent?
- Has grief been displaced or masked, e.g. by illness, drugs, alcohol or overwork?
- Was the relationship with the deceased person particularly ambivalent or dependent?
- Were the circumstances of the death unexpected or violent?

The cost of caring to the nurse

Working closely with dying patients can cause emotional distress for the nurse and can be painful. Nurses need adequate support systems in both their professional and personal lives. The nurse needs to recognize internal signs of stress and develop strategies for coping.

- Spacing of holidays and time off is important to recharge lost energy.
- Continuous training and education for stimulation.
- Take time to debrief with a colleague.
- Concise written recording can be therapeutic and help the letting go of a particularly stressful situation.
- Being honest and sharing vulnerabilities will help a

team relate and work well together.

3.2 INFECTION AND ITS CONTROL

Infection control prevents the spread of infection in hospital.

IMMUNIZATION

Immunization is based on exposure to:

- weakened or dead disease-producing microorganisms (in the form of vaccines)
- the poisons (toxins) they produce, rendered harmless by heat or chemical treatment (then called toxoids).

These will cause an individual to produce the same antibodies that would develop if the person had actually contracted the disease. Armed with the special memory that is unique to the immune system, these antibodies will 'recognize' the specific microorganisms, should they attack in the future, and destroy them.

The widely administered types of immunization are:

- diphtheria, tetanus, acellular pertussis vaccine (DTP)
- polio vaccine (OPV or TOPV)
- measles, mumps and rubella (MMR)
- varicella vaccine (chicken pox)
- haemophilus b vaccine (haemophilus influenza – Hib)
- hepatitis B vaccine
- tuberculosis (TB)
- meningitis (meningococcal c).

INFECTION CONTROL PRACTICES

Barrier nursing: the use of the single room (isolation)

When using the single room every effort must be made to ensure that instructions are kept simple and realistic. Regular assessment and evaluation of the situation must take place to ascertain whether barrier nursing continues to remain the most appropriate form of care. There are two types of barrier nursing.

- Isolation – generally used to protect staff and other patients in the ward area.
- Protective isolation – to protect the patient suffering from immunosuppression.

Isolation

A process of care whereby infectious patients and any materials that have come into contact with or been eliminated by them are isolated from others to prevent the spread of infection. This is generally determined by the availability of facilities, the infection and how the infection is transmitted:

- by direct contact
- airborne
- food or bloodborne
- by respiratory droplet
- by skin scales or excrement.

Isolation can potentially cause serious psychological effects, such as sensory deprivation, and therefore should be kept to a minimum. The principles of isolation should be based on isolation of the organism, not the patient.

Protective isolation

A process of care which provides a safe environment for patients who are susceptible to infection by isolating them from the risk of infection from all exogenous sources. It uses simple precautions which are sufficient to protect the patient, e.g. gloves and masks are not generally necessary; the most important measure is thorough hand washing.

Protective isolation is an appropriate form of care for:

- burns
- those who are immunosuppressed:
  —leukaemia, lymphoma, AIDS, SCID
  —drug therapies such as cytotoxics
  —radiotherapy
  —trauma
  —age
- patients receiving bone marrow transplantation.

Infection risk generally relates to the absolute level of circulating granulocytes. The frequency of infection rises as the granulocyte count drops below $0.5 \times 10^9/l$, with a dramatic increase in the risk of infection as the granulocyte count reaches zero.

Informing the patient and visitors

Giving careful explanation to the patient and visitors is essential so they understand why the barrier nursing restrictions are necessary and can cooperate fully with the procedures.

When a relative visits a patient in a single room there is usually no reason to ask them to wear protective clothing. Visitors do not generally go from patient to patient and as such are not in contact with other patients. Visitors do not handle infectious material and an instruction to wash their hands before and after they leave the room is all that is necessary.

> ⚠️ **Staff and visitors who have an infection, such as a sore throat or cold, must not come into contact with the patient.**

Hand washing

The process of hand washing is uncontroversial and is the single most important procedure for preventing the spread of nosocomial (hospital-acquired) infection. Hands have been shown to be an important route of transmission and responsible for a large proportion of crossinfection.

The skin, especially the hands, is a common habitat for some bacteria such as *Staphylococcus epidermidis* (Gram-positive coccus), micrococci and diphtheroids. The majority of the resident organisms are harmless but may become pathogenic if allowed to penetrate through the skin via a wound, during surgery or other invasive procedures.

Other organisms which do not generally multiply on healthy intact skin can be acquired transiently from:

- other sites on the person's own body
- another person
- the external environment.

Transient organisms that can survive for several hours on the hands unless washed off include *Staphylococcus aureus*, *Escherichia coli* and *Pseudomonas*.

Thorough hand washing before attending to a patient will ensure the majority of microorganisms acquired transiently from other patients are removed. Never let the business of the ward interfere with this important procedure.

- Transient bacteria are mostly removed from the skin by washing with soap and water.
- Resident skin bacteria, e.g. *Staphylococcus aureus*, are best removed by rubbing the hands with a bactericidal alcoholic solution, e.g. chlorhexidine.
- Alcoholic hand rubs are as effective as the more time-consuming, conventional antiseptic detergent hand-wash methods and may be used on clean hands immediately before carrying out an aseptic procedure.

Hand washing should be carried out:

- before and after patient contact
- before an aseptic procedure.

Procedure

1. Roll up sleeves, remove rings and wrist watches.
2. Use soap under continuously running water.
3. Position the hands so that water flows downwards, to avoid contaminating the arms.
4. Use friction on all surfaces and rub hands together well.

5. Rinse thoroughly and hold hands down whilst doing so.
6. Always ensure that hands are dried thoroughly, preferably using paper towels.

No-touch technique

A no-touch technique is essential to ensure that hands, even though they have been washed, do not contaminate sterile equipment or the patient. This can be achieved by the use of either forceps or sterile gloves. It must be remembered, however, that gloves can become damaged and allow the passage of bacteria. This may give a false sense of security when providing wound care, whilst forceps may damage tissue.

The use of gloves can encourage the rapid growth of skin flora on nurses' hands so it is essential to wash hands following removal of gloves.

Protective clothing

The transmission of microorganisms on staff clothing is theoretically possible but is unlikely to occur. This reduces the need for protective clothing. Bacteria can spread from white coats worn by doctors; if this does occur it is more likely to arise on the front. If uniforms are in danger of becoming contaminated with body fluids, plastic aprons provide adequate protection as they are impermeable. Fabric gowns cover more of the carer's clothing but do not prevent the passage of microorganisms, especially when wet. It is recommended that if spillage is likely, e.g. in theatres or for other sterile procedures, plastic aprons should be worn underneath sterile gowns.

Disposable gloves should be worn for any activity where body fluid may contaminate the hands and for procedures involving direct contact with mucous membranes, e.g. for mouth care. Aprons and gloves must be discarded and hands washed before caring for another patient, as the hands are easily contaminated during their removal.

Nurses may leave the room when wearing protective clothing, as long as it is understood that it is contact spreads infection and not the act of leaving the room. As long as there is no direct contact with other patients, infections are unlikely to be spread if the nurse leaves the isolation room to carry out a specific task.

Masks and eye protection

Masks are often recommended for infections that are spread by respiratory droplets. The disadvantages are that:

- they do not work when wet – damp masks do not filter microorganisms effectively
- their efficiency diminishes when worn for long periods
- they become easily contaminated by the hands during repositioning or removal.

They are now recognized as unreliable against airborne infections, especially viral.

There have been reports of acquiring HIV as a result of blood splashing into the face and masks and eye protection should be worn for any activity where there is a risk of body fluid splashing into the face.

Waste material

Waste material that is contaminated with blood or body fluids should be discarded in a yellow waste bag, in the patient's room. The outer surface of waste bags does not become significantly contaminated and there is no reason to enclose the waste in a second bag. If leakage of body fluids is likely, a second bag or a special impervious container should be used.

> ⚠ **All body fluids should be safely discarded directly into a bedpan washer or macerator.**

Excreta (urine, faeces, vomit)

Infected excreta should be disposed of immediately down a heat-disinfected bedpan washer. Ideally a toilet should be kept solely for the patient's use. If this is not possible and disposable items are not available, a separate bedpan, urinal and commode should be left in the patient's room/anteroom. Bedpans and urinals should be bagged in the isolation room, emptied and then washed in the bedpan washer, then dried and returned immediately to the patient's room. On discharge bedpans/urinals must be sent to the central sterite supplies department (CSSD) for disinfecting.

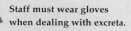

> ⚠ **Staff must wear gloves when dealing with excreta.**

Linen

Infected linen must be placed in a red alginate polythene bag. The bag is tied shut and then placed in a red linen bag to be sent in a safe manner to the laundry for washing. The alginate bag dissolves in the wash and allows the disinfectant to clean the linen. In this way staff and the environment are protected from contamination.

Domestic staff and cleaning

The domestic manager must be informed as soon as barrier nursing is commenced. The ward domestic must understand clearly why barrier nursing is required and should be instructed on the correct procedure, as scrupulous daily cleaning of the barrier nursing room is essential. All furniture must be damp dusted, the floor vacuum cleaned (containing a filter) or damp mopped with hot, soapy water. Using a broom is not recommended as it disperses organisms into the air. Cleaning equipment must be kept for the patient's sole use, preferably in an anteroom.

Aseptic technique

This method is used to prevent the introduction of microorganisms into the patient's body via contamination of wounds and other susceptible sites. It can be achieved by ensuring that only sterile equipment and fluids are used during invasive medical and nursing procedures.

There are two types of asepsis.

1. Medical or clean asepsis reduces the number of organisms and prevents their spread.
2. Surgical or sterile asepsis includes procedures to eliminate

microorganisms from an area and is practised in the operating theatre and treatment areas.

An aseptic technique is used whenever there is an invasive procedure that bypasses the body's natural defences. Examples necessitating the use of an aseptic technique are:

- application of dressings to a wound, e.g. following surgery or trauma
- caring for any broken area of skin, e.g. pressure sores, leg ulcers
- invasive procedures such as catheterization and injections or the insertion of intravenous cannulae.

Guidelines for the use of an aseptic technique when carrying out nursing procedures are given very clearly in the *Royal Marsden Manual of Clinical Nursing Procedures* (Mallet & Dougherty 2000).

Staff allocation
A minimum number of staff should be involved in caring for an infectious patient. The nurse caring for an infectious patient should not attend to other susceptible patients. If barrier nursing is for an infectious disease such as chicken pox, it is preferable that only personnel who have already had the disease attend the patient. If there is doubt, then contact the occupational health department who may offer immunization.

Notification of specific infections
If a patient develops signs and symptoms of specific infection or if

bacteriological analysis identifies an organism which necessitates barrier nursing, swift communication and action may be needed as some infections are notifiable by law. If you are unsure which infections require notification, then contact the hospital microbiology department for advice. Any problems may be discussed with the infection control team.

Equipment
This includes the instruments used and any fluids or materials, which must all be sterile. Dressing packs, which have been autoclaved to ensure sterility, are obtained from the CSSD.

Any procedure should be explained to the patient beforehand and his understanding checked. Reassurance should be offered and on completion of the procedure the patient must be made comfortable and all equipment disposed of in a manner that will reduce any health hazard.

Patient hygiene
The patient's skin flora is an important source of infection following invasive procedures but good patient hygiene will reduce this hazard. Washing with chlorhexidine solution has been shown to decrease bacteriuria. It can be used pre- and postoperatively to reduce the incidence of wound infections. Anaerobic organisms such as *Clostridium perfringens* colonize the skin around the thighs and buttocks; hence the need for appropriate hygiene following surgery in this area. For areas that

should not get wet, e.g. indwelling intravenous central catheters, stitches should be covered with transparent film dressings as protection against wetting during showering.

3.3 FLUID AND ELECTROLYTE BALANCE

The constant motion of fluid and electrolytes around the body contributes to the maintenance of equilibrium. The major body electrolytes are sodium, potassium and calcium and management of patients' fluid balance requires an understanding of fluid, sodium, potassium and calcium homeostasis. Fluid and electrolyte balance is maintained by the renal system with some help from other organs. Fluid and electrolyte balance is closely associated and a disturbance in one is rarely seen without some disturbance in the other.

To maintain fluid and electrolyte balance, water, sodium and potassium are in constant motion between intracellular (ICF) (about 25 l) and extracellular (ECF) compartments (divided into interstitial fluid – 12 l and plasma volume – 3 l).

TOTAL BODY WATER

The principal component of all body fluids is water. There are complex aqueous solutions in which biochemically distinct compartments are divided by the plasma membrane (between the ICF and ECF compartments) or by specialized cell layers (between intravascular, interstitial and transcellular compartments).

Body water accounts for between 50% (females) and 60% (males) of an adult's total body weight. Men normally have less body fat than women and thus have a higher percentage of body weight as water. The percentage of body water is higher in the emaciated than the obese for the same reasons. A newborn baby is approximately 73% water. In old age the body may be only about 45% water.

The average adult has a normal fluid intake of 2–2.5 l/day obtained by drinking and from food, either as actual water in the food or by oxidation of the food during metabolism which gives rise to some 200–300 ml per day. The normal routes of fluid loss are via the kidneys, gastrointestinal tract, respiratory tract and skin. In the healthy adult:

- the kidneys excrete approximately 1500–2000 ml of fluid daily, depending on intake
- faecal loss amounts to some 300 ml of fluid per day
- losses from the skin and respiratory passages account for approximately 600–1000 ml daily.

INTAKE AND OUTPUT

In health there is near-perfect fluid balance and the amount of fluid taken into the body daily is equal to that which is lost from the body. In illness there may be excessive loss of fluid, possibly accompanied by an inability to take in fluid by the normal routes. This may necessitate the administration of fluids by intravenous infusion.

RECORDING FLUID BALANCE

In almost every severe illness or surgical operation fluid balance can be disturbed and an accurate 24-hour record of all the fluid entering the patient and all the fluid output has to be recorded.

ELECTROLYTE COMPOSITION OF BODY FLUID COMPARTMENTS

The solute compositions of the ECF and ICF compartments are the major electrolytes, i.e. products of ionic compound dissociation in solution, and are markedly different in each compartment. *Cations* carry a positive charge and *anions* carry a negative charge. The main cations in body fluids are:

- sodium (Na^+)
- potassium (K^+)
- calcium (Ca^{++})
- phosphorus (HPO_4)
- magnesium (Mg^{++}).

The main anions in body fluids are:

- chloride (Cl^-)
- bicarbonate (HCO_3^-).

Thus, the main cation of the ECF is sodium whereas the main cation of the ICF is potassium. The main anions of the ECF are chloride and bicarbonate and those of the ICF are proteins (which are predominantly negatively charged) and organic phosphates. In body fluids the total number of positive ions equals the total number of negative ions, thus maintaining electrical neutrality.

The concentration of electrolytes is measured in mmol/l milliequivalents per litre (mEq/l) which is a measure of the number of electrical charges in 1 l: 1 mmol/l or mEq/l = 1 mmol/l for ions carrying a single charge. Non-electrolytes are also present, i.e. molecules such as glucose or urea which are uncharged in solution.

Movement of electrolytes between compartments

Several factors contribute to and maintain the differences in solute composition between the ECF and ICF. In order to pass between the ECF and ICF, a solute must cross the plasma membrane. Some move freely across the membrane due to their concentration differences, the majority require some form of assistance.

Table 3.1 A possible average daily intake and output			
Intake (ml)		Output (ml)	
Fluids	1700	Urine	1500
Food	1000	Breathing	500
Metabolic water	300	Faeces	200
		Sweat	800
Total	3000	Total	3000

Measuring electrolytes

Serum electrolytes are measured in the laboratory from a sample of blood taken from the patient. This is therefore from the ECF. The levels of the various electrolytes in the blood aid diagnosis of many conditions and can also be used to monitor the progress of an ill patient.

Sodium

Sodium is the main cation in the blood and is an important indication of daily fluid loss. Obligatory sodium loss via the skin, gut and kidneys is less than 10 mmol/day. The average intake of sodium in the Western world is 100–200 mmol/day. This is much more than is needed and excess sodium intake may be linked to hypertension. Sodium excretion is controlled by the hormone aldosterone, which is produced by the adrenal cortex and causes sodium to be retained.

Sodium and water losses are linked together as are sodium and water retention. This means that the plasma sodium is dependent on the amount of ECF and high sodium levels in the blood may be a sign of low fluid volume rather than sodium excess. The normal range for sodium in venous blood is 135–145 mmol/l.

Hyponatraemia is associated with an excess of water and develops when the serum sodium concentration decreases to below 135 mmol/L. Hyponatraemia is caused by a sodium deficit or water excess, leading to an intracellular overhydration. This can occur due to fluid regimes when fluid loss is replaced with excess intravenous 5% dextrose in water. When the body is functioning normally it is almost impossible to produce an excess of fluid by administering 5% dextrose.

Hyponatraemia is observed in conditions such as:

- inadequate sodium intake or diuretic therapy
- excessive sweating stimulating thirst and intake of large amounts of water which dilutes ECF sodium
- vomiting, diarrhoea, gastrointestinal suctioning or burns
- congestive cardiac failure
- hepatic cirrhosis
- diuretic phase of acute tubular necrosis
- adrenal insufficiency
- compulsive water drinking
- oversecretion of antidiuretic hormone (ADH)
- overhydration.

Hypernatraemia is defined as a serum sodium greater than 145 mmol/l. Excessive serum sodium may be caused by an acute gain in sodium or a loss of water. It is always associated with hyperosmolality. The main cause of high sodium levels is inappropriate administration of saline solutions (as sodium bicarbonate, for treatment of acidosis during cardiac arrest, or sodium chloride). This is often due to therapeutic misadventure.

Because of the high concentration of sodium, large infusions of saline solutions may increase blood osmolality, resulting in an increased load onto the circulation due to the response of compensatory mechanisms (ADH production and the renin- angiotensin-aldosterone mechanism). These processes cause movement of water to the ECF and signs of fluid overload may be evident, weight gain, pallor, breathlessness, convulsions and pulmonary oedema being the most obvious.

Though 0.9% saline is much better than 5% dextrose (which causes water retention and dilutional hyponatraemia if infused in excess), for resuscitation/operative purposes (i.e. correction of hypovolaemia or hypotension) it is still not ideal.

Other causes of hypernatraemia are:

- excess sodium and loss of water
- general fever or respiratory infections which increase the respiratory rate, enhancing water loss from the lungs and sweating
- diabetes insipidus and mellitus
- polyurea
- severe vomiting and diarrhoea
- insufficient water intake can also cause hypernatraemia, particularly in individuals who are comatose, confused or immobilized
- oversecretion of aldosterone, as in primary hyperaldosteronism, or Cushing's syndrome caused by excess secretion of adrenocorticotrophic hormone (ACTH), which also causes increased secretion of aldosterone.

Potassium

Potassium is the main intracellular cation. Only 2% of the body's potassium is in the ECF compartment and thus free to be measured. The healthy kidney is less able to conserve potassium than sodium and potassium depletion can occur occasionally on a normal diet if there are increased losses from the body. The kidney controls the potassium balance in the blood. Aldosterone is released in hypovolaemia and hyperkalaemia and aldosterone stimulates potassium excretion. The normal range for potassium in venous blood is 3.3–4.7 mmol/l.

Hyperkalaemia is a high level of potassium in the blood. The clinical features of hyperkalaemia may be very few but if there are any symptoms there will be characteristic changes in the ECG. This will show peaking of the T waves, followed by loss of P waves and then abnormal QRS complexes.

Potassium levels are increased in:

- renal failure
- the use of potassium-sparing diuretics
- adrenal insufficiency
- acidosis (potassium increase tends to cause acidosis).

> ⚠️ **Hyperkalaemia can kill without warning. Cardiac arrest with ventricular fibrillation may be the first sign of hyperkalaemia.**

Hypokalaemia is a low level of potassium in the blood. The clinical features of hypokalaemia are decreased excitability of the nervous system and muscle weakness. In addition there may be:

- depression
- confusion
- arrhythmias
- ECG changes
- susceptibility to digoxin toxicity
- polyuria
- alkalosis.

Blood potassium levels are decreased in:

- diarrhoea and vomiting
- other gastrointestinal losses
- excessive sweating
- use of diuretics (loop and thiazide-like diuretics)
- steroids
- salbutamol and other B_2 agonists
- nephrotic syndrome
- diabetes
- Cushing's syndrome
- excessive renin secretion
- alkalosis (potassium depletion tends to cause alkalosis)
- overhydration
- laxative abuse.

> ⚠️ **Severe hypokalaemia may be asymptomatic. Muscular weakness, constipation and paralytic ileus are the most common problems.**

Calcium
Calcium is a necessary ion for many fundamental metabolic processes:

- the structure of teeth and bones
- muscle contractions (including the heart)
- blood coagulation
- transmission of neural impulses
- maintaining cell membrane stability and permeability.

The bones contain more than 99% of the body's calcium; the rest is in the serum and exists in two forms:

1. ionized or free calcium (found in foods and the only type that the body can use)
2. bound to albumin – which accounts for about half of the serum calcium

Serum levels of free calcium are normally 4.5–5.5 mmol/l and total serum calcium, including bound and free, is usually 8.5–10 mg/dl.

Hypocalcaemia is usually associated with inadequate dietary intake of calcium or vitamin D, which is essential for optimal calcium use by the body. There are some diseases which interfere with calcium absorption from the gut.

- Pancreatitis.
- Respiratory alkalosis due to hyperventilation; calcium binds to bicarbonate so less calcium is available for use.
- Renal failure on loop diuretics because of excessive calcium loss.
- Patients suffering from burns – calcium can become trapped in burned tissue.
- Blood transfusion of banked blood.
- Hypoparathyroidism – lack of parathyroid hormone leads to a drop in calcium levels.
- Low magnesium, which inhibits parathyroid function.
- A high level of phosphorus (hyperphosphataemia) as phosphorus is calcium's reciprocal.

Hypercalcaemia is defined as total serum calcium above 10 mg/dl or a free calcium level above 5.5 mmol/l. The condition is most often related to malignant tumours and prolonged immobility. Other conditions that can increase bone reabsorption include:

- adrenal insufficiency
- hyperparathyroidism
- hypophosphataemia
- hyperproteinaemia
- hyperthyroidism
- renal dysfunction
- thiazide diuretics
- vitamin D intoxication
- tuberculosis.

Phosphorus

Phosphorus is the primary anion, or negatively charged ion, in the ICF. Adults who get enough calcium usually get the daily dietary requirement for phosphorus of 800–1300 mg. This is because both electrolytes are present in many of the same foods.

Phosphorus is vital for:

- formation of stored energy in the cells (adenosine triphosphate, ATP)
- formation of bones and teeth
- interacting with haemoglobin to promote oxygen release to the tissues
- contributing to the phagocytic action of white blood cells
- helping to metabolize proteins, carbohydrates, fats
- normal platelet structure and function.

The serum phosphorus level is normally 2.3–4.4 mmol/l.

Hypophosphataemia is most commonly caused by diseases that raise the renal excretion of phosphorus. These include:

- hyperparathyroidism
- hypokalaemia
- administration of PN solutions as they often do not contain enough phosphorus
- overuse of certain antacids, e.g. those containing aluminium, calcium or magnesium inhibit GI absorption of phosphorus
- chronic alcohol abuse because of the associated diarrhoea, vomiting and malnutrition.

Hyperphosphataemia occurs when serum phosphorus exceeds 4.5 mmol/l. The most common cause is renal dysfunction but it can also result from:

- overuse of laxatives that contain phosphorus
- a diet too rich in phosphorus
- increased GI absorption of phosphorus related to excess vitamin D intake
- hypo/hyperparathyroidism
- metabolic acidosis
- rhabdomyolysis
- use of cytotoxic agents
- chemotherapy.

Magnesium

A serum range of 1.5–2.5 mmol/l determines magnesium levels. It is the most abundant intracellular cation. Calcium and magnesium often interact in reactions at the cellular level. Magnesium is stored around the body:

- 53% of the body's magnesium is in the bones
- 27% is in the muscles
- 19% is in the soft tissues

- 0.5% is contained in the erythrocytes
- 0.3% is free in the serum.

Magnesium is vital to several body functions; it:

- is involved in enzyme reactions that result in the production of ATP or energy
- plays a major role in maintaining and correcting electrical excitability in the nerves and muscle cells, including the heart and cardiac conduction system
- helps maintain the structural integrity of the heart.

The maintenance of normal magnesium levels is determined by dietary consumption, e.g. 280–350 mg/day.

Hypomagnesaemia is a rare condition but occurs most commonly in:

- increased renal excretion related to the use of loop diuretics (Frusemide) or some antibiotics (garamycin, nebcin); both types of drugs speed magnesium loss by inhibiting its reabsorption in the loop of Henle
- alcohol abuse, which increases renal magnesium loss
- renal tubular dysfunction
- diarrhoea and vomiting as magnesium is not absorbed properly from the lower GI tract
- pancreatic insufficiency
- pancreatitis
- malnutrition, malabsorption syndromes and ulcerative colitis.

The most common signs are leg and body cramps, lethargy, weakness, nausea, abdominal distension, constipation, anorexia, confusion and arrhythmias.

Hypermagnesaemia is also a rare condition, with a level above 2.5 mmol/l, and is generally unrelated to magnesium replacement as the kidney can usually excrete magnesium excesses. It is nearly always linked to renal failure. The condition can also be caused by overuse of magnesium-containing antacids and cathartics like Milk of Magnesia and magnesium citrate.

In excess, magnesium depresses skeletal muscle contraction, nerve function and the cardiovascular system, acting like a calcium channel blocker. These patients will experience:

- nausea and vomiting
- drowsiness
- hypotension
- muscle weakness
- hot flushes
- reduced deep tendon reflexes
- bradycardia, complete heart block
- respiratory depression, coma and cardiac arrest.

Chloride
This is the major anion in the ECF and ranges between 95 and 106 mmol/l. It provides electrical neutrality, particularly in relation to sodium, and facilitates the release of carbon dioxide and oxygen from the haemoglobin (the *chloride shift*). The transport of chloride is generally passive and follows the active transport of sodium, so that increases or decreases in chloride are proportional to changes in sodium.

Because bicarbonate is the other major anion in the ECF, the concentration of chloride tends to vary inversely with changes in bicarbonate concentration.

Hyperchloraemia occurs clinically when there is an excess of sodium or a deficit of bicarbonate. Greater than normal amounts of chloride can be expected with hypernatraemia or metabolic acidosis.

Hypochloraemia is the loss of chloride and is usually the result of hyponatraemia or elevated bicarbonate concentration, as in metabolic alkalosis. Hypochloraemia develops with:

- vomiting
- loss of hydrochloric acid from the stomach
- sodium deficit related to restricted intake
- the use of diuretics
- cystic fibrosis.

Alterations in chloride levels are usually secondary to pathophysiological processes and treatment is usually related to management of the underlying disorder. Therefore, there are no specific symptoms associated with chloride deficit or increase.

Bicarbonate
Bicarbonate forms part of one of the major buffering systems in the body, which operates in the lung and kidney: the carbonic acid–bicarbonate buffer pair. It maintains acid–base balance of the ECF; as carbon dioxide is an acid, the greater the carbon dioxide content, the more carbonic acid and conversely, the

more hydrogen ions, the more carbonic acid is formed.

$$CO_2 + H_2O \leftrightarrow H_2CO_3 \leftrightarrow HCO_3^- + H^+$$

The lungs can decrease the amount of carbonic acid by blowing off CO_2 and leaving water. The kidneys excrete the excess hydrogen ions, reabsorb the bicarbonate or regenerate new bicarbonate from CO_2 and water. The renal mechanism does not act as rapidly as the lungs but the two systems are very effective together because the lungs can rapidly adjust acid concentration and bicarbonate is easily reabsorbed or regenerated by the kidneys to maintain acid–base balance.

Changes in either bicarbonate or hydrogen ion levels will change the pH. If the amount of bicarbonate is decreased, the pH will also decrease, causing a state of acidosis. The pH can be returned to normal range if the amount of carbonic acid also decreases, known as *compensation*. Conversely, if the bicarbonate increases, the pH will also increase, and compensation will include the increase of carbonic acid (see p. 67).

Treatment
Most of the treatment for electrolyte imbalances is to treat the underlying cause, replace any loss of electrolyte until normal values are reached or symptoms are improved, flush out the extra high concentration via increasing urine output or dilute it with carefully monitored fluid regimes or removal by dialysis.

MAINTAINING CIRCULATING VOLUME AND FLUID BALANCE

To maintain circulatory fluid volume, people consume liquids. However, in instances where there is a decrease in circulating fluid volume, this needs to be replaced. The main aetiologies of fluid loss are as follows.

- *Increase in temperature* – this leads to vasodilatation and may lead to symptoms of reduced circulating volume, as fluid space has increased.
- *Dehydration* – more common in the elderly but if severe, it can lead to reductions in circulating volume and hypovolaemia.
- *Loss of whole blood* – the most common cause of circulation loss; leads to decreases in the oxygen-carrying capacity of the blood and contributes to hypoxia.
- *Loss of plasma* – occurs in large partial-thickness or full-thickness burns or burns over more than 20–25% of the total body surface area.
- *Bleeding disorders* – platelet (thrombocytopenia, thrombocytosis) and coagulation (vitamin E deficiency, liver disease, DIC) disorders can cause or fail to prevent an internal or external haemorrhage.
- *Third space fluid shift* – any type of trauma or cell damage (surgery, MI, pancreatitis, head injury) will automatically stimulate the inflammatory immune response. Capillaries dilate and become more permeable, causing localized swelling and lymphatic blockage, leading to loss of circulating volume.

The decline in blood volume produced by continued bleeding, plasma loss, water or fluid shifts decreases venous return and cardiac output. Replacement therapy might be required.

Colloid therapy

Colloid solutions (human albumin solution, Gelofusin, plasma protein fractions, salt-poor albumin, Haemacel and Hespan) are used to restore plasma volume and improve or maintain oxygen transport, providing adequate oxygen and nutrients which are needed for the maintenance and restoration of cellular function. Administering plasma expanders produces an improvement in oxygen availability, oxygen consumption, circulating volume, haemodynamic status and tissue perfusion.

Crystalloid therapy

Crystalloid therapy (5% dextrose, normal saline and dextrose saline) during hypovolaemic states is necessary due to sodium leaks into the surrounding cells. There needs to be a balanced use of a salt solution, to restore extracellular fluid volume. Haemodilution occurs when the blood becomes so dilute that the measured blood haematocrit is

> ⚠ The sole use of crystalloids to avoid blood transfusions in low circulating states can lead to haemodilution.

reduced to 17–21% (normal range 38–46%). Haemodilution decreases colloid osmotic pressure, reduces haemoglobin content and coagulation factors as there is less of these elements in relation to fluid contained within blood. This increase in fluid in relation to solutes in the blood will serve to dilute body sodium, increase blood osmolarity and, via the osmoreceptors, stimulate the release of ADH. Consequently, more sodium and water will be reabsorbed from the renal tubules, causing a net increase in extracellular fluid volume and total body weight.

In hypovolaemic states, it seems necessary to administer a combination of blood, colloids and crystalloids. Blood to maintain clotting factors, haemoglobin levels and to prevent haemodilution, colloids to maintain the overall circulating volume, and crystalloids to maintain fluid and electrolyte balance and prevent the movement of water and sodium into the cells.

> It is imperative that the patient's cardiopulmonary dynamics be monitored in a way that is reliable to determine physiologic trends and responses to whichever therapy is finally chosen.

Blood transfusion therapy

The human cardiovascular system is designed to minimize the effects of blood loss but the body can only compensate for a finite loss. Losses of 15–30% cause pallor and weakness while a loss of more than 30% of blood volume results in severe shock and can be fatal. To treat haemorrhage whole blood is generally used as routine, especially when blood loss is substantial.

Packed red cells (whole blood from which most of the plasma has been removed) is generally only used to treat anaemia. Fresh frozen plasma (FFP) is used for patients with bleeding disorders, whereby there is a deficiency in platelets or clotting factors, e.g. in disseminated intravascular coagulation (DIC), warfarin overdose, trauma or thrombotic thrombocytopenia. Blood transfusions can cause serious reactions, some of which arise from the changes that occur in stored blood (Table 3.2).

Autotransfusion

To minimize the need for blood transfusion by blood donor, during or following procedures, blood can be salvaged through an autotransfusion device. This blood can either be reinfused back into the patient during surgery if blood loss is great or saved for transfusion at a later date.

Synthetic blood products

Recently artificial blood substitutes, or perfluorochemicals, have become available and are often used in cases of severe anaemia when transfusion of blood products is not an option. Oxygen is dissolved in the perfluorochemical microdroplets (which have a high solubility of oxygen) and transported to

Table 3.2 Changes that occur in stored blood

Changes that occur	Causes	End result
Acid–base changes	Stored blood is in an air-free container and aerobic metabolism cannot take place but anaerobic metabolism does.	This gives rise to lactic acid production. The longer the unit of blood is stored, the greater amount of acid it will contain.
	The citrate phosphate dextrose (CPD) solution added to blood reduces the pH from a normal pH of 7.4 to about 7.0.	These two processes accumulate metabolic acids and the unit of blood pH decreases to about 6.6–6.8 after 14–21 days of storage.
Alterations in electrolyte concentration	When blood is stored the sodium and potassium undergo alteration. It can be expected that a unit of blood will contain approximately 75 mmol of sodium and 5–7 mmol of potassium.	Patients with normal cardiac and renal functions are able to handle the increase in sodium and potassium. In patients with profound trauma and shock with cardiac and renal dysfunction, the sodium and potassium content may have profound effects.
	There is also a progressive loss of red cell viability and the red blood cells tend to take up water.	This causes a leftward shift in the oxyhaemoglobin dissociation curve and thus transfused blood cells are less capable of releasing oxygen to the tissues.
The microaggregate load in stored blood	During storage there is an increased aggregation of platelets and leucocytes. To prevent these from entering the blood, it is always filtered.	It is recommended that microfilters with pore sizes of 20–90 microns are used.
Depletion of clotting factors	Stored blood is deficient in the factors necessary for coagulation, e.g. factors V, VIII, IX and platelets.	Clotting screens and bleeding status should be closely monitored, and platelets and FFP administered when required.
The temperature of stored blood	Blood is stored at a temperature between 1 and 6°C.	Large quantities of cold blood can cause a hypothermia. This compromises heart rate, blood pressure, cardiac output and coronary blood flow. Cold blood should be warmed prior to being transfused.

capillaries for diffusion across capillary walls.

These blood products do have side-effects, which include:

- pulmonary oedema
- arrhythmias
- chest pain
- respiratory distress
- the positive effects of perfluorochemicals do not endure beyond 24 hours after infusion due to their short half-life.

These synthetic blood products may in the future:

- reduce blood recipient adverse reactions from donor blood
- minimize the use of and improve the cost effectiveness of blood transfusions
- reduce the risk of spread of infections such as HIV/AIDS and hepatitis B.

Colloid versus crystalloid therapy

The use of colloid and crystalloid therapy to replace circulating volume is disputed. If crystalloids are to be used as the primary resuscitative agents in hypovolaemia, the volumes required to achieve normal haemodynamic values are 2–4 times those required with colloids. Massive crystalloid fluid resuscitation predisposes the patient to the adult respiratory distress syndrome (ARDS) or pulmonary oedema, which is alleged to be negligible with colloid therapy.

An overuse of crystalloids to avoid blood transfusions can lead to haemodilution (see p. 125).

Infusion devices

An infusion device is designed to deliver a measured amount of drug or fluid (either intravenously or subcutaneously) over a period of time with no adjustment to 'catch up'. It is set at an appropriate rate to achieve a desired therapeutic response and to avoid:

- over/underinfusion
- metabolic disturbances
- air embolism
- phlebitis
- toxic concentrations or below therapeutic doses of medications.

Gravity infusion devices

Gravity flow. These depend entirely on gravity to drive the infusion. They consist of an administration set containing a drip chamber and a roller clamp to control flow, which is usually measured by counting drops. They are useful for infusing fluids which do not need absolute precision. Flow rate is calculated using a formula, which requires the following information:

- the volume to be infused
- the number of hours the infusion is running over
- the drop rate of the administration set (20 drops/ml crystalloid administration set, 15 drops/min blood giving sets).

The rate can be calculated from the following equation.

$$\frac{\text{Volume to be infused}}{\text{Time in hour}} \times \frac{\text{Drop rate}}{60 \text{ minutes}}$$
$$= \text{Drops per minute}$$

Gravity controllers These operate by gravity and there is no pumping action.

- Drip rate controllers detect and count drops in the drip chamber and contain an automatic clamping mechanism to control the flow.
- Volumetric controllers calibrate millilitres per hour and the accuracy of the drip flow is dependent mainly on the size of the drop formed.

Infusion pumps

These pumps do not rely on gravity and an alarm will sound if the catheter becomes occluded or displaced. There are two types.

Volumetric pumps. Used when a large volume of infusion needs to be administered, e.g. during parenteral nutrition. They work by calculating the volume delivered. All are mains or battery powered, with the rate selected in ml per hour. The accuracy is usually within 5% when measured over a period of time. These pumps:

- are able to overcome resistance to flow by increased delivery pressure and do not rely on gravity
- are capable of accurate delivery over a wide range of flow rates
- incorporate a wide range of features, e.g. air-in-line detectors, alarms, etc.
- are usually expensive and some are complicated to use.

Syringe pumps. These are low-volume, high-accuracy devices designed to infuse at low flow rates.

The rate is controlled by the drive speed of the piston attached to the syringe driver. These devices are:

- useful where small volumes of highly concentrated drugs need to be infused
- limited to the size of the syringe, usually a 60 ml syringe, but most will accept different sizes and brands
- mains and/or battery powered
- easy to operate and tend to cost less than volumetric pumps.

Specialist pumps

Patient-controlled analgesia (PCA) pumps. These are syringe pumps but the distinguishing factor is that the pump can deliver doses on demand, when the patient pushes a button. Patient-controlled analgesia (PCA) pumps are usually categorized into three types.

1. *Basal* – a baseline rate is set but can be accompanied by intermittent doses requested by the patient.
2. *Continuous* – designed for the patient who needs maximum pain relief without the option of demand doses, e.g. epidural.
3. *Demand* – drug is delivered by intermittent infusion and can be used alone or supplemented by the basal rate.

This method of delivering analgesia increases patient satisfaction as less sedation is required, anxiety is reduced and so is nursing time and stay in hospital.

Ambulatory infusion devices. These are small devices which allow the patient more freedom to continue normal activity. These pumps are used for small volumes of a variety of drugs and fall into two categories.

- Mechanical infusion devices
  —Elastomeric balloons
  —Spring mechanism
  —Gas powered hydrogen or carbon dioxide
- Battery-operated infusion devices
  —Ambulatory volumetric infusion pump – works the same as the larger volumetric pumps but is smaller and portable
  —Syringe drivers – for subcutaneous medications

3.4 NUTRITIONAL SUPPORT

Recording and monitoring this area of nursing care can affect the patient's recovery and as such it is an essential part of the nurse's survival on the ward.

NUTRITION

Food contains nutrients, which are digested by enzymes, which are controlled and regulated by hormones. There are six principal classes of nutrients.

- Minerals
- Vitamins
- Carbohydrates
- Fats
- Proteins
- Water

The essential function of minerals and vitamins (*micronutrients*) is the regulation of physiological processes. The energy-yielding nutrients are carbohydrates, fats and protein or *macronutrients*. These provide primary and alternative sources of energy. Water is the overall vital nutrient sustaining all life processes. Nutrients produce and maintain the human body, build and rebuild tissue, provide energy and regulate metabolic processes.

Guidance on the adequacy of nutrition is required and standards have been devised against which measured intakes can be compared. These standards are known as Recommended Daily Amounts (RDA). In 1991 the Department of Health, in the COMA Report, updated the dietary reference values (DRVs). These are not intended to be used in evaluating the adequacy of an individual's daily diet, as we do not need to eat the DRV of every nutrient every day, but to establish the wide variety of foods that patients can eat as part of a healthy diet.

MALNUTRITION

The maintenance of health depends upon the consumption and absorption of appropriate amounts of energy and all the necessary macro- and micronutrients. Too little of some over a period of months may lead to malnutrition. Malnutrition is defined as a state which occurs when there is an imbalance between nutritional intake and nutritional requirements. When nutrition ceases during periods of fasting, there is a loss of energy stores and malnutrition will ensue.

The physiological effects of malnutrition

Carbohydrates are the first source of energy utilized by the body (*glycolysis*) and are needed to maintain a normal blood glucose level.

- During starvation carbohydrates are not available directly from the gut but the body can utilize carbohydrates stored as glycogen in the liver and skeletal muscles as a source of energy.
- During approximately the first day of fasting, low glucose levels stimulate glucagon secretion by the pancreas. As a result, glycogen is converted to glucose (*glycogenolysis*) and released from the liver. This restores blood glucose levels to normal. Glycogen can be lost without any physiological consequences.
- These mechanisms supply blood glucose but cannot maintain blood glucose levels for very long.
- Fat stores may be used for energy. This requires a major body adjustment, as all other body tissues must reduce their oxidation of glucose and switch over to fat as their energy source.
- As the liver metabolizes fat, ketone bodies are produced in large quantities. These are oxidized by the body into carbon dioxide, water and adenosine triphosphate (ATP). As a result of fat utilization as a source of energy, an individual can fast for several weeks, provided water is consumed.

If fasting continues, the brain, having become deprived of glycogen stores, has to gradually adapt to the use of ketone bodies as the major source of energy. When this occurs, depression of the central nervous system may ensure, leading to coma. Since other body cells are also limited in the amount of ketone bodies they can metabolize, excess ketone bodies appear in the blood, resulting in ketosis which, if food intake is not initiated, can lead to a metabolic acidosis.

When fat reserves are completely depleted, the body will break down large quantities of muscle protein as a source of energy, to maintain cellular functions. Large amounts of amino acids can be released and converted to glucose in the liver by *gluconeogenesis* or the amino acids may be oxidized directly. It is estimated that once protein stores are depleted to about one-half of their normal level, death results. During fasting, amino acids contribute to blood glucose only after liver glycogen and fat stores are depleted.

IMPROVING DIETARY INTAKE

The success of nutrition is largely dependent on the nurse's interest, knowledge and understanding. Improving dietary intake may prevent further invasive treatments, e.g. parenteral nutrition or nasal gastric feeding, to improve nutritional intake.

To improve dietary intake a thorough nutritional assessment needs to take place. Then an individual personal food plan must be decided, in partnership with the patient, to cover the following factors.

- It should fulfil basic nutritional needs, in increased amounts to meet additional metabolic demands.
- It should encompass 'comfort foods' or familiar ethnic dishes and well-liked foods.
- The patient's cultural and religious beliefs, likes and dislikes, appetite and motivation should be considered.
- Variety in food texture, colour and flavour.
- Build-up foods may be negotiated with the patient and added in between meals.
- Timing and frequency of food and drink.

A strict record of all food, offered and eaten, must be kept. Evaluation of the personal food plan must be implemented to determine whether there is a need for further changes or adjustments to the diet or knowledge base of the patient.

Nurses may have to discuss changing eating habits and attitudes to food due to surgery or illness. This may be very complex and difficult to accomplish due to issues such as culture, religion, socioeconomic status, age, physical disability or psychological problems. Nurses should try to discuss dietary matters with patients and how they may be able to maintain an adequate diet following discharge from hospital.

PARENTERAL NUTRITION (PN)

Parenteral Nutrition (PN) is 'the provision of all nutritional requirements via the intravenous route'. Instead of food being fed into and absorbed from the gastrointestinal tract, nutrients are infused directly into the venous circulation, thus bypassing the gut. PN contains essential nutrients in quantities to meet all the daily needs of patients. It is administered using an aseptic technique into a central line, which is situated usually in the subclavian or internal jugular vein.

PN is indicated for patients with:

- prolonged ileus
- uncontrolled vomiting
- chronic diarrhoea or malabsorptive states
- severe radiation enteritis
- short bowel syndrome
- gastrointestinal obstruction
- severe pancreatitis with fistula
- hypercatabolic states
- critical illnesses
- multiple trauma or burns
- hepatic or renal failure
- inflammatory bowel disease.

The type of patients selected for PN are as follows.

- Patients who are unable to eat or absorb orally for a period > 5 days.
- Patients who are malnourished and unable to eat or absorb food.
- Unconscious patients who may aspirate if fed orally.
- Patients who are hypercatabolic or have multisystem failure and are unable to maintain adequate nutritional intake.
- Bowel rest for patients with fistulae, pancreatitis or inflammatory bowel disease.

There are generally two routes of administration.

1. Central venous line, usually subclavian vein; this may lead to problems with infection.
2. Skin-tunnelled catheter for long-term nutrition or a peripherally inserted central catheter (PICC).

The PN solution contains the following.

- Amino acids – both essential and non-essential, 1–2 g/kg/day.
- Glucose – carbohydrate energy source, provides 3.75 kcal/g. Use 25–50% dextrose and increase the insulin to prevent liver complications.
- Fat emulsion – fat energy source, generates 9 kcal/g. Use 10–20% solution plus increased insulin to prevent liver complications.
- Electrolytes, e.g. sodium, potassium, magnesium, calcium and phosphorus.
- Vitamins, minerals and trace elements are required.

There are many choices of PN regime.

- Premixed
- Either prepared by hospital pharmacy or purchased
- A regime for a particular patient formulated to the patient's needs for energy and nutrition

Standardized PN regimes are available and depend on body weight. They are ordered daily as the patient's requirements change. They can last up to 7 days but must be kept in the fridge. Some require mixing prior to administration.

The nurse's role in delivery
- Administration sets need to be changed every 24 hours.
- Feeding line should never be used for the administration of additional medicines – PN is incompatible with numerous other medicines.
- Separate lumen should be used for other medicines, blood products or CVP readings.
- Volumetric infusion pumps should be used.
- Never attempt to 'catch up' if the infusion is running slowly.
- Incomplete bags should be discarded.

The nurse's role in management
- Aseptic conditions
  —Tubing
  —Dressings
  —Connections of feeding solution
- Site of the subclavian catheter observed for inflammation/infection
- No blood products should be infused through the line
- Monitoring of PN
  —TPR and BP
  —Body weight – increases
  —Fluid balance – positive balance
  —Urine testing – sugar and ketones
  —Blood testing – urea, nitrogen, creatinine, urea, glucose, sodium, potassium
- Mouth care due to nil-by-mouth state

Complications
These are many and should be detected by appropriate monitoring.

Central line complications
- Pneumothorax
- Arterial puncture
- Air embolism
- Sepsis
- Vein thrombosis
- Catheter blockage and accidental removal

Metabolic complications
- Fluid overload
- Hyperglycaemia
- Hypoglycaemia
- Translocation of bacteria/ sepsis
- A reduction in trace elements and vitamins
- Metabolic acidosis – chloride/CO_2
- Refeeding syndrome
- Electrolyte disturbances
  —Hyperammonaemia
  —Hyponatraemia
  —Hypernatraemia
  —Hypokalaemia
  —Hypocalcaemia
  —Hypophosphataemia
  —Hypomagnesaemia

Some of these may require a review of the PN solution, rate of administration, additional fluids, blood products and drugs. Parenteral nutrition should not be terminated until oral or enteral feeding is well established.

ENTERAL FEEDING (EF)

Enteral feeding (EF) includes any method of delivering nutrients for absorption by the gastrointestinal tract. This generally includes feeding via the nasogastric route, even though this type of feeding can be achieved through the nasoenteric route (i.e. placed in the duodenum or jejunum).

There is clear evidence that long periods of time without enteral nutrition can produce detrimental gastrointestinal responses and serious complications. It is advocated that the use of EF be initiated early, when oral diet is insufficient. Early EF immediately following any type of surgery is possible (i.e. within 6 hours of insult) and is only generally to be contraindicated in complete gut failure, which is apparently very rare.

Types of tubes

Nasogastric/nasoduodenal tubes are the most commonly used and are suitable for short-term use such as postoperatively or during radiotherapy. The wide-bore tube is used initially to allow easy assessment of gastric contents, e.g. aspiration of the nasal gastric tube 4 hourly to determine gastric content and pH. When feeding is commenced aspiration is continued until it is evident the patient is successfully absorbing. The narrow-bore tube should replace the wide-bore for long-term feeding needs and should be used whenever possible as it is more comfortable for the patient and less likely to interfere with swallowing or cause oesophageal irritation. It collapses when aspirated and is not suitable during the initial assessment stage, but has many benefits following effective assessment.

A *gastrostomy* tube may be more appropriate than a nasogastric tube when:

- long-term feeding is anticipated, as it avoids delays in feeding and discomfort associated with tube displacement and is cosmetically more acceptable
- there is upper gastrointestinal obstruction.

The tube of choice is the percutaneous endoscopically guided gastrostomy (PEG). These are made from polyurethane or silicone and are held in place with an inflatable balloon. The one disadvantage of this method is that it requires some form of sedation and radiological support to ensure that it is in place and may need an anaesthetic for insertion.

A *jejunostomy* tube is placed into the jejunum and is the preferable method if a patient has undergone upper gastrointestinal surgery or severe delayed gastric emptying.

Methods of administration
1. Bolus feeding – indicated in situations when the patient is restless or confused, as the tube may become displaced and the patient is at risk of pulmonary aspiration.
2. Intermittent continuous feeding – feeding needs to be interrupted to allow gastric emptying prior to positioning and intense physiotherapy due to the risk of pulmonary aspiration, reducing the nutrition that the patient receives. It is not suited for restless or confused patients.
3. Gravity drip – whereby it is just allowed to flow through over a given period of time.

4. Pump-assisted feeding – connected to a pump for the majority of the day. The pump can be set at various flow rates per hour from 1 ml to 300 ml.

The complications of EF
These complications can be easily recognized and prevented if the nurse understands and anticipates the potential problems:

- pulmonary aspiration
- nausea and vomiting
- diarrhoea
- blockage of tube
- trauma to the nose
- overfeeding.

It is important to ensure that patients are able to meet their nutritional requirements orally before terminating EF. It may be useful to maintain an overnight feed while the patient is establishing oral intake.

Overfeeding
Excess carbohydrate and lipid intake can cause hepatic steatosis and abnormal liver function. Lipid may also be deposited in the lung and impair diffusion of gases and produce infusional hyperlipidaemia. Overfeeding with excess carbohydrate can lead to excess carbon dioxide production, which can precipitate respiratory failure.

The energy requirements of disease have often been overestimated. The recommendation that more energy should be provided to counter the effects of pyrexia (13% of basal metabolic rate per degree Centigrade rise in temperature) is inappropriate. It is also recommended not to account doubly for the energy cost of breathing; for patients with acute respiratory distress, their resting energy expenditure may represent only 20–30%, rather than 50%, and a normal subject with no respiratory problems will only be 2–3%.

The energy requirements of patients who are unwell are usually similar to or less than those of healthy subjects, the reason being that the basal hypermetabolism often seen in inpatients is offset by the decrease in physical activity. The normal daily energy expenditure in adults is generally 1700–2500 kcal (30–35 kcal/kg) (1 kcal is 4.184 j). It is recommended that hypocaloric feeding be the current practice in hospital feeding regimes, especially in the early stages of injury (e.g. 1500 kcal/day for up to a week). This would reduce the risk of liver and lung complications and metabolic instability and their consequences.

An increase in calorie intake should take place in the recovery phase, when nutrition level is normal and the patient is no longer at risk. This regime, to reduce prescribed energy intake initially in patients with acute illnesses and/or malnutrition, should be followed irrespective of whether the patients are preoperative or postoperative, receiving parenteral or enteral nutrition or are in intensive care units.

A SYSTEMS APPROACH

4.1 The cardiovascular system 138

4.2 The respiratory system 159

4.3 The blood 172

4.4 The gastrointestinal system 189

4.5 The renal system 221

4.6 The nervous system 230

4.7 The endocrine system 249

4.8 Diseases of bones and joints 266

4.9 The immune system 283

4.10 Cancer 291

4.11 Surgery 305

In this section some common medical and surgical conditions that you will meet on the wards are considered. The care and management of the patient are looked at and in some cases a problem-solving approach has been used and the care planned in a little more detail following the activities of living. Using these examples as a guide, you will be able to plan the care for other patients using this section.

4.1 THE CARDIOVASCULAR SYSTEM

More than 40% of patients admitted to medical wards in the United Kingdom have some form of heart disease. This includes:

- hypertension
- angina
- myocardial infarction
- cardiac arrhythmias
- heart failure.

Hypertension, angina and myocardial infarction are all due to ischaemic heart disease (IHD), caused by an inadequate blood flow to the heart. IHD is due to a narrowing or blockage in the coronary circulation and accounts for 40–50% of all deaths in the developed world.

HYPERTENSION

Many of the clients that you nurse on medical wards will have a raised blood pressure and are likely to be on medication for this. A blood pressure of 140/85 or below is regarded as normal by the WHO.

Hypertension is the *most important risk factor* for diseases of the cardiovascular system, including stroke and coronary heart disease. Diseases of the cardiovascular system kill more people in Britain than all other causes of death combined and hypertension may be known as the 'silent killer'.

Patients have raised blood pressures and feel well. They may have no symptoms but the raised blood pressure may be slowly damaging their bodies. The patients that you nurse with cardiovascular disease may have had raised blood pressure for many years.

The control of hypertension can lead to the prevention of its cardiovascular complications.

Mild hypertension	140/85–160/100
Moderate hypertension	160/100–180/115
Severe hypertension	over 180/115

Only in 2–3% of patients can a definite cause be found for the raised blood pressure. This is called *secondary hypertension*.

Causes
- Phaeochromocytoma (tumour of the adrenal medulla)
- Conn's syndrome (hyperaldosteronism)
- Cushing's disease (overactivity of the adrenal cortex or due to administration of long-term steroids)
- Hyperthyroidism

- Hyperparathyroidism
- Renal hypertension.

For the vast majority of cases where there is no definite cause, the term *essential hypertension* is used.

Treatment

In mild hypertension lifestyle changes alone may be recommended at first and these may include weight loss, reduction in salt intake, safe exercise, stopping smoking and stress reduction.

Medication

The drugs used to treat hypertension include the following.

- *Diuretics*–bendrofluazide is the commonest and a small dose of 2.5 mg daily is usually prescribed.
- *Beta-blockers*–these are especially suitable where the patient also has angina but should not be given to patients with airway obstruction. The commonest drug used is atenolol which is a cardioselective beta-blocker.
- *Angiotensin-converting enzyme (ACE) inhibitors*–these drugs block the formation of angiotensin II from angiotensin I that is manufactured from renin, produced by the kidney. Examples of these drugs are captopril and enalapril. Captopril may cause a very sudden drop in blood pressure when first prescribed. The first dose should be given when the patient is in bed for the night and blood pressure may be monitored in some patients for the first 2 hours after administration.

- *Calcium antagonists*–nifedipine and diltiazem are examples. These drugs cause vasodilatation and are also useful in clients with angina. Side-effects include headache and flushing.

Clients admitted with a very raised blood pressure will usually have this controlled slowly rather than giving drugs to act quickly by the intravenous route. The aim is to reduce the diastolic blood pressure to <110 mmHg over approximately 24 hours.

LOW BLOOD PRESSURE

Often a fall in blood pressure is more significant than the absolute value and monitoring of blood pressure is an activity that as a nurse you will be performing daily.

A low blood pressure (hypotension) will:

- lead to reduced tissue perfusion throughout the body
- reduce the blood supply to the heart
- reduce renal blood flow and thus reduce urine output
- reduce blood flow to the brain and eventually lead to unconsciousness.

Causes of hypotension

- Depletion in blood volume
  —Blood loss as a result of trauma, a leaking aneurysm, bleeding from the gastrointestinal tract or postoperatively.
  —Dehydration from any cause such as diabetic ketoacidosis and diarrhoea or vomiting

—Loss of serous fluid from severe burns
- Pump failure
  —Myocardial infarction
  —Pulmonary embolism (if very large)
  —Depression of the myocardium due to acidosis or septicaemia
  —Drugs that depress the contractility of the heart, e.g. beta-blockers
- Large fall in peripheral resistance
  —Septicaemia
  —Peritonitis
  —Pancreatitis
  —Anaphylactic shock
  —Neurogenic shock

Management and care
- This will depend on the cause of the hypotension.
- Record observations of blood pressure, pulse and respirations as prescribed.
- When the blood pressure is low, the pulse rate will usually be increased (*tachycardia*).
- The respiratory rate may also be increased, as in acidosis or haemorrhage, but in severe instances the rate may be reduced and respirations may be shallow.
- Fluid replacement may be commenced by intravenous infusion and a plasma expander such as Gelofusin or Haemaccel may be given.
- If blood has been lost the doctor will group and crossmatch the patient and order a transfusion.
- The urine output has to be closely monitored as hypotension can lead to impaired renal function. It may be necessary to catheterize the patient if the urine output falls and it should remain above 30 ml per hour.
- Oxygen may be prescribed.
- The patient may be anxious and will need reassurance.
- Investigations such as an electrocardiogram, chest X-ray and blood cultures to identify infection may be ordered.

ANGINA PECTORIS

This is pain, usually in the chest, felt as a result of lack of blood supply (*ischaemia*) to the heart. There is a narrowing of the coronary vessels, usually due to deposits of atheroma but sometimes due to spasm.

Clinical features
- The pain is usually in the chest but may extend down the left arm or both arms or into the neck.
- Some patients may experience pain just in the arm, the neck or the back.
- It is usually described as a tightness or squeezing pain or discomfort.
- The pain is brought on by exertion.
- The pain fades fairly rapidly on rest.
- A glyceryl trinitrate (GTN) tablet sublingually usually gets rid of the pain.
- The pain will always occur after a similar amount of physical exertion.
- The distribution of the pain will be the same each time but in more severe attacks it may extend further.

• Sometimes the pain of angina is mild and the patient confuses it with heartburn or ignores it.

Unstable angina

• This is a more ominous symptom and may be a sign of an impending heart attack.
• The episodes of pain are more frequent.
• They may occur without obvious cause and at rest.
• The patient is usually admitted to hospital.
• Sometimes it is difficult for the doctor to differentiate between unstable angina and a myocardial infarction.

Management of stable angina

This patient is likely to be treated in the community. General advice will aim to restore normal exercise capacity and will include:

• cessation of smoking
• weight loss if necessary
• treatment of hypertension if present
• treatment of raised cholesterol levels if necessary
• low saturated fat intake
• low salt intake.

Drugs, including nitrates, may be needed to treat the angina. These may be given in several forms and relieve the pain of angina by causing vasodilatation. All nitrates may produce a troublesome headache. GTN may be given as a tablet sublingually or as an aerosol spray. The spray has a longer storage life. Its onset of action is very rapid, 1–2 minutes, and its duration of action is under 10 minutes.

GTN may also be given in the form of a sustained-release transdermal patch and the GTN is absorbed through the skin over the whole period of time the patch is in situ. In 24 hours there should always be a 'patch–free' period or tolerance to the drug may result. Some patches now have a nitrate-free period built into them.

Isosorbide mononitrate and isosorbide dinitrate are both longer acting nitrates that are given two or three times daily.

Beta-blockers

Contraindicated in asthma, beta blockers reduce the heart's demand for oxygen and also reduce pulse rate and blood pressure.

An example of a beta-blocker is propranolol. A cardioselective beta-blocker is atenolol. This drug blocks the beta–1 receptors in the heart in preference to the beta–2 receptors found in other parts of the body, e.g. the bronchi.

Calcium antagonists

These vasodilate and may be used in angina or hypertension. An example is nifedipine.

Surgical treatment of angina

Coronary artery bypass grafting

The narrowed coronary artery that is causing the angina is replaced by a graft taken from the saphenous vein in the leg although the internal mammary artery may also be used. The mortality is 2–3%. Symptoms are alleviated in 80–90% of cases and improved in a further 5–10%.

Coronary angioplasty

A procedure in which a segment of narrowed artery is stretched by a balloon that has been introduced by cardiac catheterization.

Angioplasty is suitable only for some narrowed segments of the coronary arteries and may be used in the arteries of the leg also.

MYOCARDIAL INFARCTION

This is a heart attack or coronary thrombosis. A blood clot (thrombus) occurs in one of the coronary arteries supplying the heart muscle with oxygen. The lack of blood supply leads to death of the area supplied by that artery. The word 'infarct' means death.

About 100 000 people die in Britain each year from heart attacks and approximately half of these die in the first hour following infarction. Death is usually due to cardiac arrhythmias and in hospital the patient will usually be nursed in a coronary care unit where staff are experienced and equipment is available. Any arrhythmia can be treated immediately and DC countershock administered if needed.

Clinical features

- Chest pain which is tight or crushing in nature; 80% of patients have this.
- The pain may be similar to that of angina, but more severe.
- The pain lasts longer than angina – usually more than 20 minutes.
- Pain may radiate to the arms, throat and jaw.
- The pain is not relieved by sublingual GTN.
- Nausea and vomiting may occur.
- Sweating.
- Pallor.
- Hypotension.
- Tachycardia.
- Anxiety.

> ⚠️ The elderly or diabetic patient may sometimes have a 'silent' MI where no chest pain is experienced

Always ask patients about the type of pain they have – their vocabulary may help to confirm the diagnosis.

Management and nursing care

The patient is likely to be very frightened so the nurse will need to offer reassurance, using a calm and confident manner.

On admission to the coronary care unit (CCU):

- the patient will be connected to a cardiac monitor for detection of cardiac arrhythmias
- analgesia will be given as needed to try and keep the client pain free. This is likely to be IV diamorphine 2.5–5 mg and an antiemetic such as prochlorperazine (Stemetil)
- an intravenous cannula will be inserted to allow drugs to be given easily and immediately
- the patient will be made comfortable using the headrest and pillows
- oxygen may be prescribed and given if circulation is inadequate

- observations of blood pressure and pulse will be monitored half hourly at first
- a 12-lead ECG will be done. In the early stages of an MI the ECG may be normal
- blood will be sent to the laboratory so that cardiac enzyme levels may be assessed
- a 'clotbuster' such as streptokinase will be commenced as soon as possible unless there are any contraindications.

Cardiac enzymes

These are enzymes released by the damaged myocardium. They rise following an MI and this may confirm the diagnosis. The degree to which they rise may also aid assessment of the severity of the infarct (see Table 2.4).

- *Creatine kinase* peaks within 24 hours of MI and falls back to baseline by 48 hours.
- *Aspartate aminotransferase* peaks at 24–48 hours and falls to baseline by 72 hours.
- *Lactate dehydrogenase* peaks at 3–4 days and remains raised for 10–14 days. It is useful when the patient has not been diagnosed immediately as having had an MI.

Streptokinase and rt-PA (alteplase)

- These are the fibrinolytic (thrombolytic) drugs that are most frequently used to break down a blood clot.
- Given by infusion as soon as possible in the first 12 hours following a heart attack.
- Any delay will lessen the effectiveness of the treatment.

Contraindications for their use include recent haemorrhage, trauma or surgery, history of cerebrovascular disease, severe hypertension, history of peptic ulceration and pregnancy. Therapy with streptokinase from 5 days to 12 months previously means the drug cannot be used and an alternative may be sought. This is due to the presence of antibodies in the circulation.

> ⚠ It is important to observe for any signs of bleeding when the patient is on thrombolytics

Aspirin

Aspirin 75–150 mg daily has been shown to reduce mortality following an MI and also to work in an additive manner with streptokinase in the prevention of a second MI. Aspirin reduces platelet 'stickiness'.

Heparin

Heparin is an anticoagulant that works rapidly but has a short duration. It is used in the treatment of pulmonary embolism and deep venous thrombosis but may also be used in MI and unstable angina.

It may be given as a continuous intravenous infusion or by subcutaneous injection. The patient receiving heparin will need laboratory monitoring, usually by determination of the activated partial thromboplastin time (APTT). You will also see heparin being used on surgical wards to prevent the occurrence of DVT and pulmonary embolism in high-risk patients.

Low molecular weight heparins (LMWHs) are used more frequently now and they are given once daily by subcutaneous injection. Examples include dalteparin (Fragmin) and tinzaparin (Innohep).

Cardiac arrhythmias

Cardiac arrhythmia is the commonest and most lethal complication of an MI. The most dangerous irregularity is ventricular fibrillation (VF) which constitutes a cardiac arrest. This is shown in Figure 4.1. Immediate treatment of VF using defibrillation (DC shock) may be lifesaving and paramedics as well as qualified staff in CCUs are trained to defibrillate.

Drugs used to treat cardiac arrhythmias include the following.

- *Lidocaine* (*lignocaine*) – used in ventricular arrhythmias, including ventricular tachycardia.
- *Digoxin*–used in atrial fibrillation.
- *Amiodarone*–used in atrial fibrillation and other supraventricular arrhythmias but also ventricular arrhythmias. Amiodarone must always be given by a central line when given intravenously.
- *Adenosine*–short-acting drug useful in supraventricular tachycardia but often used as an aid to the diagnosis of broad or narrow complex supraventricular tachycardias.
- *Verapamil*–a calcium antagonist that may be used in supraventricular tachycardias. It must not be given to a patient who is being treated with a beta-blocker as both drugs reduce the force of cardiac contractions.

> There are many different cardiac arrhythmias which may follow an MI. When you work in CCU, collect the rhythm strips from several patients, label them correctly and point out their identifying features. Note the treatment of the arrhythmia.

Acute MI is commonly associated with fatal dysrhythmias and the

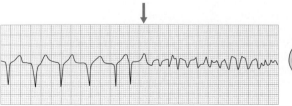

Fig. 4.1 Ventricular fibrillation. From Hampton/The ECG Made Easy, reproduced with permission.

detection and treatment of these was the primary reason for the creation of CCUs. Dysrhythmias may occur because of abnormal impulse formation, abnormal conduction or ectopic activity.

Following an MI patients invariably show overactivity of the autonomic nervous system. Parasympathetic overactivity is common after an inferior or posterior MI. Sympathetic overactivity (tachycardia and transient hypertension) may be present in nearly half of all patients (especially with anterior MI) and lowers the threshold for ventricular fibrillation.

Different cardiac arrhythmias and their causes are shown in Table 4.1.

Consequences of cardiac dysrhythmias
- Impairment of circulation or myocardial oxygenation has consequences.
- They are extremely variable but are more pronounced in the presence of cardiac disease.
- The healthy heart can withstand many abnormal rhythms.
- The diseased heart cannot and sustained tachycardias may lead to circulatory collapse or ischaemic pain.

Management of acute dysrhythmias Aim:
- to restore normal sinus rhythm
- to prevent recurrence of the dysrhythmia.

Establishment of sinus rhythm is not always possible (e.g. in atrial fibrillation) and treatment is then

Table 4.1 Causes of different cardiac arrhythmias

Abnormal impulse formation and ectopic beats	Conduction disturbances
At the sinus node Sinus arrhythmia Sinus bradycardia Sinus tachycardia Sinus arrest	**In the sinus node** SA block
In the atria Atrial ectopic beats Atrial tachycardia Atrial fibrillation Atrial flutter Wandering atrial pacemaker	**In the AV node** First, second and third degree AV block
In the AV node Nodal ectopic beats Junctional rhythm Junctional tachycardia	**In the bundle of His** Left bundle branch block Right bundle branch block Left anterior and posterior hemiblocks
In the ventricles Ventricular ectopic beats Idioventricular rhythm Ventricular tachycardia Ventricular fibrillation	**Others** Intra-atrial block Ventricular pre-excitation Atrioventricular dissociation

designed to slow the ventricular rate and improve cardiac output.

Sinus bradycardia
- Sinus rhythm slower than 60 beats per minute during the day or 50 beats per minute in the night.
- Bradycardia occurs in about 30% of patients following MI.
- Normally indicates parasympathetic overactivity, with release of acetylcholine from autonomic fibres in the atria and AV node.
- Afferent vagal fibres are more common on the inferior surface of the heart and inferior MI is complicated more by this. Slowing of the heart is useful and protective in that it limits myocardial work but may result in hypotension secondary to a reduced output. Coronary perfusion may also be reduced.
- Usually symptomless but sudden onset of bradycardia may result in hypotension with dizziness or syncope.

Causes include:
- hypothermia, hypothyroidism, raised intracranial pressure
- drug therapy with beta-blockers, digitalis or other antiarrhythmics
- acute ischaemia and infarction
- chronic degenerative causes.
- fit young persons

Junctional bradycardia
- If the sinus node fails to initiate an impulse and there are no other focuses in the atria, the AV junction takes over the pacemaker function.

- Most commonly occurs after acute MI, particularly if the patient is hypoxic or acidotic.
- Relatively slow (40–60 beats per minute) but sometimes may speed up and junctional tachycardia (>100) may occur.

Ventricular standstill and asystole
- Occurs when impulses fail to reach the ventricles or impulse formation ceases.
- If the problem is in the conduction system, atrial P waves may continue to occur.
- There will be no ventricular activity unless a ventricular pacemaker takes over.
- The ventricles are left without electrical stimulation and ventricular standstill occurs.
- No cardiac output and cardiac arrest results.
- More often, no electrical activity (either atrial or ventricular) is seen and the term *asystole* is used.

This form of arrest has a poor prognosis and has several causes:

- metabolic acidosis
- electrolyte imbalance
- hypoxia and drugs
- acute MI.

About 25% of arrests in hospital and 10% out of hospital are of this type. Mortality exceeds 90%.

Tachycardias
- An increase in rate is the normal response of the heart to increased work. This occurs so that cardiac output will increase.

- However, abnormal tachycardias are frequently associated with a diminished cardiac output.
- Increase in heart rate is at the expense of diastole and the heart has less time to fill.
- If ventricular filling is reduced, cardiac output will be reduced.
- Coronary blood flow takes place in diastole and therefore ischaemia may result.
- Symptoms provoked by tachycardia may include angina, dyspnoea, palpitations or syncope.
- Most tachycardias are produced by reentry or enhanced automaticity.
- Narrow complex tachycardias include junctional tachycardias (SVTs), atrial flutter and atrial fibrillation.
- Each may present as sustained or paroxysmal tachycardia.

Atrial flutter
- Rate 220–350/min (usually about 300).
- ECG shows flutter waves which have a saw-tooth appearance in the inferior leads.
- There may be some AV blockade resulting in a ventricular rate of about 150 (i.e. 2:1 block).
- Atrial flutter is always unstable and should be converted to sinus rhythm.

Atrial fibrillation
- One of the commonest cardiac arrhythmias.
- Affects 2% of those over 60.
- Complicates 10–15% of MIs and is associated with a poor prognosis.

- Normal atrial contraction is replaced by a series of irregular fibrillation waves (350–600/min) caused by multiple and changing micro reentry circuits.
- Myocardial contraction is ineffective for atrial emptying and the atria remain functionally in diastole.
- Reduces cardiac output by 10–20%.
- Although AF makes the heart less efficient, the most important consequence is thrombo-embolism, especially stroke.

Sinus tachycardia
- Sinus rhythm greater than 100 and commonly between 100 and 150.
- P waves are normal and have a 1:1 relationship with the QRS.
- Found in one-third of patients with MI – an attempt to maintain cardiac output when there is reduced stroke volume.
- May be worsened by fear, pain or anxiety.
- Adequate analgesia will often settle this post MI.
- Mortality for those with MI is higher in sinus tachycardia than for those with sinus bradycardia.

Atrial ectopic beats
- Common in health and disease.
- Seen as premature P waves on ECG.
- Very common after an MI. May indicate sympathetic overactivity, hypoxia or anxiety.
- Usually asymptomatic and cause no haemodynamic upset.

Ventricular dysrhythmias

- These include ventricular ectopics, ventricular tachycardia, ventricular flutter and ventricular fibrillation.
- Myocardial ischaemia predisposes to ventricular dysrhythmias as normal electrical conduction pathways may be disturbed.
- Myocardial irritability following an MI is the commonest cause of ventricular arrhythmias.
- Necrotic myocardial tissue is a focus for this ectopic activity.
- Predisposing factors following an MI include potassium imbalances or drugs.

Ventricular ectopics

- These are premature ventricular complexes which can occur at any time in diastole.
- The QRS complex is premature and widened. Danger is progression to VT.
- Drugs, such as lidocaine (lignocaine), used to reduce ectopics post MI have not been shown to reduce mortality.
- Amiodarone may be the exception to this (CASCADE 1993).
- Beta-blockers post MI seem to reduce serious dysrhythmias as well as limiting infarct size.

Ventricular tachycardia (VT)

This is a life-threatening reentry dysrhythmia. QRS complexes are wide and regular at a rate of 100–220 beats per minute. The atria continue to beat and dissociated P waves may be seen. The atrial rate is usually slower as it arises from the SA node.

There are four types of VT.

- The commonest is *monomorphic VT* and the complexes are of uniform appearance (monomorphic). Each episode of VT continues for a variable time and usually terminates in a long pause before sinus rhythm returns.
- *Polymorphic VT (torsades de pointes)* is a dangerous dysrhythmia. The QRS undulates around the isoelectric line, with a marked change in amplitude every 5–30 beats. Episodes may be precipitated by drugs that prolong the QT interval or by electrolyte imbalances. Usually terminates spontaneously but may lead to VF.
- *Ventricular flutter* is characterized by a rapid ventricular rate of about 180–250 beats. The ECG has been likened to a row of hairpins. It often precedes VF.
- *Accelerated idioventricular tachycardia* is an escape rhythm which is slow, usually about 60 and not exceeding 120. After about 30 beats, sinus rhythm usually returns but may occasionally be replaced by sustained VT or VF.

Ventricular fibrillation (VF)

- Electrically and mechanically, the heart is completely disorganized and cardiac arrest ensues.
- The ECG shows fine and coarse waves of irregular size, shape and rhythm.
- Fine VF may mimic asystole and produce an apparently flat line on the ECG.
- About 90% of deaths following acute MI are due to VF. Nearly half occur in the first half hour.

- Primary VF is that which occurs in the first 12 hours after MI. Usually associated with a good prognosis as the heart is usually still functioning well.
- Reperfusional VF may occur following thrombolysis, but this probably reflects a good prognosis as the infarct related artery has been reopened.
- Secondary or late VF occurs when function has been severely compromised by the infarct and prognosis is poor.

CARDIAC FAILURE

Heart failure occurs when the heart is no longer acting as an efficient pump and thus cannot respond to the demands made upon it.

The heart is really two pumps in series – the right side of the heart and the left side – and either side may fail independently. There may, however, be a failure of both sides together or left heart failure may lead to right.

The term *congestive cardiac failure* is usually taken to mean combined right and left heart failure but may be used to mean just right-sided heart failure. Due to this confusion, this term is best avoided although you will certainly still meet it on the wards.

Left heart failure

Commonly known as left ventricular failure (LVF), thus results from damage to, or overload of, the left ventricle. This could be due to an increased load on the left side of the heart or reduced muscular power. Causes include:

- hypertension
- mitral and aortic valve disease
- cardiac arrhythmias
- overtransfusion
- myocardial infarction.

Figure 4.2 shows that if the left ventricle is not pumping adequately there will be a build-up of blood in the left side of the heart. This will cause a backlog in the left atrium and then the pulmonary veins and also in the blood vessels within the lungs themselves. The raised pressure in the vessels will cause fluid to leave the blood vessels and enter the lung tissue, causing *pulmonary oedema*.

Symptoms depend on the severity of the failure but it is commonplace in an accident unit for patients to come in as an emergency with severe dyspnoea due to LVF. This most commonly occurs during the night and in the early hours of the morning when the patient has been lying in bed.

The patient on the ward can also suddenly develop a worsening LVF and need rapid treatment.

Clinical features of severe pulmonary oedema (acute LVF)
- Severe breathlessness
- Moist, wheezy breathing
- Anxiety – feeling of suffocation
- Tachycardia
- Cold, clammy skin
- White, frothy sputum – may be pink in terminal stages

Care and management
- Aid the patient to sit up in bed and thus allow maximum lung expansion.

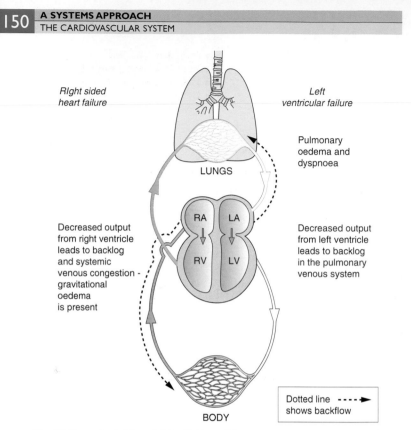

Right sided heart failure

Left ventricular failure

LUNGS

Pulmonary oedema and dyspnoea

RA   LA

RV   LV

Decreased output from right ventricle leads to backlog and systemic venous congestion - gravitational oedema is present

Decreased output from left ventricle leads to backlog in the pulmonary venous system

Dotted line - - - - ▶ shows backflow

BODY

Fig. 4.2 Congestion in left- and right-sided heart failure.

- Reassure him that this terrible suffocating feeling will be relieved.
- Administer oxygen as prescribed – this is likely to be a high concentration.
- A portable chest X-ray may be performed.
- Urgent diuretics are needed to relieve the pulmonary oedema. It is likely that the doctor will administer furosemide (frusemide) intravenously. This will start to work rapidly and in about 30 minutes or less the

patient should start to feel better.

⚠ Do warn the patient that he will need to pass urine more than once and that this is just what we want him to do. If he is not aware of this he will worry about his constant need to urinate

- A small dose of diamorphine (2.5 mg) is often administered intravenously. This relieves the panic and anxiety but also helps to reduce the strain on the heart.

- Occasionally you may see venesection performed on these patients; 500 ml of blood is removed rapidly to reduce the strain on the heart. This is done if other treatment is failing.

In a milder and more chronic form LVF will cause shortness of breath on exertion and perhaps some breathlessness in the night with a cough that occurs on lying down. The patient will be treated with oral diuretics such as furosemide, which is likely to be given as frumil. This is furosemide combined with amiloride. The latter is potassium sparing and so prevents excess potassium loss from the furosemide.

Right heart failure

Failure of the right side of the heart is usually secondary to lung disease. It may also occur following a large pulmonary embolus or in those with right-sided valvular disease.

You will nurse many clients with right-sided heart failure because of the high incidence of chronic respiratory problems in Britain.

Clinical features

- When the right ventricle cannot pump adequately the backlog of blood occurs in the right atrium and then the vena cavae. This causes the venous system to become congested.
- Due to the raised pressure in the veins, fluid leaves the capillaries

and enters the tissues, giving rise to gravitational oedema.

- The earliest sign of right-sided heart failure is pitting oedema. This will occur in the feet and legs of those who are ambulant and in the sacrum if the patient is in bed and may spread to the groin.
- The fall in cardiac output results in salt and water retention by the kidneys, which causes a raised blood volume and more oedema.
- Ascites (fluid accumulated in the peritoneal cavity) may occur.
- Pleural effusion (fluid in the pleural space) may add to the breathlessness.
- All the abdominal organs are engorged with blood and in the liver this may cause abdominal pain.
- Loss of appetite.
- Lethargy and fatigue.

Management and care

Breathlessness. The patient will usually be more comfortable sat upright in bed or in a chair. Some clients prefer to even sleep sitting in a chair.

Oxygen should be administered if it has been prescribed. This is usually at a low concentration because the patient is likely to have chronic lung disease.

Oedema

- An accurate record of fluid intake and output is kept.
- To assess the oedema, daily weighing may be done.
- Diuretics will be prescribed – examples are Frumil or, if the oedema is not so severe, bendrofluazide.

- Reduced salt intake will help to prevent further accumulation of fluid in the tissues.
- Fluid restriction may become necessary if diuretics fail.

Fatigue. The patient will feel tired as the heart cannot respond to any increased demands made upon it. Rest is important to reduce the strain on the heart and also to promote a diuresis as this allows more cardiac output to flow to the kidneys.

> ⚠️ This client is very susceptible to deep venous thrombosis whilst resting and active leg movements must be encouraged.

Abdominal discomfort

- Venous congestion can cause problems throughout the gastrointestinal tract.
- Loss of appetite and constipation are common.
- Straining to go to the toilet should be avoided and so a laxative may be ordered.
- Congestion of the liver may lead to slight jaundice.

Skin care. Poor circulation, oedema and rest in bed all increase the risk of pressure sores developing.

Orientation. If circulation is very poor, cerebral hypoxia may occur and the patient may become confused and disorientated. Conscious level may deteriorate.

Administration of medication.
Diuretics are essential to help to reduce the oedema. On long-term diuretic therapy it is necessary to supplement potassium intake and the patient could be advised to eat fresh fruit or drink fruit juice to help this process. (This advice no longer holds if the patient is prescribed ACE inhibitors – see below.) Diuretics such as furosenide are now often given combined with a potassium-sparing diuretic such as amiloride. The two come in one tablet, e.g. Frumil.

Digoxin may be prescribed to increase the force of the cardiac contractions. It is especially useful if the patient has atrial fibrillation as well as heart failure.

The toxic level of digoxin in the blood is close to the therapeutic level and the nurse should be aware of the signs of digoxin toxicity. These include:

- slow pulse rate – below 60 beats per minute (bpm)
- anorexia
- nausea and vomiting
- diarrhoea
- blurred vision
- arrhythmias.

> ⚠️ The pulse rate is checked before digoxin is administered and the dose is usually omitted if the pulse rate is below 60 bpm.

ACE inhibitors such as captopril are now commonly prescribed in heart failure.

They help to take the strain off the heart by causing vasodilatation and also have a slight diuretic action. They do cause some retention of potassium and when they are prescribed any potassium-sparing diuretic will be omitted from the drug regime.

> ⚠ A reduced potassium level leads to increased cardiotoxicity of digoxin.

Anticoagulants, e.g. heparin may be ordered for some clients if the risk of thromboembolism is assessed as severe.

Principles of nursing management using activities of living
Communicating. The patient needs constant reassurance, clear explanations regarding care and a calm atmosphere.

Breathing. The patient may be very breathless and should be sat up in bed or in a chair, well supported with pillows and given a bedtable to rest his arms upon. Oxygen may be given if prescribed.

Maintaining a safe environment. Hypoxia may lead to confusion. The nurse needs to be with the patient should this occur.

Eating and drinking. There may be reduced appetite and small attractive meals should be offered. Dietary advice should be followed.

Eliminating. Urine output must be measured accurately because of the diuretic therapy and the oedema. Constipation may be present and a laxative may be needed.

Personal cleansing and dressing. The patient may have a dry mouth and ice cubes may be appreciated. Mouth care may also be needed.

Mobilizing. Initially the patient will need to rest but beware of the risk of

DVT and the need for passive or active leg movements.

Sleeping. The breathlessness may appear worse at night. Ensure the patient is comfortable and he may need to sleep in a chair. Sedation should be avoided if possible. An open window may help if the ward is rather airless.

Right-sided heart failure or congestive cardiac failure is a chronic condition and the patient will need to be on medication for the rest of his life. He will need a varying degree of support to live in the community.

STROKE

A stroke (cerebrovascular accident – CVA) is an acute event, in which a neurological deficit appears over a few minutes or hours, sometimes in a step-wise fashion, persists for more than 24 hours and is presumed to be due to impairment of the blood supply to one part of the brain.

The interruption of blood flow to the brain may be due to an embolus or thrombus (80% of cases) or a haemorrhage into the brain (20% of cases) from a weakened intracranial arterial wall. Motor and sensory loss or disturbance will ensue. Recovery is variable but in many cases can be complete.

Stroke is the third most common cause of death in Britain.

Transient ischaemic attack (TIA)

An episode of acute neurological deficit, of presumed vascular origin, which resolves completely in 24 hours. The patient may present with the features of a stroke but these resolve over this short period. There may be a small infarction and this will show up on a CT scan.

Predisposing factors
- Incidence increases with age.
- Higher in men at all ages (male : female = 1.5:1).
- Hypertension is the major predisposing factor.
- Atheroma of part of the cerebral circulation, causing narrowing of the blood vessels.
- Disease of the heart valves and atrial fibrillation may instigate the formation of emboli in the heart which may then break off and travel to the brain.
- Other factors include diabetes mellitus, smoking and hyperlipidaemia.

Management of stroke is often difficult and may have disappointing results. Primary prevention is cheaper and more effective. Health education and lifestyle changes are the way forward.

Control of hypertension is also essential. It has been estimated (O'Brien et al 1995) that if the blood pressure of the whole population of Britain was reduced by 5 mmHg, the community risk of stroke could be reduced by 30%.

Clinical features of stroke
- Depend on the position and extent of ischaemia or haemorrhage.
- Abrupt onset.
- Vary enormously in severity and symptoms and signs.
- Slow worsening over hours, or a stepwise deterioration over days, may occur (evolving stroke).

- Loss of consciousness may occur.
- Headache, dizziness.
- Fitting.
- Vomiting.
- Motor disorders (hemiplegia or hemiparesis).
- Aphasia (difficulty in speech) – may be partial or complete loss of the ability to communicate. If the stroke affects the dominant hemisphere of the brain where the speech centre is located (left side in right-handed people), aphasia is likely to occur.
- Sensory disorders – visual impairment, loss of sensation (hemianaesthesia).
- Consciousness may deteriorate as cerebral oedema increases.
- Affected muscles are flaccid at first (the limbs on the affected side feel floppy; if the arm is lifted and released, it falls back onto the bed). After about 48 hours, the muscles become spastic – rigid and difficult to move.

> ⚠ A stroke affecting the right side of the body has originated in the left side of the brain and vice versa.

Initial management
Refer to Section 2.2 on assessment of the unconscious patient.

Maintaining a safe environment
- Swiftly assess and record the patient's level of consciousness (see p. 31) and respirations (see p. 45). Position in bed accordingly, insert airway if necessary and have suction fitted and working nearby.

- Record pulse, blood pressure and respirations. The blood pressure may be high in the initial stages of the stroke.
- Note any irregularity of the pulse.
- An ECG and chest X-ray may be ordered.
- A CT scan may be done to differentiate between a blood clot or a bleed.

Breathing
- Carefully monitor the respiratory rate and observe for any cyanosis.
- Respirations may be slow and stertorous.
- Chest physiotherapy may be needed.

Communicating
- Provide continuous reassurance to the patient, even if he appears unconscious.
- Provide accurate information for relatives.

Eating and drinking
- The patient must not be given anything by mouth until the swallowing reflex has been assessed and is present.
- If the patient cannot drink, a nasogastric tube may be passed or an intravenous infusion commenced.

Eliminating
- A catheter may be inserted if the patient is unconscious.
- This will prevent retention or incontinence and allow the urine output to be measured accurately.

Personal cleansing and dressing
- Carry out frequent mouth care, especially if the patient is breathing through his mouth, receiving oxygen or not drinking.
- Keep the skin clean and dry.

Mobilizing
- If immobile, the patient will need to be turned frequently (at least every 2 hours) and carefully to prevent pressure sores developing.
- Carry out gentle passive exercises to flaccid limbs, under the guidance of a physiotherapist.
- Correctly position the limbs after turning the patient.

Dying
- Provide continual reassurance.
- Ensure that accurate information is provided to the relatives, without disguising the serious nature of the illness.

Continuing care and rehabilitation
In the convalescent and rehabilitative phase the goals are to prevent complications, to aid maximum independence and to provide support for the family.

Maintaining a safe environment
- Keep the surrounding floor area free from obstructions.
- Ensure the patient wears shoes rather than slippers for walking practice.
- Keep the bed at a suitable height for the patient.

Communication

- Continually encourage both the patient and the relatives.
- Repeat information as necessary to ensure understanding.
- The patient may not be able to respond and the nurse will need to liaise with the speech therapist and use picture boards or the alphabet where appropriate.
- Observe for emotional lability (weeping outbursts are common with stroke patients).

Breathing

- Ensure the patient is positioned carefully in the bed or chair to permit maximum lung expansion.
- Encourage breathing exercises as taught by the physiotherapist.
- Observe for signs of a chest infection.

Eating and drinking

- Avoid foods that could cause choking (e.g. crumbs).
- Remember that food may lodge in the mouth on the paralysed side.
- Help to make mealtimes interesting and a time to look forward to.

Eliminating

- Help the patient to achieve continence without the aid of a catheter.
- Avoid constipation by providing high-fibre foods if appropriate and the use of a gentle laxative if necessary.

Personal cleansing and dressing

- Frequent mouth care and washes, watching again for any food debris in the mouth.
- Assist with washing and dressing as necessary.
- Do not leave the patient unattended in the bath.
- Use appropriate lifts and hoists.
- Try out adaptations to clothing, e.g. Velcro instead of buttons.
- Seek the advice of the occupational therapist regarding dressing and suitable clothes and aids.
- Appreciate that progress may be by very small steps and give the patient praise for any advances he makes in self-care.

Mobilizing

- With the physiotherapist, make achievable short-term goals for the patient to work towards.
- Carry out exercises in the physiotherapist's absence, using aids and equipment provided and as taught by her.
- Maintain the limbs in a straight position when the patient is at rest.

Working and playing

- A positive attitude demonstrated by all caring professionals will encourage the patient to believe that progress can be made.
- If the patient cannot communicate do ask the relatives if he usually likes to listen to the radio and do provide such distractions some of the time.
- Occupational therapy workshops may be available to practise therapeutic activities.
- The social worker may be able to give advice concerning possible employment changes.

Sleeping
- Keep the limbs carefully positioned at night.
- Observe for an increase in depression or anxiety at night.
- Provide company when possible if the patient is awake.

Dying
- Stroke carries a mortality of about 20% within the first month.
- Forty percent of patients make a full recovery.
- Provide accurate information, in a sensitive manner, to both the patient and his relatives, to enable them to plan for the future.
- Listen to the worries of both the patient and his relatives and to any anger and bitterness they may feel.
- Arrange a visit from the hospital chaplain where this is appropriate.

PERIPHERAL VASCULAR DISEASE

This usually presents as a chronic ischaemia of the legs due to atheromatous disease involving the aorta, iliac or femoral arteries. It is more common in men over 50 years who are smokers.

Clinical features
- Ischaemia – a cramp-like pain in the calves during exercise and relieved by rest (intermittent claudication).
- Rest pain.
- The limb will be cold to the touch, lack hair and the skin will be dry.

- Non-healing ulcers or gangrene may occur.
- Absent pulses in severely diseased areas.

Both limbs are usually affected but one may be worse than the other.

Investigations
- X-rays may show calcification.
- Doppler ultrasound may help to define the severity.
- Arteriogram using contrast media to show the narrowing.

Care and management
- Reduce risk factors such as smoking, treat hypertension and diabetes if present, lose weight if obese.
- Keep limbs warm but do not apply heat.
- Avoid infection and trauma to the feet.
- Regular exercise – encourages new vessel formation.
- Low-dose aspirin.
- Bypass surgery may be considered.

Acute ischaemia of the legs
- May be due to an embolism.
- Extremely painful, pale, pulseless limb.
- Treatment is removal of the clot.
- If gangrene develops, amputation may be necessary.

AORTIC ANEURYSMS

An aneurysm is a bulge in the vessel wall usually due to atheroma. It is a weak point and the danger is that it will leak or rupture. It may be asymptomatic and found as a pulsatile mass on examination or as calcification on an X-ray. An ultrasound will show how large the aneurysm is and if a leak has occurred.

Rupture causes intense pain in the back and the patient is shocked due to blood loss. A dissecting (splitting) aortic aneurysm usually starts in the ascending aorta and pain is severe and central, often radiating to the back. It may feel similar to a myocardial infarction.

Emergency surgery may be necessary.

DEEP VEIN THROMBOSIS (DVT)

- Venous thrombosis often occurs in normal vessels.
- Important causes are stasis and hypercoagulability.
- The majority occur in the deep veins of the leg.
- A thrombus forms in the vein and inflammation of the vein wall follows.
- Can occur in any vein in the leg but most often in the calf.
- Often undetected and at autopsy is present in over 60% of hospitalized patients.

Risk factors

- Trauma or surgery, especially of the pelvis, hip or lower limb.
- Immobility – increased in bedrest of over 4 days' duration.
- Varicose veins.
- Obesity.
- Previous DVT.

- Pregnancy.
- High doses of oestrogens (slight increased risk with oral contraception).
- Polycythaemia, sickle cell anaemia, thrombocytopenia, nephrotic syndrome, cardiac failure, recent myocardial infarction and malignancy are all conditions that increase the risk of a DVT.

Clinical features

- May be asymptomatic and the features of a pulmonary embolism may be the first sign.
- Pain in the calf – may be swelling, redness and engorged superficial veins.
- Affected calf may be warmer.
- Ankle oedema may be present.

Medical management

- Diagnosis is by ultrasound or Doppler ultrasound.
- Venography will detect practically any thrombosis but is not usually necessary.
- Main aim of treatment is to prevent pulmonary embolism.
- All patients with thrombi above the knee should be anticoagulated as these are the ones that usually cause a pulmonary embolism.
- Anticoagulation of below-knee thrombi is controversial.
- Bedrest is advised until fully anticoagulated and then mobilization with an elastic stocking.
- Heparin is usually given for 48 hours.
- Warfarin may be given for 4 weeks to 3 months.

- The international normalized ratio (INR) should be at 2.0–3.0.
- Anticoagulants do not affect the thrombus that is already present.

Prevention

- Subcutaneous low-dose heparin is given to those at specific risk, e.g. surgery to the leg or pelvis or immobility and cardiac failure.
- Early mobilization after surgery as most cases occur in the first 72 hours postoperatively.
- Leg exercises should be encouraged.
- Patient should not sit on a chair with his legs immobilized on a stool.
- Elastic support stocking for those at risk.

4.2 THE RESPIRATORY SYSTEM

There are some clinical features that are common to many disorders of the respiratory tract. These include:

- cough
- dyspnoea – a subjective sensation of shortage of breath
- orthopnoea – breathlessness when lying flat
- wheeze
- sputum
- haemoptysis – coughing up blood.

ASTHMA

Asthma is a common and chronic inflammatory condition of the airways. As a result of the inflammation the airways are hyper-reactive and narrow easily in response to a wide range of stimuli. While initially reversible the inflammation may lead to an irreversible obstruction of airflow. The bronchoconstriction that occurs is an abnormal narrowing of the airways caused by bronchospasm, mucosal oedema and increased secretion of sticky mucus. Alveoli can become blocked with plugs of mucous. Expiration becomes an active rather than a passive process. Precipitating factors may include exercise, house dust mites, pollens and spores, pets, smoke, chemicals, certain foods, drugs (especially beta-blockers and non-steroidal anti-inflammatories) and emotional factors.

Extrinsic asthma

- Commonly develops during childhood.
- Identifiable factors provoke wheezing.
- Often associated with other features of atopy such as hay fever and eczema.
- Sometimes nocturnal cough may be the only symptom.

Intrinsic asthma

- Begins in adult life.
- Airflow obstruction is more persistent
- Most exacerbations have no obvious stimuli other than a respiratory tract infection.

In an asthma attack there is:

- dyspnoea
- cough
- wheezing
- sense of tightness in the chest.

It may be precipitated by exposure to one or more of a wide range of allergens.

> ⚠️ **Asthma can produce symptoms of all grades** varying from very mild to life-threatening. Its danger should never be underestimated and several hundred people die each year from asthma.

Recording airflow obstruction
- Mini peak flow meters are a cheap and reliable way of doing this.
- They are used in hospital and patients will use them at home to assess the control of asthma and the response to treatment.
- Peak flow recordings in a diary allow patients to see a deterioration in airflow although they may be asymptomatic.
- Peak flow recordings are taken in hospital before salbutamol is administered and repeated about 20 minutes after administration to assess improvement. An increase of 15% is considered to be significant.
- In hospital when the patient is very breathless it may not always be appropriate to immediately measure the peak flow rate.

Medication in asthma
The British Thoracic Society (BTS) published revised guidelines in 1999 now known as the British Guidelines on Asthma Management (Box 4.1). These recommend a stepwise treatment but do emphasize that treatment can begin at any step on the ladder. If that step does not control the asthma, the treatment moves up to the next step. The aim is to totally control symptoms and reduce medication to a level that will maintain this control.

The patient's inhaler technique should always be checked, as should his compliance.

Aerosols
The duration of action of an aerosol inhaler depends on the dose administered and the drug it contains. Rimeterol usually lasts 1–2 hours, salbutamol 3–5 hours and salmeterol around 12 hours.

Short-acting bronchodilators are used to treat an attack, long-acting are taken regularly to prevent an attack.

Steroid inhalers are widely used to prevent attacks of asthma and decrease the inflammatory process within the lungs. Oral candida is a common complication and the risk may be minimized by using mouthwashes after administration and using a spacer.

Advantages of aerosols
- Provide more rapid relief.
- Administered directly to the bronchioles, therefore smaller doses required.
- Fewer side-effects.

The dose needs to be stated explicitly – the number of inhalations at one time, the frequency and the maximum number of inhalations allowed in 24 hours.

Box 4.1   British Thoracic Society Guidelines on Asthma Management

Step 1
Salbutamol inhaler on demand.
If needed more than once a day, move onto step 2.

Step 2
Inhaled short-acting steroid such as beclometasone or budesonide 100–400 μg twice daily or fluticasone 50–200 μg twice daily.
Cromoglycate may be used as an alternative to steroids.

Step 3
Higher dose inhaled steroids or a long-acting beta-agonist twice daily are added. Theophylline may be added to step 2 medication or cromoglycate may be tried.

Step 4
Inhaled short-acting bronchodilator plus regular high-dose inhaled steroids via a large-volume spacer.
In addition one or more of the following may be tried: long-acting beta-agonist, e.g. salmeterol, sustained-release theophylline, inhaled ipratropium (Atrovent), high-dose inhaled bronchodilators or cromoglycate.

Step 5
Regular prednisilone tablets in a single daily dose are added to the other medication.

If the patient is using his aerosol excessively this is usually due to undertreatment of his asthma. *Nebulized salbutamol* is used frequently in the treatment of acute asthma both in hospital and in general practice.

Acute severe asthma
- The patient may be very anxious and a calm atmosphere is essential.
- Speed of onset varies – some attacks come on over minutes, in some deterioration occurs slowly over days.
- Breathlessness – may lead to inability to hold a conversation.
- Wheezing.
- The respiratory rate is raised >30/min.

- Cyanosis.
- Tachycardia >110/min.
- Peak flow <33% normal.

Management and nursing care
- A calm and reassuring atmosphere will help the patient.
- Sit the patient up.
- Administer oxygen as prescribed.
- Administer salbutamol nebulizer.
- Ipratropium bromide (Atrovent) nebulizer may also be used.
- Aminophylline may be prescribed intravenously in a continuous infusion of dextrose 5%.
- Hydrocortisone intravenously or oral prednisilone may be given.
- Antibiotics in case of infection – may be intravenously administered.
- Chest X-ray may be ordered.

- Blood pressure measurement – if hypotensive, this is a sign of deteriorating condition.
- Pulse and respiratory measurements – bradycardia is a very severe sign. Usually there is a rapid pulse rate.
- Pulse oximetry measurement (see p. 72).
- If oximetry is poor blood gases may be measured (see p. 67).
- Occasionally artificial ventilation is needed, dependent on the blood gas analysis and if the patient is exhausted.

CHRONIC OBSTRUCTIVE AIRWAYS DISEASE (COAD)

Although this term is still widely used, chronic airflow limitation (CAL) is regarded as more accurate. Chronic obstructive pulmonary disease (COPD) is also used.

In Britain the most common causes of COAD are chronic bronchitis and emphysema, which often occur together. They are linked closely to cigarette smoking and patients are usually diagnosed as having both chronic bronchitis and emphysema.

> *Chronic bronchitis* **is said to be present when there is a *productive cough* for most days of 3 consecutive months for more than 1 year. The disorder is characterized by excessive mucus production.**
>
> *Emphysema* **is characterized by *permanent enlargement of the air sacs* within the lung tissue. There is destruction of pulmonary tissue and a loss of elastic recoil.**

The breathlessness is caused by the limitation of expiratory airflow that causes the residual volume to be increased. The thorax is overinflated and inspiratory capacity is now impaired.

Predisposing factors
- The dominant cause of this condition is cigarette smoking.
- Atmospheric pollution and occupational dust exposure are minor factors in Britain.

Clinical features
- Chronic bronchitis and emphysema develop over many years and patients are rarely symptomatic before middle age.
- Minor symptoms at first – morning cough and a little sputum.
- Breathlessness initially occurs on exertion but gradually increases so that eventually dyspnoea will occur even at rest.
- If bronchitis predominates, periodic chest infections often occur.
- Cyanosis may be present – 'blue bloater'.
- If emphysema predominates there is extreme breathlessness but the patient is often not cyanosed–'pink puffer'.
- Respiratory wheeze.
- Use of accessory muscles of respiration.
- 'Pursed lips' during expiration (makes breathing out easier).
- Often dyspnoea at night, causing wakefulness and leading to exhaustion.

- Extreme anxiety during very breathless periods.

Correction of hypoxaemia to achieve an arterial oxygen tension of at least 7.3–8.0 kPa is the immediate priority of management in acute exacerbations of COPD.

Often low-flow oxygen administered by nasal prongs (1–2 litres/minute) or Venturi-type facial masks (28%) is sufficient.

Administration of oxygen and arterial blood gases is carefully monitored over time as in a few patients arterial PCO_2 may increase and acute respiratory acidosis may occur. It is not understood why this happens. It used to be believed that in many sufferers of COAD, the respiratory centre became relatively insensitive to increased carbon dioxide levels and relied upon a decreased oxygen level in the blood to drive respirations. Evidence now suggests that drive to breathe does not decrease with oxygen administration.

> ⚠ It is essential to always check the percentage of oxygen prescribed for these patients and never exceed it.

Management and nursing care
- Reduce mucosal irritants and encourage the patient to stop smoking.
- If very breathless, complete rest may be needed.
- Provide oxygen as prescribed, usually at 24–28%.
- Ensure the patient is sat up in bed, well supported with pillows and his arms resting on a bedtable to allow maximum lung expansion.
- Administer the prescribed bronchodilators via nebulizer.
- Obtain sputum specimen for culture and sensitivity.
- Administer antibiotics if prescribed.
- Refer for chest physiotherapy to loosen and help to expectorate sputum.
- Observe the patient for increased breathlessness and cyanosis or any changes in mental state.
- Provide reassurance as needed when breathlessness is extreme.
- Carry out the prescribed pulmonary function tests – this may include measurements taken with a peak flow meter.
- Steam inhalations may be tried to loosen secretions. Cough mixtures are of little benefit.

> ⚠ Try and demonstrate empathy with this very frightened, breathless patient. Stay with him and offer reassurance during his worst periods.

Drug therapy
Restoration of normal function is not possible. The aim of therapy is to reduce the disability.

Bronchodilators
- Selective beta-2 agonists such as salbutamol and terbutaline are the most useful. They are best given by inhalation and a nebulizer may be used.
- Atropine analogues such as ipratropium bromide (Atrovent)

may be helpful, given by nebulizer.

- Long-acting preparations such as theophylline may be prescribed.

Corticosteroids

- A trial of corticosteroids may be indicated. There may be a reversible element to the disease and airway function may improve.
- Prednisilone 30 mg daily for 2 weeks may be prescribed and lung function will be assessed before the course is commenced and after the treatment period.
- If there is improvement (at least 15% increase in FEV_1) the oral steroids will be tailed off and a steroid inhaler may be prescribed.

Antibiotics

- Antibiotics given promptly in an acute attack may shorten the exacerbation.
- Patients may be given a supply of antibiotics to keep at home and to take when their sputum turns green.
- Some bacteria are resistant to ampicillin and a cephalosporin such as ceflaclor may be used more.

Diuretics

If oedema is present (lung disease may cause right-sided heart failure), diuretics may be prescribed.

Advice for healthy living

- Stop smoking.
- Influenza vaccine each autumn.
- Keep warm and dry during the winter months.

- Advice on the effective use of an inhaler.
- Antibiotics available for an exacerbation.

BRONCHIECTASIS

> ⚠️ Bronchiectasis is a dilatation of the bronchi, which may be localized in one tree or generalized.

The dilatation leads to impaired clearance of bronchial secretions and these become infected.

Causes

Most cases arise in childhood but the incidence has decreased as pneumonia has been treated more successfully with antibiotics.

- Inflammatory due to pneumonia or whooping cough.
- Obstruction of an airway due to inhalation of a foreign body or enlarged lymph nodes.
- Cystic fibrosis.

Clinical features

- Cough.
- Sputum production – the sputum may be copious and thick, green and foul smelling.
- Wheeze and breathlessness.
- Haemoptysis.

Management and nursing care

- Physiotherapy and postural drainage are very important. These must be done on a daily basis and the patient or family is taught to do this at home.

- Antibiotics when there is an acute exacerbation.
- Bronchodilators if necessary.
- Family support.

RESPIRATORY FAILURE

Respiratory failure occurs when pulmonary gas exchange is sufficiently impaired to cause hypoxaemia (reduction of oxygen in arterial blood) with or without hypercarbia. The PaO_2 is <8 kPa or the $PaCO_2$ is >7 kPa. It can be divided into Type I and Type II.

These patients are usually nursed on an intensive care ward.

Causes of respiratory failure are shown in Table 4.2.

PNEUMONIA

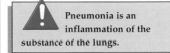

Pneumonia is an inflammation of the substance of the lungs.

It is usually due to bacteria but may also result from chemical causes, aspiration of vomit, radiotherapy or an allergic mechanism.
Pneumonia is an acute illness characterized by:

Table 4.2 Classification of causes of respiratory failure		
Mechanism	Acute causes	Chronic causes
Reduced ventilation Restrictive Neuromuscular diseases (failure of respiratory muscles)	Tetanus, botulism, poliomyelitis, polyneuritis, spinal cord injury	Muscular dystrophy Myasthenia gravis
Chest wall diseases (failure of chest expansion)	Pneumothorax Flail chest (trauma)	Kyphoscoliosis Obesity Pleural effusion Mesothelioma Ankylosing spondylitis
Lung diseases	Radiation pneumonitis	Interstitial fibrosis Sarcoidosis
Obstructive	Foreign bodies Epiglottitis Angio-oedema Bronchiolitis Asthma	Chronic obstructive pulmonary disease Bronchiectasis
Abnormal perfusion	Pulmonary embolism Fat embolism	Recurrent emboli Vasculitis
Impaired diffusion Interstitial disease	Shock Interstitial pneumonitis	Sarcoidosis Pneumoconiosis Interstitial pneumonitis Interstitial fibrosis
Pulmonary oedema	Acute left ventricular failure Toxic gases Mitral stenosis	Chronic left ventricular failure

- a cough – may be dry at first
- purulent sputum – haemoptysis sometimes
- fever
- raised respiratory rate
- pleuritic pain
- confusion may occur in the elderly and may be the only sign.

There will be changes on the chest X-ray to show consolidation of the lung.

> ⚠️ Pneumonia may be localized and affect one lobe – *lobar pneumonia*.
> It may be diffuse and affect the lobules of the lung and the bronchioles – this is *bronchopneumonia*.

Some bacteria causing pneumonia:

- *Streptococcus pneumoniae*
- *Mycoplasma pneumoniae*
- *Haemophilus influenzae*
- *Staphylococcus aureus*
- *Legionella pneumophilia*
- *Myobacterium tuberculosis*

There are viral, fungal and protozoal pneumonias as well.

Aspiration pneumonia

- Aspiration of gastric contents into the lungs can cause severe illness, which may be fatal. Gastric acid in the stomach contents is very destructive.
- Aspiration material enters the right lung more readily than the left due to the wider right bronchus.
- Infection is usually with an anaerobic organism derived from the upper respiratory tract.

Factors predisposing to aspiration pneumonia include:

- altered consciousness – drug overdose, anaesthesia, epilepsy, cerebrovascular accident, alcoholism
- dysphagia and oesophageal disease – stricture, fistula, hiatus hernia, reflux
- Neurological disorders – myasthenia gravis, motor neuron disease
- nasogastric tubes
- terminal illness.

Pneumonia in the immunocompromised patient

- With the use of immunosuppressive drugs and the emergence of HIV infection, these types of pneumonia have become much more common.
- These are the so-called 'opportunistic' infections.
- These may be rapid pneumonias that are extensive and life threatening.
- They may be viral, fungal, protozoal or bacterial in origin.
- *Pneumocystis carinii* is the most common opportunistic infection.

Management and nursing care in pneumonia

- Mild cases will not be admitted to hospital.
- Rest in bed.
- The patient in hospital should be made comfortable, sitting up in bed.
- Sputum should always be sent for culture.
- Chest X-ray will be performed.
- A white blood cell count may be done.

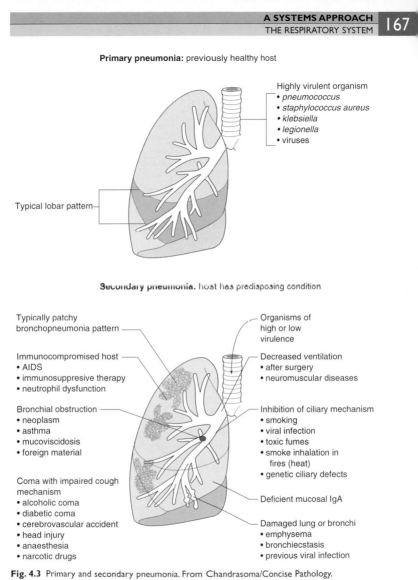

Primary pneumonia: previously healthy host

Highly virulent organism
• *pneumococcus*
• *staphylococcus aureus*
• *klebsiella*
• *legionella*
• viruses

Typical lobar pattern

Secondary pneumonia: host has predisposing condition

Typically patchy
bronchopneumonia pattern

Immunocompromised host
• AIDS
• immunosuppresive therapy
• neutrophil dysfunction

Bronchial obstruction
• neoplasm
• asthma
• mucoviscidosis
• foreign material

Coma with impaired cough
mechanism
• alcoholic coma
• diabetic coma
• cerebrovascular accident
• head injury
• anaesthesia
• narcotic drugs

Organisms of
high or low
virulence

Decreased ventilation
• after surgery
• neuromuscular diseases

Inhibition of ciliary mechanism
• smoking
• viral infection
• toxic fumes
• smoke inhalation in
  fires (heat)
• genetic ciliary defects

Deficient mucosal IgA

Damaged lung or bronchi
• emphysema
• bronchiecstasis
• previous viral infection

Fig. 4.3 Primary and secondary pneumonia. From Chandrasoma/Concise Pathology.

● Antibiotics will be prescribed –
these will depend on the type of
pneumonia. Cefuroxime and
erythromycin are examples.

● Fluids should be encouraged to
avoid dehydration – in the very
ill, intravenous fluids may be
necessary.

- Physiotherapy may be needed to help expectoration.
- Pleuritic pain may need analgesia.
- Oxygen may be prescribed in severe hypoxia.
- Temperature and respirations will be monitored.

LUNG ABSCESS

A cavity occurs and fills with pus.

Causes
- May follow a severe pneumonia.
- More likely to occur with TB, *Staphylococcus aureus*, *Klebsiella*, aspiration pneumonia or septic emboli.

Clinical features
- Pneumonia that is persistent or worsening.
- Foul-smelling sputum in large amounts.

Patient management
- Antibiotics may be given intravenously.
- Sometimes surgery is necessary.

PULMONARY TUBERCULOSIS

- An infection due to *Myobacterium tuberculosis*.
- The primary infection is usually symptomless, most commonly involves the lungs and heals leaving dormant tubercle bacilli in about 20% of old calcified lesions.
- When the host's immune system is at an ebb the tubercle bacilli may be reactivated and spread to all organs of the body

including the lungs, the kidneys and bones.
- There is a high incidence in patients infected with HIV.
- Pulmonary tuberculosis is the commonest form of tuberculosis.
- There are approximately 7000 new cases each year in Britain at present (Kumar & Clark 1998).

Clinical features
- Gradual onset of symptoms over weeks or months.
- Tiredness, malaise, anorexia and weight loss.
- Fever.
- Cough.
- Sputum may be mucoid, purulent or bloodstained.
- May be a dull ache in the chest.
- There may be a pleural effusion (fluid in the pleural cavity).
- Chest X-ray will show shadows and perhaps fibrosis.

Care and management
Sputum is sent for culture of acid-fast bacilli (AFB). The growth in culture is slow. The nursing management depends on the severity of the illness.

> ⚠ The most important factor in the treatment of tuberculosis is compliance with a drug regime for 6 months.

Drug therapy
- Rifampicin and isoniazid are given daily as a combination tablet 30 minutes before breakfast for 6 months.

- For the first 2 months pyrazinamide is also given.
- Drug resistance after initial drug sensitivity tends to develop in those who do not comply with regimes.
- Multidrug resistance occurs particularly in patients with HIV and carries a high mortality. At least three drugs to which the organism is sensitive are used in these instances and therapy is continued for up to 2 years.

PULMONARY EMBOLISM (PE)

This is the obstruction of one of the pulmonary arteries by an embolism, which is usually in the form of a blood clot originating from a DVT in the leg. There is often a history of DVT or of tenderness in the calf.

Pulmonary embolism should be suspected in a patient who collapses suddenly 1–2 weeks after surgery.

> ⚠️ A large pulmonary embolus is a medical emergency and can result in death.

Clinical features

These depend on the size of the embolus but include:

- sharp, knife-like pain in the chest, usually well localized in a small embolus
- if the embolus is large the pain may be more central
- shortness of breath
- anxiety and distress
- haemoptysis

- hypotension
- tachycardia
- pallor or cyanosis – cyanosis suggests a large embolus
- collapse.
- Massive PE may present as a cardiac arrest or shock.

Care and management

Again, this will depend on the severity of the episode and may include the following.

- Reassurance of the patient.
- Monitoring of vital signs – blood pressure, pulse and respirations.
- Cardiac monitor.
- Continuous pulse oximetry.
- Administration of oxygen.
- Pain relief – opiates may be needed.
- Investigations – chest X-ray, ECG, arterial blood gases.
- Anticoagulation – usually with heparin. The doctor may give an intravenous bolus of 5000–10 000 units followed by an infusion of 1000–2000 units per hour regulated by monitoring the APTT, which will be kept about 2–3 times that of the control.
- Analgesia – non-steroidal antiinflammatory drugs may work well. Diamorphine may be given but there is sometimes a reluctance to give opiates in a large embolus as these may lower the blood pressure more.
- Warfarin is introduced as an oral anticoagulant in the first few days and an INR of 2–2.5 is aimed for.
- Thrombolytic therapy may be used in a large embolism.

CARCINOMA OF THE LUNG

This is the most common cause of cancer death in the UK and there has only been a minimal improvement in 5-year survival in the past 15 years.

The incidence in women is increasing and it is the second most common cancer (breast cancer being the most common) in women.

It is probably caused by smoking in 90% of cases (Barr et al 1997). The risk increases with the number of cigarettes smoked each day.

There are four main types of lung cancer:

- squamous cell (35% of cases)
- adenocarcinoma (21% of cases)
- large cell (19% of cases)
- small (oat) cell (25% of cases).

Clinical features
- May be unspecific
- Cough
- Haemoptysis
- Dyspnoea
- Chest pain (may be mild)
- Wheeze
- Malaise
- Weight loss
- Hoarseness
- Anaemia
- Clubbing of the fingers
- Enlarged supraclavicular lymph nodes
- Direct spread may involve the pleura and there may be a pleural effusion

Metastatic complications
- The growth frequently metastasizes to bone, giving severe pain and sometimes pathological fractures.
- The liver is frequently involved.
- Secondary deposits in the brain may lead to personality changes or epilepsy.
- May metastasize to the adrenal glands.

Investigations
- Diagnosis is usually by chest X-ray and 90% of tumours will show on presentation. At this point, the tumour has sometimes been present for many years and there have been no symptoms until recently. A CT scan is more sensitive but time consuming and expensive.
- A bronchoscopy and biopsy may be done.
- A specimen of sputum will be sent for cytology.
- Bone scan and abdominal ultrasound may be used to detect metastases.

Care and management
The prognosis in lung cancer is very poor. In small cell carcinoma it is 3 months survival from diagnosis if untreated and a year median survival with treatment. In others there is a 50% 2-year survival without spread and a 10% 2-year survival with spread.

- In the early stages surgery may benefit the patient and excision may be attempted. This can consist of removal of a lobe of a lung or a whole lung and may be followed by chemotherapy or radiotherapy.
- In small cell carcinoma combination chemotherapy prolongs survival.

- For most patients the aim is symptom relief.
- Radiotherapy is used for bronchial obstruction or haemoptysis and to relieve bone pain.
- Pleural effusion may need draining if it is troublesome.
- Palliative care is vitally important in these patients (see p. 107).
- Effective assessment and relief of pain are essential.
- Morphine will probably be used for pain relief, in slow-release tablet form or elixirs. A syringe pump may be used to administer continuous morphine.
- Morphine is constipating and laxatives should be prescribed.
- Oxygen may be given for attacks of breathlessness.
- Relief of other symptoms such as nausea or confusion.
- The patient and relatives will need much emotional support during this distressing time.

THE PLEURA

Dry pleurisy

- Pleurisy is inflammation of the pleura.
- In dry pleurisy there is no effusion.
- There is a sharp pain, worse on inspiration or coughing.
- Causes include pneumonia and carcinoma.

Pleural effusion

This is an excessive collection of fluid in the pleural space. The fluid may be serous fluid, blood, pus or lymph.

 A collection of blood in the pleural space is a *haemothorax*.

A collection of pus in the pleural space is an *empyema*.

Causes
- Heart failure
- Hypoproteinaemia
- Pneumonia
- Carcinoma bronchus
- Tuberculosis

Clinical features
- Dyspnoea which is variable dependent upon the size of the effusion.
- Dull chest pain.
- Symptoms due to the underlying cause, e.g. carcinoma of the lung.

The effusion will be seen on a chest X-ray as a water-dense shadow with a concave-upwards upper border.

If the effusion is causing dyspnoea it should be drained. The fluid is best removed slowly and an indwelling chest drain may be inserted.

PNEUMOTHORAX

A pneumothorax is an accumulation of air in the pleural space.

Causes

It may occur spontaneously, most often in young thin men. Other causes include:

- trauma
- asthma
- COAD
- Tuberculosis

- pneumonia
- lung carcinoma
- cystic fibrosis and any diffuse lung disease.

Clinical features
- May be no symptoms if small and in a young fit man.
- Dyspnoea dependent on the size of the pneumothorax. Varies from mild to very severe.
- Pleuritic pain, sometimes transient.
- The pain usually begins abruptly and the patient may have felt 'something snap' before the onset of the pain and the dyspnoea.

The pneumothorax will show on the chest X-ray as an area devoid of lung markings.

Management
- Analgesia
- Oxygen (care if COAD)
- A small pneumothorax will resolve without treatment and analgesia and rest may be the only prescribed care with a repeat chest X-ray next day.

- A larger pneumothorax may be aspirated or a sealed underwater chest drain inserted.

 Tension pneumothorax is an emergency.

A breach in the lung surface acts as a valve, admitting air into the pleural cavity when the patient breathes in but preventing its escape when he breathes out. Unless the air is rapidly removed, cardiopulmonary arrest will occur.

4.3 THE BLOOD

Blood consists of red cells, white cells, platelets and plasma. Plasma is the liquid component and contains clotting factors and proteins as well as carrying nutrients and waste products.

THE RED CELL
Anaemia
Anaemia is present when there is a decrease in the level of haemoglobin (Hb) in the blood below the

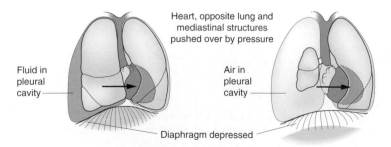

Heart, opposite lung and mediastinal structures pushed over by pressure

Fluid in pleural cavity

Air in pleural cavity

Diaphragm depressed

Fig. 4.4 Pressure collapse of the lung. From Govan/Pathology Illustrated, reproduced with permission.

reference range for the age and sex of the individual. Usually there is also a decrease in the red cell count (RCC) and packed cell volume (PCV). Normal values for the cells in blood are shown in Table 4.3.

Clinical features
- May have an insidious onset
- Lethargy
- Faintness
- Breathlessness
- Tachycardia
- Angina if atherosclerosis is present
- Pallor of skin and mucous membranes
- Cardiac failure may occur in the elderly or those with compromised cardiac function
- Confusion in the elderly

Classification of anaemias
Terms that refer to cell size end with 'cytic', whereas terms that describe the red cell colour end with 'chromic'. The classification of anaemias is shown in Table 4.4. In microcytic anaemia the red blood cell is smaller and paler than usual.

Iron deficiency anaemia
Iron is needed for the formation of the red oxygen-carrying pigment in the erythrocyte. It is present in the diet and is absorbed from the small intestine. Green vegetables, red meat, eggs and milk all contain iron.

Deficiency is commoner in premenopausal women as they have an additional loss of iron in the menstrual flow.

Causes
- Blood loss from menstruation
- Chronic blood loss, usually from gastrointestinal tract. May be the only clue in cancer of the colon
- Inadequate intake in the diet
- Increased demands in pregnancy or growth
- Decreased absorption with small bowel disease or following gastrectomy

Additional symptoms include brittle hair and nails due to decreased epithelial cell iron, a red smooth tongue (atrophic glossitis), spoon-shaped nails (koilonychia) and, rarely, pharyngeal webs at the back of the throat which cause difficulty in swallowing (dysphagia)

Treatment
- Treat the underlying cause.
- Oral iron, e.g. ferrous sulphate 200 mg three times daily for about 6 months.
- Side-effects include gastrointestinal disturbance –

Table 4.3 Normal values for adult peripheral blood		
	Men	Women
Hb (g/dl)	14–17	11–16
RCC ($\times 10^{12}$/l)	4.5–6.0	3.9–5.1
WCC ($\times 10^{9}$/l)	4.0–11.0	4.0–11.0
Platelets ($\times 10^{9}$/l)	150–400	150–400

Table 4.4 Classification of anaemia		
Microcytic	Macrocytic	Normocytic
Iron deficiency	Vitamin B_{12} deficiency	Aplastic anaemia
Anaemia of chronic disease	Folate deficiency	Haemolytic anaemia

usually constipation but may be diarrhoea. This can be reduced by changing to a different iron preparation, e.g. ferrous gluconate.

- Some patients may need iron injections if absorption is so poor.

Anaemia of chronic disease

This starts as a normochromic (erythrocytes are normal colour), normocytic (cells are normal size) anaemia and occurs in a variety of chronic diseases, e.g. rheumatoid arthritis, chronic infections, renal and liver failure, neoplasia (malignancies) and inflammatory disease, e.g. Crohn's disease. There is a slightly reduced survival of the red cell (normal survival about 120 days) and a low level of erythropoietin release (hormone produced by the kidney that stimulates the production of red cells). Iron stores tend to be normal or increased.

Treatment

- This type of anaemia only responds to treatment of the underlying disease and not to the administration of iron.
- Erythropoietin may improve some patients.

Macrocytic anaemia

Here the red cells are large and immature. They have defective DNA synthesis. The most common causes are deficiencies in either vitamin B_{12} or folate, both of which are needed to synthesize DNA.

Vitamin B_{12} deficiency

This vitamin is obtained from animal sources (meat, fish, eggs and milk). To

be absorbed in the gastrointestinal tract it has to bind to the intrinsic factor, which is secreted by the gastric parietal cells in the stomach.

Vitamin B_{12} is stored in the liver, where there is sufficient supply for 2 years or more.

Causes

- Low dietary intake – usually vegans
- Impaired absorption
- Intrinsic factor deficiency
- Pernicious anaemia
- Following gastrectomy
- Small bowel malabsorption:
  —ileal disease or resection
  —tropical sprue
  —coeliac disease
- Pancreatic disease
- Chronic pancreatitis

Pernicious anaemia

This is an autoimmune disorder in which there is atrophy of the gastric mucosa and a failure of intrinsic factor and gastric acid production that leads to a decreased absorption of B_{12}. It is the commonest cause of vitamin B_{12} deficiency in Western countries.

- Commoner in late adult life and the elderly.
- In Britain, women are affected more commonly than men.
- Commoner in those with blue eyes and fair hair.
- Associated with other autoimmune disorders, e.g. hypothyroidism.

Clinical features

- Onset insidious with increasing symptoms of anaemia.

- Usually quite severe by the time it is diagnosed.
- Lethargy, tiredness and weight loss.
- Pallor and sometimes slight jaundice due to the increased breakdown of the immature red cells.
- Glossitis may occur.
- Neurological features include subacute combined degeneration of the cord with peripheral neuropathy and symmetrical paraesthesia of the hands and feet. Ataxia may follow and eventually paraplegia. Higher cerebral function may be affected, leading to dementia.

Investigations
- Blood count and film.
- Measurement of serum vitamin B_{12}.
- Serum bilirubin may be raised.
- Parietal cell antibodies are present in 90% of cases.
- The Schilling test differentiates pernicious anaemia from malabsorption as the cause of vitamin B_{12} deficiency.

Treatment
- Intramuscular hydroxycobalamin (B_{12}).
- Injections are needed because the vitamin cannot be absorbed orally; 1 mg is given twice weekly for 3 weeks to replenish body stores and then 3 monthly for life.
- Treatment can reverse early neurological signs and stop the progress of later changes.

Folate deficiency
Folic acid is a B vitamin and its role is interdependent with B_{12} as both are needed by rapidly dividing cells. It is found in liver, yeast extract and green vegetables. There is an increased requirement in pregnancy and supplements should be given to prevent neural tube defects (e.g. spina bifida).

Causes
Decreased intake:
- elderly
- alcoholism
- milk-fed premature infants.

Malabsorption:
- coeliac disease
- tropical sprue
- gastrectomy
- Crohn's disease.

Drugs:
- phenytoin

Increased requirement in pregnancy, lactation, prematurity, growth in childhood.

Clinical features
Those of anaemia.

Treatment
- Underlying cause must be treated.
- Deficiency corrected by oral administration of folic acid 5 mg daily.
- If the cause of the macrocytic anaemia is not known, folate must not be given on its own as it may aggravate the neuropathy of B_{12} deficiency.

Aplastic anaemia
This is very rare and is due to suppression of the bone marrow leading to failure in production of

all blood cells. This means there is a shortage of white blood cells and platelets as well as erythrocytes. It may be inherited but is more commonly acquired.

Many drugs have been associated with aplastic anaemia. Some anticancer drugs cause this in a dose-related manner but with some drugs it may be an idiosyncratic reaction, e.g. chloramphenicol.

A blood count shows pancytopenia (low count of all blood cells).

Treatment
- Elimination of the cause if possible.
- Supportive care with transfusions and antibiotics.
- Bone marrow transplant may be possible in some patients – the young or those older with a very severe form of the disease.
- Immunosuppressive therapy may be used for older patients with a less severe form of the disease.

Haemolytic anaemia
- This is due to the rapid breakdown of red cells before the natural end of their normal lifespan.
- There is evidence of both increased red cell production (*reticulocytosis*) and increased red cell destruction.

Causes of haemolytic anaemia are shown in Box 4.2.

Clinical features of increased haemolysis
- Pallor
- Jaundice
- Splenomegaly (enlarged spleen)

Red cell membrane defects
- Most common in this country is hereditary spherocytosis. This is inherited in an autosomal dominant manner. Found in 1–2 per 10 000 of the population.
- There is a defect in the production of the protein spectrin which results in the production of

---

Box 4.2   Causes of haemolytic anaemia

Inherited	Acquired
Red cell membrane defect	*Immune*
Hereditary spherocytosis	Autoimmune haemolytic anaemia
Hereditary elliptocutosis	Haemolytic transfusion reactions
Haemoglobin abnormalities	*Non-immune*
Thalassaemia	Rare cases of nocturnal
Sickle cell disease	haemoglobinuria
	Mechanical haemolytic anaemia
Metabolic defects	*Miscellaneous*
Glucose-6-phosphate dehydrogenase	Infections (e.g. malaria)
deficiency	Drugs/chemicals
	Hypersplenism

spherical red cells, which are more rapidly destroyed.

- Most patients can live a normal life, although being slightly anaemic.
- An acute haemolytic crisis may occur at certain times (e.g. an acute infection) and require a blood transfusion.
- There is an increased need for folic acid as more red cells are being manufactured.
- Diagnosis is by the blood film.

Treatment
- The treatment of choice is a splenectomy. This is usually delayed until after childhood to minimize the risk of overwhelming pneumococcal infection.
- Following splenectomy, all patients should receive pneumococcal vaccine and long-term prophylactic penicillin.

Haemoglobin abnormalities
Normal adult haemoglobin is made up of two polypeptide globin chains (alpha and beta) and an iron-containing pigment (haem). The haemoglobinopathies are abnormalities of the polypeptide chains.

Thalassaemia
- These are a group of disorders arising from one or more gene defects and resulting in reduced production of one or more of the globin chains.
- This leads to precipitation of the globin chains in the red cells and ineffective erythropoiesis (red cell

manufacture) and haemolysis (red cell breakdown).
- There are two main types:
  —alpha – thalassaemia: reduced alpha-chain synthesis
  —beta – thalassaemia: reduced beta-chain synthesis.

In both types there are several clinical forms of the disease varying from asymptomatic and mild to severe with presentation in the first year of life. In the most severe form of thalassaemia there is complete absence of alpha-globin and infants may be stillborn (*hydrops fetalis*).

Thalassaemia trait (thalassaemia minor)
- The most common abnormality.
- Heterozygous form of the disease.
- Very mild defects of the red cells.
- Commoner in certain parts of the world and affects 20% of people from certain areas of Africa, Asia and the Mediterranean.
- No treatment is required but need to check for any anaemia.

Treatment of thalassaemias
- Detection of severe forms in the fetus means that termination can be offered. This would be tested for if the mother was found to have thalassaemia trait.
- Blood transfusion is the mainstay of treatment.
- Iron overload may result from repeated transfusions. This may lead to damage to endocrine glands, liver, pancreas and heart, with death in the second decade from cardiac failure.

- Treatment with desferrioxamine (an iron-chelating agent) may prevent iron loading.

Sickle cell syndromes
- This results from the production of an abnormal haemoglobin – haemoglobin S.
- It is a hereditary defect due to the substitution of the amino acid valine for glutamic acid in the beta-chain.
- It is found most commonly in those of African origin (25% carry the gene). It may confer a biological advantage against infection with malaria and so natural selection has increased the incidence of the HbS gene in this group.
- When deoxygenated, HbS molecules link together and this causes increased rigidity of the red cells and the characteristic sickle shape.
- The sickled cell has a shortened survival and is unable to pass through the very small capillaries (microcirculation). This may cause a chronic anaemia and chronic organ damage from vascular occlusion. Sickling may be precipitated by infection, dehydration, cold or hypoxia.

Clinical features
Sickle cell trait
- Those heterozygous for HbS (one gene HbS and one normal Hb gene) have sickle cell trait and are asymptomatic unless the oxygen tension is reduced (at high altitude, in an aircraft or under general anaesthesia).

- Still get renal microinfarcts due to obstruction of small capillaries and may complain of haematuria. May develop renal impairment.

Sickle cell disease
- Homozygous patients (both genes are HbS) suffer from chronic haemolysis but this is usually compensated. Hb usually between 5 and 10 g/dl.
- Usually mild jaundice.
- Acute haemolytic crises are precipitated by infections, pregnancy, drugs, surgery and anaesthesia.
- This may precipitate microvascular occlusion and tissue death.

Sickle cell crisis
- Associated with fever, malaise and severe pain.
- Can occur in most parts of the body.
- Organs affected include eyes, brain, bone, muscle, lung, spleen, liver, kidney and skin.
- May have pleuritic chest pain.
- Cerebral infarction leading to fits and hemiparesis.
- Priapism (prolonged erections).
- Carries a high mortality in young children and death is usually from renal failure or overwhelming infection.
- Management is aimed at prevention of infections and other situations leading to a crisis.

Treatment of an acute crisis
- Oxygen
- Rehydration
- Antibiotics

- Adequate pain relief – opiate analgesia often required
- Anaemia can be treated by blood transfusion

Metabolic defects
- Commonest is glucose-6-phosphate dehydrogenase deficiency (G6PD).
- G6PD is a vital enzyme to combat oxidative stress in the red cell.
- Deficiency is a heterozygous X-linked trait (carried on the female chromosome).
- Found predominantly in African, Mediterranean and Middle Eastern populations.
- Red cell breakdown occurs, precipitated by some oxidizing drugs (e.g. sulphonamides), oxidants in foods and infection.
- Usually presents with haemolysis and anaemia.
- Large number of foods and drugs may be implicated and should be avoided.
- To diagnose, the enzyme activity can be measured.

Acquired haemolytic anaemias
- Most common type is due to the presence of autoantibodies (against self). These attach to the red cells and reduce their survival time.
- Diagnosed by a positive Coombs' test.

Polycythaemia
- A group of disorders in which there is an increased Hb concentration in the blood. There is a raised red cell count and packed cell volume (PCV).

- In true polycythaemia there is an absolute increase in the red cell mass. In apparent polycythaemia the red cell mass is normal and the rise in PCV is secondary to a decrease in plasma volume.
- Stimulus for increased red cell production is hypoxia and polycythaemia may occur secondary to oxygen lack, as at altitude or in chronic lung diseases.
- Associated with thrombotic (blood clot) disorders such as myocardial infarction, stroke, peripheral vascular disease and DVT.
- There is increased viscosity (thickness) of the blood which results in reduced flow.

Polycythaemia rubra vera (primary polycythaemia)
- A defect that arises in the stem cell and causes an overproliferation of red blood cells.
- Usually in the middle aged and elderly.
- Often found by chance when an elevated Hb is recorded.
- There is an enlarged spleen and this may be the first finding.
- Sometimes it may only be diagnosed after an acute thrombotic event.
- Plethoric (ruddy) complexion.
- Diagnosis is confirmed by blood tests.
- About 60% of patients die from thrombotic events.
- Treatment is to lower the Hb often by repeated venesection (withdrawal of blood).
- Chemotherapy with hydroxyurea may help.

- Radioactive phosphorus is used in severe cases.
- Untreated cases – the mean survival is 2 years. May be increased to about 14 with treatment.

Myelofibrosis

Increased fibrous tissue is formed within the marrow cavity. This disturbs normal manufacture of red blood cells which now occurs in the spleen and liver. It may be a consequence of other myeloproliferative disorders such as polycythaemia and acute myeloid leukaemia.

Clinical features
- Weight loss – thin arms and legs with enlarged abdomen.
- Usually grossly enlarged spleen.
- Anaemia.
- There may be ascites.
- Purpura and bleeding may result from thrombocytopenia (low platelets).

Treatment
- Supportive and symptomatic.
- Blood transfusion may be necessary for severe anaemia.
- Death usually occurs from gradual marrow failure with bleeding and overwhelming infection.

THE SPLEEN

- Largest lymphoid organ in the body.
- Situated in the left hypochondrium.

- Main functions are destruction of old red cells and immunological defence.
- Splenomegaly is enlargement of the spleen and this can lead to hypersplenism – a decrease in the number of red cells due to pooling and destruction by the enlarged spleen.

Causes of splenomegaly

Haematological
- Chronic myeloid leukaemia – may be massive and extend into right iliac fossa
- Other leukaemias
- Lymphomas
- Haemolytic anaemia
- Myelofibrosis

Infections
- Chronic malaria
- Schistosomiasis
- Septicaemia
- Glandular fever (infectious mononucleosis)
- Tuberculosis
- Brucellosis

Inflammation
- Rheumatoid arthritis
- Sarcoidosis
- Systemic lupus erythematosus

Portal hypertension

Splenectomy

Removal of the spleen, performed mainly for:
- trauma
- haemolytic anaemias
- idiopathic thrombocytopenic purpura
- hypersplenism.

The main short-term complication is thrombophilia and the main long-term complication is overwhelming infection. The main infective organisms are *Streptococcus pneumoniae*, *Haemophilus influenzae* and the *meningococci*. Vaccines against these bacteria must be given to all who undergo a splenectomy.

Prophylactic antibiotics need to be given for the first 2 years following the splenectomy. In children antibiotics should be continued prophylactically until the age of 16 years. Some recommend lifetime antibiotics following splenectomy.

PLATELETS

Platelets are small disc-shaped structures, 1–2 µm in diameter, present in the blood. Their functions are related to haemostasis (stopping bleeding).

Essential thrombocythaemia
- There is an overproduction of platelets, which may be functionally impaired. This is associated with other myeloproliferative disorders such as polycythaemia, chronic myeloid leukaemia and myelofibrosis.
- Normal platelet count is $250–400 \times 10^9/l$. Diagnosis is on a platelet count of $1000–2000 \times 10^9/l$.
- Thrombotic occlusion of arteries, leading to myocardial infarction, stroke or gangrene, is common.
- Treatment is aimed at reducing the platelet count by using cytotoxic drugs such as busulfan

or cyclophosphamide or radioactive phosphorus.

Thrombocytopenia
This is a reduction in platelet count and is discussed under bleeding disorders.

Bleeding disorders
A bleeding disorder is suggested when the patient has unexplained (i.e. no history of trauma) bleeding or bruising or prolonged bleeding following injury, surgery or tooth extraction.

> ⚠️ Haemostasis is the process of stopping bleeding following damage to a blood vessel. It is a complex process that involves platelets, coagulation factors (increase blood clotting) and anticoagulation factors (decrease blood clotting).

Coagulation defects
- Inborn defects have been described in all coagulation factors but are mostly extremely rare.
- The two commonest are haemophilia (factor VIII) and Christmas disease (factor IX). Both of these are transmitted as sex-linked recessive characteristics. This means that females carry the disease but only males actually have the full disease.
- They are both associated with an increased bleeding tendency.
- There is a wide range of severity.
- Bleeding may occur into any tissue of the body but the most common bleeding site is into the

joints (*haemarthrosis*). The joints most frequently involved are knees, elbows, ankles, shoulders and hips.

- Haemarthrosis leads to the sudden onset of acute pain and swelling. Movement is restricted by the patient.
- Recurrent episodes lead to chronic degenerative joint disease with chronic pain, deformity and limitation of movement.
- The most common cause of death from bleeding is cerebral bleeding.
- Internal bleeding may also occur leading to obstruction of the ureter and haematuria. Intestinal obstruction is one manifestation of bleeding into the bowel.

Investigations
- There is a prolonged APTT.
- The individual clotting factors then need to be measured.

Treatment
- Specialized units are best.
- The deficient clotting factor (found in plasma) is infused intravenously both as prophylaxis, before and after surgery, and to treat acute bleeding.
- Many patients have supplies of the missing factor at home and inject themselves at the first sign of bleeding.
- Tragically, many patients have been infected with HIV from contaminated plasma. Some clotting factors are now available synthetically (using recombinant DNA) but are extremely expensive.

Von Willebrand's disease
- This is an inherited deficiency of von Willebrand's factor, which is essential for normal platelet adhesion in the damaged blood vessel lining. It also leads to low levels of factor VIII.
- It can occur in both men and women and there is a broad range of severity from symptomless to severe.
- Presentation is usually with bleeding.
- Treatment is administration of vasopressin preparations and if severe, the administration of cryoprecipitate or plasma.

Vitamin K deficiency
Vitamin K is needed for the synthesis of several clotting factors. A deficiency of this vitamin results in a bleeding tendency.

Causes
- Haemorrhagic disease of the newborn – synthesis is defective in premature infants. They are given the vitamin at birth to reduce the risk of cerebral bleeding.
- Intestinal malabsorption, e.g. Crohn's disease, coeliac disease
- Hepatobiliary disease, e.g. liver failure, obstructive jaundice
- Dietary deficiency
- Oral anticoagulant use (warfarin inhibits the action of vitamin K)

Disseminated intravascular coagulation (DIC)
This is an inappropriate activation of the coagulation pathways leading to the inappropriate deposition of

fibrin-platelet thrombi in the arterial and venous tree. This stimulates fibrinolysis (clot breakdown) and the two processes run in parallel. This leads to:

- depletion of clotting factors
- depletion of platelets leading to thrombocytopenia and increasing the bleeding tendency
- loss of haemostasis
- excessive bleeding.

A large number of conditions may lead to acute or chronic DIC.

Causes of acute DIC
- Infections/infectious diseases such as meningococcal septicaemia and malaria.
- Obstetric causes such as preeclampsia.
- Shock due to trauma, cardiac arrest, blood loss or extensive burns.
- 60% have septic shock. The overall mortality is 50%.

Acute DIC presents as a haemorrhagic illness.

- The patient is usually severely ill.
- Fever, acidosis and hypoxia and hypotension due to severe blood loss are present.
- May be extensive petechiae or bleeding into the skin.
- May also be bleeding into the eyes, alimentary, renal, respiratory or genital tracts.

Diagnosis is made by laboratory testing.
- Platelet count is reduced.
- The partial thromboplastin time (PPT) is prolonged.

- Presence of fibrin degradation products (FDPs).

Treatment
- Treat the underlying condition.
- Restoration and maintenance of the peripheral circulation.
- Replacement therapy with plasma products.
- Use of heparin may control the thrombotic component but remains controversial.

Chronic DIC occurs in some patients with malignant conditions or chronic inflammatory diseases.

THROMBOSIS
A thrombus is a solid mass formed in the circulation from the constituents of blood.

Arterial thrombosis
Usually the result of atheroma which tends to occur in areas of turbulent blood flow in the arteries, e.g. at the femoral bifurcation.

Venous thrombosis
- Unlike arterial thrombosis, this usually occurs in normal vessels (i.e. without atheroma deposition), often in the deep veins of the leg.
- It originates around the valves as red thrombi.
- There is a risk of propagation and embolization to the pulmonary vessels.

More detail on p.158. The risk factors for venous thrombosis are shown in Box 4.3.

Box 4.3   Risk factors for a deep vein thrombosis

Patient factors	**Disease or procedure**
Age	Trauma – especially pelvis or hip
Obesity	Surgery – especially pelvis or hip
Varicose veins	Malignancy
Immobility (bedrest, long-haul flights)	Heart failure
Pregnancy	Recent myocardial infarction
High doses of oestrogens	Infection
Previous DVT	Inflammatory bowel disease
Thrombophilia	Polycythaemia
	Thrombocythaemia
	Nephrotic syndrome

WHITE BLOOD CELLS

Leukaemias

Neoplastic disorders of the blood-forming tissues. There is an unregulated proliferation of white cells or accumulation of white cells in the bone marrow. These replace the normal cells.

- There may be proliferation at any stage of development from the stem cell.
- Normal cells are replaced by malignant cells and this leads to a low white cell, haemoglobin and platelet count.
- There may also be damage to normal white cells so they cannot function properly. There is a fall in antibody production.
- There is infiltration of other tissues including the spleen, liver and central nervous system.
- Divided into acute and chronic forms.

Causal factors

- No evidence of inheritance pattern
- Some genetic disorders are associated with it, e.g. Down's syndrome

- Radiation
- Chemicals
- Therapeutic drugs – cytotoxics
- Viruses
- Philadelphia chromosome

Diagnosis

- Blood picture
- Bone marrow puncture

Classification

Acute leukaemias

- Uncontrolled clonal proliferation and accumulation of blast cells in the bone marrow and other body tissues.
- Clinical features are a result of anaemia, neutropenia and thrombocytopenia.

Acute lymphatic/lymphoblastic leukaemia (ALL)

- Most common in childhood – peaks between 4 and 5 years.
- More common in developed countries.

Acute myelogenous leukaemia (AML)

- Commonest in middle to old age.

- Males over 65 with a minor peak under 5.
- Seven types, according to cell type predominating.

Chronic leukaemias
- Very few normal cells but the abnormal do differentiate to a degree and thus marrow failure is not a feature.
- Mass of cells produced give the clinical symptoms, e.g. splenomegaly, lymphadenopathy.

Differ from acute in that:

- the time course is longer
- the onset is more insidious
- the cells are more mature
- the treatments required are less intensive.

Chronic lymphatic leukaemia (CLL)
- Commonest leukaemia in Europe and the USA. Accounts for 30% of leukaemic deaths.
- Rare below 30 then increases sharply with age. Mean age at diagnosis is 60 years.
- Less common in Asians than whites or blacks.
- More common in men.

Chronic myeloid/granulocytic leukaemia (CML)
- Predominantly middle age – mean age at diagnosis is 45 years.
- Small peak in white boys under 5.
- Presence of the Philadelphia chromosome in about 95% of cases.

Pathophysiology

Acute leukaemias. Cause morbidity and mortality through:

- deficiency in numbers of normal blood cells
- invasion of vital organs with impairment of organ function
- systemic disturbances shown by metabolic imbalances – hyponatraemia, hyperuricaemia – may be a symptom of the disease or its treatment.

Aetiology unknown but may include viruses, chemicals and radiation.

Clinical features
- Result from bone marrow failure
- History usually short
- Symptoms of anaemia and malaise – pallor and tiredness
- Repeated acute infections – fever
- Bruising and bleeding
- Painful and enlarging lymphadenopathy
- Bone pain, especially in children
- Symptoms due to infiltration of tissues – splenomegaly, hepatomegaly
- Headache, nausea, vomiting and blurred vision due to raised intracranial pressure in patients with CNS involvement

Treatment
- Induction of remission
- Consolidation
- Cranial prophylaxis
- Continuation/maintenance therapy

Relapse can occur in three sites – bone marrow, CNS, testicle.
    Treatment should be carried out in specialist centres. Chemotherapy may include combinations of steroids, vincristine, asparaginase, methotrexate, daunorubicin and

cytosine arabinoside. Cytotoxic drugs are described on p. 301.

Chronic lymphatic leukaemia. A disease of middle age and the elderly. Onset is insidious with:

- lethargy
- fever and sweating
- loss of weight
- infections
- moderate enlargement of lymph nodes in neck, axilla and groin
- splenic and hepatic enlargement.

It is often picked up at a routine blood count. Usually some anaemia, WCC $>15 \times 10^9/l$, of which more than 40% are lymphocytes. Patients may not need any treatment in the early stages when asymptomatic.

Single drug therapy is used, e.g. chlorambucil, cyclophosphamide. This can induce partial remission in 50% of cases and complete remission in 10–15%.

Patients are very susceptible to infections which are often the cause of death.

Chronic myeloid leukaemia

- Deceptive to call it chronic.
- Usually associated with a chromosomal abnormality. The Philadelphia chromosome is present in 95% of patients.
- Treatment is by control of the proliferation by the use of busulfan or hydroxyurea.
- Median survival 35 months. Usually within 5 years of diagnosis there is a blast crisis and acute transformation occurs, i.e. to acute leukaemia.
- Allogenic bone marrow transplant is useful in the chronic phase in

young patients who have a compatible donor. Should be done within the first year for the best chance.

Myelodysplastic syndromes

These disorders are characterized by the liability to develop acute myeloid leukaemia.

THE LYMPHOMAS

Lymphomas are malignant tumours of the lymphoreticular system. They originate in one of the lymph nodes or other lymphatic tissues of the body. They are classified on histological appearance (appearance of the cells under the microscope) into Hodgkin's disease and various subtypes of non-Hodgkin's lymphoma (NHL).

Hodgkin's disease

The most common of the lymphomas. Early peak incidence is in the early 20s and a later peak occurs in middle age after 45 years.

Clinical features

- Seventy percent of cases arise as a painless enlargement of a lymph node in the neck, axilla or groin and it spreads to adjacent groups of lymph nodes.
- Systemic features include fever, night sweats and weight loss.
- Other symptoms include pruritus, fatigue, anorexia and alcohol-induced pain at the site of the enlarged lymph nodes.
- On examination the affected nodes are usually painless and have a rubbery consistency.

- There may be enlargement of the liver and spleen (hepatosplenomegaly).
- Staging in Hodgkin's disease is shown in Box 4.4.

Investigations
- Blood count may show anaemia and a raised erythrocyte sedimentation rate (ESR).
- Liver biochemistry may be abnormal.
- Radiological examination of the chest and CT scanning.
- Lymph node biopsy will give a definite diagnosis.
- Bone marrow biopsy may show involvement in advanced disease.

Treatment
- Radiotherapy or a cyclical combination of cytotoxic drugs or a combination of both is used.
- The prognosis is related to the stage of the disease.
- In the early stages (I and II without beta symptoms) radiotherapy may produce a cure. There is a 25% relapse rate and subsequent combination

chemotherapy produces virtually 100% cure.
- In stages III and IV, with or without beta symptoms 60% are disease free at 5 years.
- Variations depend on the presence of adverse prognostic factors such as beta symptoms, age > 40 years, bulk disease.
- Most relapses occur within 1–2 years of completion of combination therapy.

Non-Hodgkin's lymphoma (NHL)
This is a group of disorders arising from many different cell types. There are several confusing classifications but the simplest is high-grade or low-grade NHL.

Clinical features
- Rare before the age of 40 years.
- Presents in a variety of ways and almost any organ in the body can be involved.
- Peripheral lymph node enlargement is the commonest presentation.
- Systemic symptoms as in Hodgkin's may occur.

Box 4.4	Staging in Hodgkin's disease (Ann Arbor System)
Stage I	Involvement of one lymph node or extralymphatic organ
Stage II	>1 lymph node involved on the same side of the diaphragm or with localized involvement of an extralymphatic organ on same side of diaphragm
Stage III	Nodal disease on both sides of the diaphragm or with extralymphatic site or spleen
Stage IV	Involvement of extranodal sites, e.g. bone marrow, liver and lungs
Beta symptoms	Night sweats
	Fever >38°C for 3 consecutive days
	Unexplained weight loss >10% of body weight

- Bone marrow infiltration may occur and lead to anaemia, recurrent infections and bleeding.
- Investigations are similar to those for Hodgkin's.

Treatment

Low grade
- Not usually curable unless early stage I.
- Staged as for Hodgkin's. With involvement of one gland, this may be excised and followed with radiotherapy. This is, however, very rare.
- Patients may survive for many years (mean 7–10 years) and experience remissions following radiotherapy or cytotoxic therapy.
- Interferon-alpha is also used in the management.

High grade
- Rapid onset and 60–70% of cases present in stage III or IV.
- Commoner in impaired immune surveillance such as following kidney or heart transplants and treatment for another malignancy or AIDS.
- Combination chemotherapy is used for all patients, irrespective of staging.
- Some radiotherapy may be used for localized glands.
- 70% in stages I and II are disease free at 5 years.
- 40% in stages III and IV are disease free at 5 years.

LYMPHADENOPATHY

This is enlargement of the lymph nodes and has many causes.

Local
- Infection such as tonsillitis, tuberculosis
- Secondary carcinoma
- Lymphoma

Generalized
- Infections:
  —Epstein–Barr virus (glandular fever)
  —Cytomegalovirus
  —Toxoplasmosis
  —Tuberculosis
  —HIV infection
- Lymphoma
- Leukaemia
- Drug reactions, e.g. phenytoin
- Systemic lupus erythematosus
- Rheumatoid arthritis

MULTIPLE MYELOMA

This is a cancer of the antibody-producing cells (plasma cells) in the bone marrow. Antibody may be present in the urine (Bence-Jones protein) and this is diagnostic of the disease.

It only accounts for 1% of all neoplasms and is more common in the elderly (mean age of presentation is 60–70 years) and rare in those <40 years old.

Myeloma is not a curable disease and the median survival from diagnosis is 2 years.

Clinical features
- Bone pain is the commonest presenting feature.
- Anaemia, infections and bleeding occur as the bone marrow is infiltrated with the cancer cells

and cannot produce sufficient blood cells.
- Renal failure may occur due to the deposition of antibody in the kidney tubules.
- Bone cells are involved and osteoporosis, hypercalcaemia and pathological fractures may result.

Treatment
- Combination chemotherapy with melphalan and prednisilone is one treatment.
- Bone marrow transplantation – only recommended under 60 years.
- Localized bone pain may be helped by radiotherapy.
- Interferon-alpha is also used in the management.

4.4 THE GASTROINTESTINAL SYSTEM

Stretches from the mouth to the anus and is really a muscular tube that is adapted along its length to aid the digestion and absorption of nutrients.

Symptoms of gastrointestinal disease could include the following.

- *Dysphagia* – difficulty in swallowing.
- *Dyspepsia* – a term used to describe many different symptoms of indigestion such as heartburn, acidity and pain.
- *Heartburn* – a symptom of acid reflux. A retrosternal burning discomfort which sometimes is confused with coronary pain.

- *Flatulence* – excessive wind. This may present as belching, abdominal pain and the passage of flatus.
- *Vomiting* – associated with many gastrointestinal conditions, but also occurs in many other conditions. If it is without pain it is not usually GI in origin.
- *Haematemesis* – vomiting blood. May be bright red, contain dark clots or look like coffee grounds, showing that digestion in the stomach has commenced.
- *Constipation* – infrequent passage of stool or difficult passage of hard stool.
- *Diarrhoea* – the passage of increased amounts of loose stool, not small amounts of stool.
- *Malaena* – bleeding in the tract which leads to the passage of black, sticky and smelly stools composed of partially digested blood.
- *Steatorrhoea* – the passage of fatty stools, these are pale, bulky and usually float, making them difficult to flush away.

VOMITING

There are many causes of vomiting and it is likely to accompany any severe illness.

- Gastrointestinal causes include appendicitis, gastric ulcer, hiatus hernia, oesophageal carcinoma, gastritis, food poisoning, excess alcohol, pyloric stenosis, intestinal obstruction, strangulated hernia and, rarely, severe constipation.
- Metabolic disturbances such as diabetic ketoacidosis, uraemia and hypercalcaemia.

- Drugs such as chemotherapeutic agents, antibiotics, digoxin and opiates.
- Alcohol.
- Cerebral causes, e.g. raised intracranial pressure, head injury, meningitis, migraine.
- Any severe infection.
- Myocardial infarction or other trauma to the body.
- Severe pain.

Patient management and nursing care

- Ensure the patient has a vomit bowl and tissues at the bedside.
- Stay with the patient if he wishes this.
- Record the type of vomit and the amount.
- Observe for signs of dehydration.
- The doctor may take blood for U&E estimation.
- The management will depend on the cause.
- An antiemetic may be administered. Examples are metoclopramide (maxalon) or prochlorperazine (Stemetil).
- If the vomiting is secondary to chemotherapy, ondansetron may be more effective.
- Fluid replacement intravenously may be needed if the patient cannot tolerate fluid orally.

DIARRHOEA

This is the passage of loose, semi-solid or liquid stools which are passed at more frequent intervals than is normal for the patient. It may also be defined as the passage of >300 ml of liquid faeces in 24 hours.

It may be acute or chronic and is not always due to a problem in the GI tract.

Causes

- Food poisoning – *Staphylococcus aureus*, Salmonella, viruses, Campylobacter, *Escherichia coli*, etc. – often accompanied by vomiting.
- Inflammatory bowel disease – ulcerative colitis, Crohn's disease, pseudomembranous colitis (sometimes following antibiotics).
- Drugs such as antibiotics, laxatives, antacids, digoxin.
- Diverticular disease, malabsorption, thyrotoxicosis, faecal impaction with overflow, irritable bowel disease.
- If the patient has recently been abroad, tropical diseases may be responsible.

Patient care and nursing management

- This depends very much on the cause.
- Barrier nursing may be needed if infective cause.
- Stool specimens may need to be collected.
- Careful recording of fluid intake and output, including diarrhoea.
- Observation for blood or mucus in the stools.
- Rehydration may be possible orally if vomiting is not present.
- Salts as well as water are needed and preparatory brands of powder to be reconstituted are available, e.g. Rehidrat.
- If vomiting is present the patient may not be able to take oral fluids

and an IV infusion may be in progress to prevent dehydration.

- Antidiarrhoeal drugs are not usually prescribed. They can actually prolong infection.
- Antibiotics are not usually needed but in persistent infective diarrhoea the microbiologist may be consulted.

CONSTIPATION

This is the infrequent passage of hard stools with straining and difficulty. It is often a problem in the immobile and the elderly where the faeces may accumulate in the rectum and overflow incontinence of loose faecal matter may occur.

Causes
- Simple constipation due to lack of dietary fibre or dehydration and lack of exercise.
- Secondary to disease of the colon, e.g. diverticular disease, cancer, Hirschsprung's disease, painful haemorrhoids and anal fissures.
- Drug related – many analgesics, especially opioids, cause severe constipation. Antacids with an aluminium base and anticholinergic drugs slow down motility.
- Neurological diseases affecting the bowel and bladder, e.g. multiple sclerosis.
- Metabolic diseases such as hypothyroidism.

Treatment
- Simple constipation usually responds well to an increased fluid intake and more fibre in the diet.

- Bulk-forming laxatives may be used. They relieve constipation by increasing the faecal mass and their full effects may not be felt for several days. Bran is an example as are methylcellulose (Celevac) and ispaghula husk (Isogel, Regulan).
- Stimulant laxatives increase intestinal motility and often cause abdominal cramps. They should never be used in intestinal obstruction. Bisacodyl and senna are examples.
- Glycerol suppositories act as a rectal stimulant.
- Osmotic laxatives such as lactulose act by retaining fluid in the bowel.
- Microenemas are often used and are made of sodium citrate.

THE OESOPHAGUS

The oesophagus is a muscular tube, about 25 cm in length, that extends from the pharynx to the stomach, passing through the diaphragm. It is lined by a mucosa of stratified epithelial tissue and a submucosa containing glands. The muscle consists of both longitudinal and circular muscle layers that are responsible for peristalsis and the passage of food from the mouth to the stomach.

The commonest congenital abnormality affecting the oesophagus is oesophageal atresia where the oesophagus ends in a blind pouch. It is often associated with a fistula between the oesophagus and the trachea (tracheo-oesophageal fistula) and in about 50% of cases there are other congenital abnormalities present. The condition is usually diagnosed at birth and the treatment is surgical to restore continuity of the oesophagus and eliminate any fistula.

Dysphagia

This is the most common symptom of any disease of the oesophagus. It is difficulty in swallowing which depends on the action of many muscle groups, some voluntary and some involuntary. The passage of food from the mouth to the stomach is dependent on a wave of peristalsis which is also dependent on nervous control.

Causes

Neuromuscular disease
- Motor neuron disease
- Myasthenia gravis
- Cerebrovascular accident that affects the ninth, 10th or 12th cranial nerves
- Achalasia
- Diabetic autonomic neuropathy

Obstruction
- Foreign body
- Stricture due to acid regurgitation (reflux)
- Tumour
- Compression from outside by a mediastinal mass

Malignancy should always be ruled out in cases of dysphagia. A barium swallow or an endoscopy will be used for this purpose.

Achalasia

There is an absence of peristalsis and a failure of the lower oesophageal sphincter to relax. The cause is not known but vitamin deficiency, viral infection and autoimmune disease have all been implicated.

Clinical features
- Develops slowly over a period of years.
- Food and liquid accumulate in the oesophagus and dilatation occurs at the lower end.
- Dysphagia and regurgitation occur.
- Accumulation of food and fluids can lead to aspiration and chest infection.

Diagnosis
A barium swallow shows the dilated oesophagus. Endoscopy will also be done to exclude any type of tumour.

Treatment
Balloon dilatation of the lower oesophageal sphincter. If dilatation is unsuccessful, surgery is possible.

Reflux oesophagitis (gastro-oesophageal reflux)

This is a very common condition caused usually by a failure of the lower oesophageal sphincter. If the sphincter is incompetent, this allows stomach contents to reflux into the oesophagus when the person is lying flat or when the stomach is full. The mucosa of the oesophagus is not as thick as the stomach mucosa and so the acid contents cause corrosion and burning, leading to inflammation. This can lead to bleeding and ulceration followed by stricture.

Sometimes, over a long period of time the mucosa may change and there may be an increased risk of malignancy.

Clinical features

- Heartburn, regurgitation and dysphagia.
- May be pain on swallowing hot or spicy food and drink.
- Posture is important and the symptoms worsen on bending or lying down and also following a large meal or the intake of large quantities of fluid.
- Ulcers may cause some bleeding.

Treatment

- Weight loss, if overweight.
- Help to stop smoking, if a smoker.
- Reduction in alcohol intake, if heavy.
- Small and regular meals. No meal just before bedtime.
- Sleep sitting up or raise the head of the bed.

Drugs

Antacids and alginates such as Gaviscon may be used to help protect the mucosa. Proton pump inhibitors may be given to reduce the acid secretion in the stomach, e.g. omeprazole.

Gastric emptying can be helped with metoclopramide. Cisapride may be given to improve motility.

If medical management fails, surgical procedures can be used.

Hiatus hernia

This is a herniation of part of the stomach through the diaphragm. It is relatively common and is one cause of reflux oesophagitis. Figure 4.5 shows a hiatus hernia.

In a *sliding hiatus hernia* the stomach herniates into the thorax when the patient is in the supine position. Standing causes the stomach to slide back into the abdominal cavity. The hernia is exacerbated by any factors that increase intraabdominal pressure such as coughing, bending, straining and pregnancy.

In a *rolling or para-oesophageal hernia*, the fundus of the stomach herniates through the hiatus alongside the oesophagus. Reflux is less common but there is a danger of

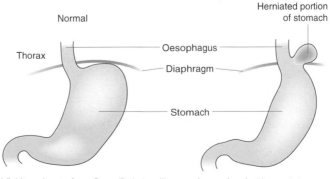

Fig. 4.5 Hiatus hernia. from Govan/Pathology Illustrated, reproduced with permission.

congestion, constriction and ulcer formation. The hernia may strangulate which is a major complication.

Diagnosis is by barium studies and endoscopy.

The usual management of a sliding hernia (the commonest type) is medical with weight reduction, antacids and sleeping in the sitting position all being important. Surgery is only contemplated when symptoms are severe. The hernia is reduced and the defect repaired. The operation is major as entry has to be made via the thorax.

Oesophageal tumours

These are usually malignant. Benign tumours of the oesophagus are rare. Ninety-five percent are squamous cell carcinomas. This occurs worldwide and has a poor prognosis. It is the leading cause of cancer death in China but accounts for only 1–2% of deaths in the West.

It has been linked to smoking, excess alcohol consumption, history of acid reflux and achalasia.

Clinical features
- Dysphagia, first with solids and eventually with liquids as well.
- Weight loss.

Investigations
- Endoscopy and biopsy.
- Barium swallow allows the length of the tumour to be assessed.
- CT scan to look for spread of the tumour into lymph nodes, mediastinum, lungs or liver.
- Endoscopic ultrasound.

Treatment
- May be curative or palliative depending on the age of the patient and the presence of metastatic disease. Most tumours are not resectable due to direct spread to the mediastinal structures, e.g. aorta, bronchus and diaphragm.
- Surgery is still the best approach in the young patient and a resection of the oesophagus or an oesophagectomy is performed. The resected oesophagus is replaced with either colon or stomach. Sometimes a surgical bypass or a palliative resection is attempted but these carry a high perioperative risk.
- There is always the danger postoperatively of anastomotic leakage and stenosis. The leaks are difficult to manage and may be fatal.
- Radiotherapy may sometimes produce long-term remission. It is used in inoperable tumours or in those too unfit for major surgery.
- In inoperable cases the obstruction can be relieved by stenting when a wire mesh tube (stent) is inserted, via endoscopy, into the lumen of the oesophagus to hold it open.

Oesophageal bleeding

May be due to Mallory–Weiss tears. These are longitudinal tears in the lower end of the oesophagus due to prolonged or violent vomiting. Occasionally the bleeding can be very severe but is usually self-limiting. The tear may be repaired surgically if necessary.

Oesophageal varices

- These occur secondary to liver disease and are due to portal hypertension causing distended and tortuous veins both in the oesophagus and in the rectum.
- Seventy percent of patients with cirrhosis will develop varices but only about one-third will bleed from them.
- Bleeding is likely from large varices and in severe liver disease.
- They are frequently the cause of life-threatening haematemesis when they rupture. This is usually painless but is extremely frightening for both the patient and the nurse. The mortality rate varies between 30% and 60%. Recurrent bleeding from varices has a poor prognosis with most patients dying within a year.

Emergency treatment of bleeding varices

- The patient will need prompt correction of hypovolaemia with plasma expanders or a blood transfusion if possible.
- Vasoconstrictor therapy may be used in an emergency to try and control bleeding. Vasopressin or glypressin may be used.
- Balloon tamponade may be needed to control bleeding. A Sengstaken–Blakemore tube is usually used. The inflated balloon presses on the bleeding veins.
- In some cases the varices are obliterated by injection of a sclerosing agent.

THE STOMACH AND DUODENUM

Peptic ulcers affect up to 10% of men and women in Britain and are the commonest disorder of the stomach and duodenum.

The stomach has a thick protective mucosa but if this should become thinner and less effective, the secretion of hydrochloric acid in gastric juice, with a pH of 1–2, and the enzyme pepsin will eat into the stomach lining and cause ulcers. The organism *Helicobacter pylori* is now known to be involved in gastritis and duodenal ulcer formation.

Helicobacter pylori

- This organism is a spirochaete and spirochaetes were first reported in the stomach of animals as long ago as 1893.
- During the 1940s human gastric spirochaetes were identified and most appeared in patients with gastric ulcers or cancer.
- In 1983 three different groups around the world reported the presence of spiral bacteria in patients with gastritis and peptic ulceration. Originally the organisms were thought to be *Campylobacter* but in 1989 it was decided they were a new species and they were named *Helicobacter*.
- It is now well accepted that *Helicobacter pylori* is the commonest cause of gastritis. It is thought to play a major part in the development of peptic ulceration and has also been associated with gastric cancer. The

WHO has classified *H. pylori* as a definite carcinogen.

- *H. pylori* infection occurs throughout the world and is commonest in developing countries.
- Infection risk increases with age.
- Low risk in childhood – below 10%
- By about 50 years of age, half the population are affected.
- The natural reservoir of *H. pylori* is not known.
- Apart from human gastric mucosa, it is not known to thrive elsewhere.
- The mode of transmission is not certain. It has been suggested that it may be transmitted by kissing and by endoscopy when instruments are not sterile.
- Water is the most likely medium for transmission, especially in the developing countries and if there is faecal contamination.

Diagnosis

Tests include C urea breath tests – very simple but not always accurate. Endoscopic musocal biopsy and culture of the organism is the most certain diagnosis.

Treatment

- The organism is resistant to single antibiotic therapy.
- The ideal treatment is still not clear but triple regimens do provide higher eradication rates (see Box 4.5) than dual therapy. These consist of a proton pump inhibitor combined with two antibiotics. One-week regimens may be preferred.

Box 4.5 An example of triple therapy: one-week regimen

Amoxicillin 500 mg 3 times daily
plus
Metronidazole 400 mg 3 times daily
plus
Omeprazole 20 mg twice daily or 40 mg once daily for 7 days

- Eradication of infection commonly results in long-term ulcer remission.

Gastritis

This is inflammation of the gastric mucosa. It can be acute or chronic. Acute gastritis is usually caused by drugs or chemicals causing injury to the protective lining of the stomach.

Alcohol, histamine, digitalis and certain metabolic disorders, e.g. uraemia, can all contribute to gastritis. Non-steroidal antiinflammatory drugs such as aspirin also cause gastritis.

Clinical features

- Abdominal discomfort
- Epigastric tenderness
- Bleeding

Usually heals spontaneously over a period of days. Any causative drugs should be discontinued and antacids may be given to combat excess acidity.

Chronic gastritis is usually associated with *H. pylori* infection. It may be associated with atrophy of the gastric mucosa and tends to occur in the elderly. There may be autoimmune attack of the parietal cells in the stomach and an inability to secrete intrinsic factor that leads to pernicious anaemia.

Peptic ulcers

The term *peptic* comes from the Greek 'to digest' and these ulcers occur as a result of the secretion of acid digestive juices.

They may occur at the following sites.

- Oesophagus – due to reflux
- Stomach – gastric ulcer
- Duodenum – duodenal ulcer

Duodenal ulcer is much commoner (five times) than gastric ulcer but the incidence has been decreasing since the 1950s. It is seen in all social groups and 80% occur in men. It is now known that *H. pylori* is the most important factor in its aetiology Surgery for ulcers used to be extremely common but now most of them are treated medically with a regime that includes eradication of *H. pylori*.

Most patients with a duodenal ulcer have excess acid secretion in the stomach. Those with a gastric ulcer have normal or low acid secretion usually.

The ulcers penetrate through the mucosa and into the muscle layer. Duodenal ulcers nearly always occur within 2–3 cm of the pylorus (where the chyme is most acidic).

Aetiology
- *H. pylori*
- Smoking
- Aspirin and NSAIDs
- Alcohol
- Stress – may lead to oversecretion of gastric acid due to stimulation of the vagus nerve. Ulcers tend to occur at times of high stress and anxiety.

- Zollinger–Ellison syndrome. This is a tumour of the pancreas that causes production of a gastrin-like hormone that stimulates the production of gastric juice, causing a hugely raised acidity in the stomach and the formation of multiple duodenal ulcers.

Clinical features
- May be similar to other acute abdominal problems.
- The pain is in the epigastrium and may be intermittent. In duodenal ulcer eating relieves the pain and so there is no loss of appetite usually. In gastric ulcer eating usually exacerbates the pain and so the patient loses weight.
- Those with a duodenal ulcer tend to be overweight and male.
- Those with a gastric ulcer tend to be thin and even emaciated.

Investigations
- Fibre-optic endoscopy. This has superseded investigation with a barium meal. The ulcer can be seen, localized and biopsied.
- The mucosa can also be tested for the presence of *H. pylori*.

Treatment
Most (over 80%) ulcers will heal with medical treatment. Treatment with either a H_2 antagonist, e.g. ranitidine, or a proton pump inhibitor, e.g. omeprazole, is used. If only this therapy is used the relapse rates are high but treating *H. pylori* infection as well has revolutionized the prognosis and reduced the relapse rate from 80% to 5–10%.

Sucralfate may be used to improve mucosal protection.

Occasionally surgery is still needed when:

- medical treatment fails to relieve symptoms (rare)
- there are complications such as uncontrolled haemorrhage or perforation
- there is a possibility of malignancy – especially with a gastric ulcer that will not heal.

Surgery

1. Bilroth I partial gastrectomy for a gastric ulcer – removes the area with the ulcer.
2. Highly selective vagotomy for duodenal ulcer – this operation reduces gastric acid secretion by dividing the part of the vagus nerve that controls acid secretion but retaining the part that controls motility of the stomach.
3. Gastrectomy – this is removal of the stomach and is only used in duodenal ulcers due to Zollinger–Ellison syndrome or as an emergency in severe bleeding.

Side-effects of partial gastrectomy

- Reduced gastric capacity – cannot eat normal-sized meals at first.
- Rapid emptying of stomach contents – dumping syndrome – causes transient hypovolaemia and faintness.
- Diarrhoea due to 'intestinal hurry'.
- Vitamin B_{12} deficiency due to lack of intrinsic factor.
- Recurrent ulceration of remnant (only 1%).

- Reduced iron absorption – may need supplements.

Complications of chronic peptic ulceration

- Perforation – causing peritonitis.
- Bleeding – causing a haematemesis; the ulcer penetrates the gastroduodenal artery.
- Pyloric stenosis due to scar tissue.
- Malignancy (gastric ulcer).

Perforation

Usually a duodenal ulcer and so this is commoner in men. There is usually a history of indigestion but sometimes no history at all.

- Sudden and excruciating epigastric pain that rapidly spreads to the whole abdomen.
- Rigid 'board-like' abdomen that is due to generalized peritonitis.
- Shock – low blood pressure, rapid pulse, cold and clammy to the touch.
- Collapse.
- Patient lies very still as any movement causes pain.

Treatment

- Intravenous infusion to combat shock.
- Analgesia for the intense pain.
- Monitoring of vital signs.
- Antibiotics.
- Nil by mouth.
- Surgery – the perforation is oversewn.
- Medical treatment is commenced after the operation.
- If it is a gastric ulcer, there is a high risk that it may be malignant and some surgeons will do

an immediate partial gastrectomy.

Haemorrhage

This may present as haematemesis or malaena and in some cases both may occur. There are many causes of bleeding from the upper gastrointestinal tract and these include:

- peptic ulcer – 90%
- oesophageal varices
- drugs – aspirin, NSAIDs and steroids, causing acute erosive gastritis
- tumours of the stomach
- Mallory–Weiss syndrome.

Treatment

- Oxygen.
- Intravenous fluids and blood replacement.
- CVP monitoring.
- Catheterization to allow careful monitoring of the urinary output.
- Most bleeding will stop spontaneously but sometimes operation is needed.

Pyloric stenosis

This is a narrowing of the muscular outlet of the stomach, which causes delay in the passage of the stomach contents to the duodenum. This results in vomiting which may be projectile and may include food eaten 24 hours earlier. The patient will lose weight and become dehydrated if the condition is not treated.

The patient does not usually give a history of ulcer pain, but just of episodic vomiting. An X-ray may show the hugely dilated stomach.

Causes

- Fibrosis and narrowing secondary to peptic ulceration
- Carcinoma of the antrum of the stomach
- Congenital pyloric stenosis in babies

Clinical features

- Vomiting – may be projectile, large amounts and containing undigested food.
- Rapid weight loss.
- Gastric peristalsis may be visible in some cases when the stomach is full.
- Mass may be felt in babies and in some cases of gastric carcinoma.
- Dehydration due to persistent vomiting.
- Electrolyte disturbance due to vomiting. Alkalosis.

Carcinoma of the stomach

Declining in incidence in the UK, it is associated more commonly with those of blood group A and is occurs more frequently in men than women. There appears to be a connection with *H. pylori* infection and atrophic gastritis.

Clinical features

- Often insidious in onset
- Increasing weakness and loss of energy
- Anaemia
- Loss of weight and anorexia
- Dyspepsia
- Pain
- Vomiting
- Perforation or haemorrhage may occur

There is a poor prognosis when diagnosed late and it should be suspected in all cases of dyspepsia that start over the age of 40.

Endoscopy with biopsy is used for diagnosis.

Treatment

Surgical when possible. A radical gastrectomy to include lymph nodes and the tail of the pancreas is more successful than less major surgery. This was pioneered in Japan.

Often the surgery is palliative as when a laparotomy is attempted there may be secondary deposits in the liver. A partial gastrectomy may prevent obstruction occurring.

Adjuvant chemotherapy or radiotherapy may be given and trials are in progress at present.

THE ACUTE ABDOMEN

This relates to a patient whose symptoms are of acute onset and the patient will usually be admitted via A&E. Abdominal pain is often the most severe feature.

The patient may have a life-threatening condition that warrants emergency surgery or may have something simple such as severe constipation or even just gas in the bowel (wind).

Common causes of acute abdominal pain in adults

- Non-specific pain that resolves without intervention
- Acute appendicitis
- Acute intestinal obstruction – strangulated hernia, adhesions, occlusion of the mesenteric artery

- Peptic ulcer – severe exacerbation of pain or perforation
- Gallstones – acute cholecystitis
- Acute pancreatitis
- Urinary tract infections
- Renal colic due to stones in the ureter
- Retention of urine
- Constipation
- Leaking or even ruptured abdominal aortic aneurysm
- Gynaecological emergencies such as ectopic pregnancy

PERITONITIS

This is inflammation of the peritoneal cavity, which includes the serosal covering of the bowel and mesentery, the omentum and the lining of the abdominal cavity. It is often localized at first as omentum is wrapped around inflammatory areas. However, this is often insufficient to prevent spread and generalized peritonitis results.

Sudden perforation of any abdominal organ leads to life-threatening peritonitis.

Common causes of peritonitis

Local

Localized peritonitis may occur in:

- appendicitis
- Crohn's disease
- diverticulitis
- cholecystitis
- salpingitis.

Appendicitis will be used as an example. Once the parietal peritoneum becomes involved, pain becomes localized to the affected area and is exacerbated by movement of the muscles in the abdomen.

The area will be tender when examined and the overlying muscles will contract – this sign is called *guarding*.

When the doctor removes his hand suddenly after applying pressure to the area, this sudden movement of the peritoneum causes intense pain which is known as rebound tenderness.

The doctor will also perform a rectal examination and anterior tenderness can be a sign of pelvic peritonitis.

There are usually signs of mild systemic toxicity that include low-grade fever, malaise, tachycardia and a slightly raised white cell count (*leucocytosis*).

Treatment

This depends on the cause. If it is appendicitis, the appendix is removed but if it is salpingitis or diverticulitis, conservative treatment with antibiotics is usually used.

General

Generalized peritonitis may occur when:

- the peritoneum is irritated by noxious materials, e.g. bile, stomach acid, pancreatic enzymes or small bowel contents due to perforation
- there is spreading intraperitoneal infection as in the rupture of an intraabdominal abscess or faecal contamination in bowel perforation, trauma or an anastomotic leak

The patient is seriously ill with generalized peritonitis. Inflammatory fluid moves into the peritoneal cavity and causes hypovolaemia. Alongside this toxaemia or septicaemia may be present.

The severity depends on the cause of the peritonitis and is most severe when contamination is by faeces, infected bile or pus. It is less severe if there is no infection, as in the early stages of a perforated duodenal ulcer.

The abdomen will be rigid and tender and because there is peristaltic paralysis, bowel sounds will be absent. A rectal examination by the doctor may reveal anterior tenderness and if so, pelvic peritonitis is indicated.

Treatment

In generalized peritonitis, the patient is extremely ill and at risk of dying from toxaemia or septic shock. High doses of antibiotics are given intravenously.

It is dangerous to operate in acute pancreatitis but in the other causes, a laparotomy will probably be done urgently to clear the contaminating material and to find the cause, if not known.

Intraabdominal haemorrhage may occur in a ruptured ectopic pregnancy, leaking abdominal aneurysm or trauma to the liver or spleen. The blood causes peritoneal irritation that is similar to peritonitis and diagnosis may be confirmed by peritoneal lavage. Saline is instilled via a peritoneal cannula and retrieval of bloodstained fluid provides the diagnosis.

INTESTINAL DISORDERS

The small intestine extends from the duodenum to the ileum and most of the nutrients are absorbed here.

Causes of bowel obstruction

- Adhesions or bands from previous surgery
- Strangulated hernia
- Volvulus
- Tumours
- Inflammatory strictures as in Crohn's disease
- Impacted faeces
- Intussusception (telescoping of the small bowel – common in children)

Management of bowel obstruction

- Nothing is given by mouth and intravenous fluid replacement is used. The volume and type of fluid depend on the fluid and electrolyte balance. If there has been severe vomiting there may be serious fluid depletion.
- If the patient is vomiting, a nasogastric tube may be passed and the stomach contents aspirated. This will help to control the nausea and vomiting and will also remove swallowed air, reducing gaseous distension. It will also reduce the risk of inhalation of gastric contents, especially if anaesthesia is needed.
- Analgesia will be needed.
- If adhesions are the cause, the obstruction may relieve itself and no further treatment may be needed. If it does not, surgery will be required.

- Large bowel obstruction due to faecal impaction can be relieved by the use of enemas or the manual evacuation of faeces.
- Operation may be necessary to relieve the obstruction. This will have to be immediate if strangulation is present and the blood supply to the bowel is threatened but may be delayed for a day or two if not, so that the patient can be stabilized and any necessary investigations can be done.

Strangulation of the bowel

This occurs when a segment of bowel becomes trapped, obstructing its lumen and disrupting its blood supply. If it is allowed to continue, there will be ischaemia of the bowel and infarction, perhaps leading to perforation.

Causes

- External hernia that may be inguinal, umbilical, femoral or incisional. The bowel becomes trapped outside the body and undergoes necrosis, often perforating within the hernial sac.
- A loop of bowel may become trapped within the abdominal cavity if there are fibrous bands or adhesions.
- A volvulus, where there is massive twisting of the bowel on its mesentery, may also be responsible.

Clinical features of bowel obstruction

- Vomiting – this may be large amounts and, depending on

where the obstruction is, may be faecal in nature.

- Abdominal pain – usually colicky in nature and more severe in strangulation.
- Absolute constipation – no flatus is passed rectally. This happens in complete obstruction but not partial obstruction.
- Dehydration due to vomiting and a lack of intake.
- Abdominal distension due to gas. The lower the obstruction, the more distension will be present.
- Abnormal bowel sounds – exaggerated, high pitched and sometimes tinkling but completely absent in some cases.

Investigations and treatment
Plain abdominal X-ray will show the gas-filled loop of bowel.

Treatment is emergency surgery to relieve the obstruction. A resection of the bowel may be necessary.

INFLAMMATORY DISORDERS OF THE BOWEL

Inflammatory bowel disease is a term that incorporates both ulcerative colitis and Crohn's disease. These are both chronic and remittent bowel disorders that share some symptoms. Diarrhoea will be present in both but recurrent bouts of abdominal pain are typical of Crohn's disease. There are periods of remission and relapse over many years.

Ulcerative colitis
First described in 1909, this is an inflammatory disorder of the colonic and rectal mucosa and submucosa. It always involves the rectum and often extends proximally to involve varying amounts of colon. In about 20% of cases the distal end of the ileum may also be involved.

Clinical features
- There are recurrent acute exacerbations and between these there may be remission or only low-grade activity.
- The acute exacerbations may last days to several months and when they have subsided they may reappear in months or not for years.
- After many episodes of inflammation the epithelium may show abnormal cellular changes (*dysplasia*) and may even develop adenocarcinoma.
- There are both systemic and intestinal symptoms, depending on the severity of the attack.
- Diarrhoea, containing both mucus and blood, may be severe and the patient may have up to 20 loose motions a day.
- The diarrhoea may be preceded by abdominal cramps.
- Incontinence is a problem for many patients if there is any delay in getting to the toilet. This may interfere with the patient's social life and some fear leaving the house at all.
- Fulminant attacks may lead to dehydration, fluid and electrolyte imbalance and blood loss.
- High fever and tachycardia occur due to systemic illness.
- Anorexia, weight loss and lethargy.

- Chronic anaemia.
- Skin lesions – rare; erythema nodosum (tender red nodules on the shins).
- Arthropathy in about 20% of cases – a large joint problem similar to rheumatoid arthritis.
- Occasionally the inflammation may spread to the muscular bowel wall causing paralysis, dilatation and some necrosis. This is known as toxic megacolon and will lead to perforation unless an emergency colectomy is performed. There is sometimes a danger of perforation when toxic megacolon is not present.
- Some patients have inflammation that is confined to the rectum (*proctitis*).

Investigations
Typically a young adult with a history of several weeks of frequent loose stools. The attack may start as traveller's diarrhoea but does not settle.

Parasitic infections need to be excluded by the collection of stool specimens for microbiology.

Barium enema and endoscopy are used to assess the extent of the disease and to take biopsies.

Treatment
- A patient with a fulminant attack will be admitted to hospital and require intravenous fluid and electrolyte replacement. Some may need a blood transfusion.
- Plain abdominal X-ray will be done to exclude toxic megacolon. Colonoscopy will not be done as there is a danger of perforation.

- Management varies not just between patients but also in the same patient for different episodes.
- Local corticosteroid preparations in the form of suppositories, enemas or hydrocortisone foam are used in all cases when the disease is active.
- If very acute, systemic steroids may be used as a short course and in severe cases may be given intravenously.
- Immunosuppressive drugs such as azathioprine are also used if there is little or no response to steroids. They may be used to allow a lower dose of steroid to be given. They do have adverse effects and skin rashes and nausea are common.
- Oral *sulfhasalazine* is used for long-term therapy and to try and prevent relapse. It is a combination of a sulphonamide and aminosalicylic acid (ASA). It appears to prevent the release of some of the inflammatory mediators and perhaps to neutralize some of the toxins present.
- Sometimes antidiarrhoeal drugs such as loperamide or codeine phosphate may be given. A bulk-forming agent such as methylcellulose may also help to reduce the frequency of bowel motion.
- Surgical removal of the colon may have to be done as an emergency but may also be done when medical treatment fails or when there is a high risk of malignancy.

Crohn's disease

This was first described in 1932 by a doctor of the same name. The incidence has risen in the last 20 years in Britain and the cause is not known.

It may affect any part of the gastrointestinal tract but usually the small bowel or the large bowel or both together are affected.

It differs from ulcerative colitis in that the inflammation involves the full thickness of the bowel wall. Chronic inflammation leads to oedema and the formation of ulcers and granulomas. Several different areas of the bowel may be affected, with bowel in between being normal (skip lesions).

The terminal ileum is the area most commonly affected so it used to be called terminal ileitis.

There are exacerbations and remissions and different areas of the gastrointestinal tract may be affected at each attack.

Clinical features

- Symptoms may be similar to ulcerative colitis, especially if the large bowel is involved, and vary according to the severity of the attack. Diarrhoea is usually less severe, containing blood less often. Abdominal pain, weight loss and lethargy are more typical and there may be nausea and anorexia.
- There is often local tenderness if the terminal ileum is affected but sometimes even with extensive disease the main feature is weight loss.
- Arthropathy can occur as in ulcerative colitis.

Complications

- Intestinal obstruction can occur due to a stricture and this may resolve spontaneously but may require surgery, especially if it is recurrent.
- The inflammation in Crohn's can spread to adjacent structures such as the peritoneum and peritonitis can occur. This may simulate acute appendicitis.
- There may be localized abscess formation following perforations, e.g. a pelvic abscess.
- Adhesions may follow from inflammatory spread.
- Fistulae may form between diseased bowel and other hollow parts:
  —stomach – gastrocolic fistula: here the patient would have faecal vomiting
  —urinary tract – leading to severe urinary tract infections
  —uterus or vagina – passage of faeces via the vagina.
- Perianal inflammation and sometimes recurrent perianal abscesses.

Investigations

Similar to ulcerative colitis for the large bowel but a barium follow-through will be done to investigate the small bowel or a 'small bowel enema' which is actually barium given via a nasogastric tube into the duodenum. Barium studies show typical narrowing of the bowel and ulceration.

Care and management

- Drug treatment is similar to ulcerative colitis and is usually effective in the acute stages but there has not been success in maintenance drug therapy. Dietary therapy has given better results long term.

- Topical steroid enemas and foams.
- High-dose oral steroids for the acute attacks. Less successful than in ulcerative colitis and of no use as maintenance.
- Elemental diets that provide all nutrients in a simple molecular form to be absorbed in the proximal bowel have reasonable success but are expensive.
- There is evidence that food intolerance may play a part in acute exacerbations and so diet is important.
- Surgery may be needed especially when some of the complications above occur. This may be a resection of the small bowel or sometimes total colectomy if the large bowel is involved. This is because there may be several lesions (skip lesions) and recurrence is very likely. Some patients require surgery on more than one occasion for complications such as fistulae and abscesses.

STOMAS

Stoma comes from the Greek word for 'mouth' or 'opening'. It is the artificial opening of a tube (the colon or ileum) that has been brought to the surface of the abdomen as a colostomy or ileostomy to allow drainage of faeces or urine (urinary stoma).

It is usually performed when the bowel below the stoma is diseased

and non-functioning. The faeces are collected in a removable plastic bag attached to the abdominal skin by adhesive.

A colostomy is fashioned to be flush with the skin, but an ileostomy has a 'spout' of bowel protruding for about 5 cm so that the irritant contents of the small bowel do not flow onto the skin. The enzymes present in the faecal content can cause destruction of the skin.

Stomas may be performed for:

- cancer of the colon – the commonest reason for having a colostomy
- diverticular disease
- inflammatory bowel disease – ulcerative colitis or Crohn's disease
- cancer of the bladder, trauma or intractable incontinence.

Types of stoma

Colostomy
Some colostomies are permanent and the stoma may be performed from any part of the large bowel, e.g. sigmoid (Fig. 4.6).

Some stomas are temporary and divert the faecal output away from a more distal part of the bowel until it heals. When healing is complete, in weeks or even months, the colostomy is closed.

Temporary colostomies are most commonly formed from the transverse colon. A loop of bowel is pulled to the surface and held there with a glass or plastic rod, shown in Figure 4.7. The distal loop of bowel has no functioning capacity and these stomas are sometimes called 'defunctioning' stomas.

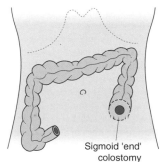

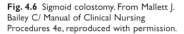

Sigmoid 'end' colostomy

Fig. 4.6 Sigmoid colostomy. From Mallett J. Bailey C/ Manual of Clinical Nursing Procedures 4e, reproduced with permission.

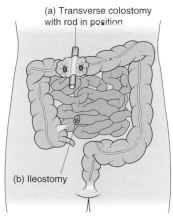

(a) Transverse colostomy with rod in position

(b) Ileostomy

Fig. 4.7 Transverse loop colostomy. From Mallett J. Bailey C/ Manual of Clinical Nursing Procedures 4e, reproduced with permission.

Reasons for a temporary colostomy

- As an emergency measure in bowel obstruction.
- To allow a difficult anastomosis to heal.
- To allow a distal part of the colon to 'rest' in an inflammatory disease such as Crohn's disease or diverticulitis.

Reasons for a permanent colostomy

- These are usually performed for cancer of the bowel.
- If there is no distal bowel remaining after a resection, as in an abdominoperineal resection of the rectum for a cancer of the lower rectum or anus

Hartmann's procedure

- This is often performed for a cancer in the rectosigmoid region of the bowel.
- The cancer is resected but the colon is not joined to the remaining part of the rectum immediately as there is a high risk of infection and breakdown of the anastomosis.
- The proximal loop of bowel is made into a colostomy and the distal part is closed with staples or sutures.
- This means that the rectum is not functioning and although there will be no faeces passing through the anus, some mucus will still pass.
- When any inflammation has settled and healing has taken place, the bowel may be reconnected.
- Some patients are very elderly and find the colostomy functions well. They may decide not to have another major operation and keep the colostomy instead.

Ileostomy

In this procedure the ileum is brought out onto the abdominal wall.

Reasons for an ileostomy
- Severe inflammatory disease of the large bowel as in ulcerative colitis.
- Familial polyposis coli – a rare disease that is genetically transmitted. Polyps first develop in adolescence and occur throughout the rectum and colon. Although the polyps are benign, invariably malignant changes occur in early adulthood. The whole colon should be removed and all close relatives should also be screened for the disease.
- An alternative to an ileostomy is a Park's pouch. A total colectomy is performed but the terminal ileum is made into a pouch and joined to the anus. The anal sphincter is preserved and thus continence is usually maintained.

Psychological preparation of the patient is of the utmost importance when a stoma is being considered and should begin as soon as possible. A specialized stoma care nurse will usually be responsible for this and will visit the patient to discuss the stoma, his lifestyle and coping with the stoma after the operation. The visits continue postoperatively and also when the patient is discharged. It is important to emphasize to the patient that his lifestyle need not change just because he has a stoma. He may be horrified and extremely anxious at the thought and it is important to involve his partner or close relatives in the discussions.

Early complications of stoma
- Sloughing or necrosis due to ischaemia (lack of oxygen due to poor blood supply) – this requires further surgery.
- Obstruction may occur due to faeces or oedema.
- Leakage onto the skin due to a badly fitting appliance may cause erosions. This may be due to poor siting of the stoma (e.g. over a crease in the skin) and if so may require further surgery to resite.

Late complications include prolapse of the bowel, parastomal hernia and retraction of a 'spout' ileostomy. All these require further surgery.

Preparation for bowel surgery
- The danger is infection and the aim is to clear all faecal material from the bowel and reduce the number of bacteria present prior to surgery.
- The patient will not be allowed solid food for a few days preoperatively and will be limited to fluids or a low-fibre diet.
- Laxatives may be given to empty the bowel.
- Enemas and distal bowel washouts are done and an antiseptic washout may be used.
- An antibiotic that is not absorbed from the bowel, such as neomycin, may be given to kill bacteria in the bowel.
- In complete bowel obstruction nothing will be given orally and only distal washouts can be performed. Great care has to be taken in partial obstruction as the use of purgatives may precipitate an acute obstruction.
- Prophylactic antibiotics are given that will hopefully prevent infection by organisms normally

living in the bowel such as *E. coli, Staph. aureus, Strep. faecalis* and *Clostridia*. The antibiotic needs to be at a high concentration at the time of operation and the first dose is usually given just prior to surgery, intravenously. A cephalosporin may be used with metronidazole.

Complications of large bowel surgery

Early complications include:

- wound infections
- pelvic or subphrenic abscess
- leak or breakdown of the anastomosis
- stoma problems, e.g. retraction.

Later possible complications include:

- diarrhoea due to short bowel
- impotence, if there has been damage to the pelvic parasympathetic nerves
- small bowel obstruction due to adhesions.

Colorectal polyps and carcinoma

Polyps

- Polyps are localized lesions protruding from the bowel wall. They are common in the colon and are actually benign neoplasms but they have malignant potential.
- They should be treated as malignant until proven otherwise.
- The patient's first symptom is usually rectal bleeding or anaemia.
- Often there are no symptoms and the polyps are found in routine investigations.

Diagnosis and treatment

- Usually made by sigmoidoscopy. With a fibreoptic sigmoidoscope the colon can be examined up to the splenic flexure, which is the area of greatest occurrence.
- The polyps can be removed using diathermy and this may be done as an outpatient procedure. Histology will always be done.
- If the result shows malignancy and the polyp has been incompletely removed then a resection will be needed.
- The patient will have to be followed up by endoscopy probably at 2-yearly intervals as there is a high risk of recurrence.

Colorectal cancer

There are about 30 000 new cases of colorectal cancer a year in Britain and it is the second or third most common form of cancer in both sexes. It is most prevalent in the Western world and is rare in developing countries.

Colorectal cancer causes about 14 000 deaths every year with incidence increasing with age and over 90% of deaths being in those over 55 years of age.

About one-third of the cancers start in the rectum.

- The cancer is usually an adenocarcinoma that starts in the glandular mucosa.
- The cancer grows outwards at first but later may ulcerate and invade the bowel wall. Narrowing of the lumen of the bowel and intestinal obstruction may occur.
- The cancer spreads via the lymphatic system and also via the bloodstream.

- Lymphatic spread tends to occur first but sometimes there is spread via the bloodstream with no obvious lymphatic involvement.
- The spread via the blood is usually to the liver as the colon is drained by the hepatic portal vein.
- At the time of diagnosis about 25% of patients already have widespread metastases.

Clinical features
- Symptomless anaemia
- Change in bowel habit
- Rectal blood loss
- Colicky pain
- Malaise, anorexia, weight loss
- Some patients may present with a bowel obstruction

Diagnosis
- Sigmoidoscopy and proctoscopy urgently performed.
- Barium enema to show any polyps elsewhere in the colon.
- CT scan or ultrasound of the liver to check for metastases.

Treatment
- Radical surgical resection. This may be an abdomino perineal resection of the rectum when the cancer is low in the rectum. The patient will have a permanent colostomy.
- A resection with an end-to-end anastomosis will be done for upper rectal or colon cancer.
- If the tumour is in the ascending colon, a right hemicolectomy may be performed and half the large bowel removed but no colostomy is needed.

- Chemotherapy has very limited success but may be used especially in an attempt to control painful liver metastases.
- Only about one in 10 patients with distant metastases at the time of operation survive 2 years.
- The metastases are usually in the liver and may be seen at operation or discovered after the operation if not found in the scan before surgery.

APPENDICITIS

The appendix is a short, thin, blind-ended tube, 7–10 cm long, situated in the right inguinal fossa and attached to the caecum (a pouch at the start of the large intestine). It has no known function in humans.

The most common abdominal emergency seen in A&E is acute appendicitis when the appendix becomes inflamed. This carries an overall mortality of about 1% and death is due to generalized peritonitis, being most common in the very young and the very old. The majority of patients do not fall in this category and are between 10 and 30 years of age.

The disease only occurs in the Western world and is probably linked to diet and lifestyle (low-fibre diets may be implicated here). Immigrants to this country become susceptible to the disease when they adopt our lifestyle.

Obstruction to the lumen of the appendix is the usual cause of appendicitis. This is commonly by faecaliths (small, hard masses of faeces). An appendix that is long, thin and retrocaecal is more prone to blockage than a short, straight appendix. Appendicitis may also be congestive and there is no obvious obstruction but inflammation is present and may have been caused by ingested organisms.

Tumours of the appendix are extremely rare

Disease process

- Resolution may occur and be complete but there is usually some scarring which makes the appendix more prone to future attacks of inflammation. This is recurrent appendicitis.
- The body may attempt to wall off the infection and an appendix abscess may result. This usually takes days to form.
- Gangrene and perforation may occur, especially in obstructive appendicitis.
- Perforation may lead to peritonitis (inflammation of the peritoneum) or local abscess formation, depending on the speed and efficiency of the body's defence mechanisms.
- Generalized peritonitis is more common in the very young and the very old where the body is less able to defend itself and the diagnosis is often delayed.

Clinical features

- Abdominal pain and tenderness in the central abdomen at first but then localizing in the lower right abdomen (right iliac fossa) over the appendix itself. The pain may be colicky at first but then becomes dull and constant.

- Unusual positions of the appendix may lead to pain in different sites, causing confusion in diagnosis.
- In congestive appendicitis development may be over a period of days and be preceded by a sore throat and flu- like illness, especially in children.
- Obstructive appendicitis has an acute onset over less than 24 hours usually.
- Anorexia, nausea and vomiting.
- Furred tongue.
- Slightly raised temperature usually.
- Diarrhoea or dysuria may sometimes occur due to irritation of the rectum or bladder.
- The white cell count is usually raised but may be normal, which can be misleading.
- The patient lies still because movement is painful.

Treatment

- Appendicectomy – removal of the appendix – is the treatment and should be carried out as soon as possible.
- Laparoscopic surgery may be performed for appendicitis.
- If the patient is very ill with generalized peritonitis and dehydration, surgery may not be immediate and intravenous fluids and antibiotic administration take precedence.
- Wound infection is common and perioperative antibiotics are usually administered.

Complications

- The patient and relatives should be made aware of the possibility of complications prior to surgery as they may view this as a simple operation that is always straightforward.

- General complications of surgery include DVT, pulmonary embolus and pneumonia.
- Wound infection is very common.
- Pelvic abscess or other collection of pus intraabdominally.
- Prolonged paralytic ileus may occur following removal of a very dirty appendix.
- Adhesive obstruction can develop months later and be the source of future problems.

THE BILIARY TRACT

Gall stones

Gall stone disease is known as *cholelithiasis*. The gall bladder is a muscular sac that stores and concentrates bile, made in the liver. The bile is released when the gall bladder contracts on the arrival of a fatty meal in the duodenum. It emulsifies fats prior to their digestion by lipase enzymes. If bile does not arrive in the duodenum, fats are not digested or absorbed and loose, foul-smelling, fatty stools are passed (*steatorrhoea*). This leads to a lack of absorption of the fat-soluble vitamins (A, D, E and K). Lack of vitamin K leads to inadequate synthesis of prothrombin and problems with blood clotting. This is very important if surgery is necessary in these patients.

Bile leaves the liver via the common hepatic duct, which is joined by the cystic duct from the gall bladder to become the common bile duct. This joins the duodenum with the pancreatic duct at the ampulla of Vater, shown in Figure 4.8. Most gall stones in the Western world are predominantly cholesterol mixed with bile pigments and calcium salts (75–90%). Some (up to 10%) are pure cholesterol. In Asia, however,

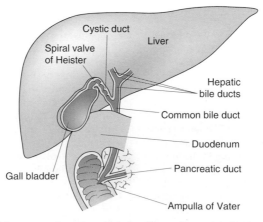

Fig. 4.8 The biliary system. From Govan/Pathology Illustrated, reproduced with permission.

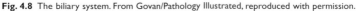

gall stones are mostly bile pigment only. Radioisotope dating shows that the average gall stone is 11 years old when it is removed!

In Britain, at least 10% of the population probably have gall stones but most remain symptom free. They are rare in childhood and increase with age. Women are affected four times as often as men and it is said that the typical patient is *fair, fat, fertile, female and forty*! However, many do not fit this description.

The Western diet is believed to play a large part in the formation of gall stones because of its high fat and poor fibre content.

Clinical features

- Most often the patient presents with pain in the epigastrium or the right hypochondrium. It is often not severe or well defined.
- May present with jaundice, if the gall stone passes into and blocks the common bile duct, thus obstructing the flow of bile into the duodenum.
- Transient obstruction of the gall bladder by a stone may cause episodes of severe pain that are called *biliary colic*. These may be accompanied with nausea and vomiting.
- The obstruction may cause inflammation of the gall bladder which is called *cholecystitis* and in its acute form this is a common cause of attendance to A&E.
- If the infection persists an abscess may develop and is called an *empyema* of the gall bladder.

Investigations

Ultrasound will identify the presence of stones and the thickness of the gall bladder wall. It is not reliable in identifying stones in the duct, especially at the lower end.

Gall bladder function can be demonstrated by an oral *cholecystogram*. A plain film is taken (control film) and may demonstrate the presence of stones, although only 10% of stones are radiopaque. Immediately after this a contrast medium is taken orally and is excreted by the liver, concentrating in the gall bladder. Twelve hours later, further films are taken. Filling defects can be identified that may be due to stones and the gall bladder may fail to opacify, which may mean a non-functioning gall bladder due to inflammatory damage.

Endoscopic retrograde cholangiopancreatography (ERCP) involves the use of an endoscope to view the biliary duct system (see p. 81).

Small gall stones can be removed by slitting the sphincter at the lower end and using a balloon catheter or Dormia basket to retrieve them. This may make a potentially dangerous operation unnecessary.

Percutaneous cholangiography is used if ERCP is not available or is unsuccessful. A fine needle is inserted through the skin into an intrahepatic duct under X-ray control. Contrast medium is then injected and a stone may be identified as a filling defect.

Care and management

- *Cholecystectomy* (removal of the gall bladder) is the usual treatment for low-grade obstructive gall bladder disease.

- A low-fat diet is prescribed preoperatively and this may help to relieve symptoms, probably by not stimulating the gall bladder to contract as much. It may also lead to some weight loss and this is good in the overweight patient.

Biliary colic

This is caused by sudden and complete obstruction of the cystic duct by a stone. There is severe pain, rising to a crescendo in a few minutes and continuing relentlessly. The pain may last several hours and may end spontaneously or may be relieved by opiate analgesia. The patient may vomit.

There is usually a history of similar attacks. No fever is present.

Care and management
- Patients may be managed at home with opiate analgesia.
- Ultrasound examination should be performed as soon as possible and a cholecystectomy will be done either as an emergency or booked electively.

Acute cholecystitis

This is acute inflammation of the gall bladder. The patient is unwell and often has a fever and is tachycardic. The right upper outer quadrant of the abdomen is tender.

The pain usually lasts for several days before subsiding.

Care and management
- Ultrasound may show stones and a thickened gall bladder wall.

- Analgesia in the form of pethidine or an alternative opiate is usually needed.
- Fluids only should be given orally.
- The patient may be nauseous and vomiting and an intravenous infusion may be needed.
- An antiemetic may also be administered if needed.
- Antibiotics are usually administered and are given intravenously.
- Cholecystectomy will be needed and some surgeons keep the patient in hospital and perform the operation early. Others prefer to allow the acute episode to settle and bring the patient back for elective surgery in about 6 weeks.

Empyema of the gall bladder

This often presents with a swinging pyrexia, as do other abscesses. The gall bladder may become necrotic and perforate, leading to a subphrenic abscess or generalized peritonitis.

Immediate surgery is needed in empyema.

Bile duct stones

These originate in the gall bladder and pass down the cystic duct. Often they may be small enough to pass through the bile duct and into the duodenum. They may produce some biliary colic and mild jaundice on their way. This means that recurrent gall bladder disease is common as there may be many stones in the gall bladder. The stone may become lodged in the narrowest part of the common bile duct, just before its entry into the duodenum. It may act as a sort of valve and lead to intermittent jaundice or may become lodged and lead to progressive jaundice. Some stones start off small and develop whilst actually in the bile duct system, becoming larger all the time.

Sometimes the stones in the bile ducts do not cause symptoms so the surgeon will investigate the bile ducts prior to surgery and will explore the common bile duct and remove any stones whilst removing the gall bladder. Following exploration of the bile duct, a latex T-tube drain will be inserted to allow drainage of bile and remain in situ for at least a week so that another cholangiogram can be done to ensure that all stones have been removed. If there are no stones in the common bile duct at operation, it will be closed without a T-tube drain.

Complications of biliary surgery

- Retained stone in the common bile duct.
- Biliary peritonitis caused by bile leaking into the peritoneal cavity.
- Bile duct damage.
- Haemorrhage.
- Ascending cholangitis. This is an infection ascending from the gall bladder and bile ducts upwards to involve the intrahepatic ducts. There will be swinging fever, intermittent pain and jaundice. Drainage is needed as an emergency.

LIVER DISEASE

May be acute or chronic. There may be few signs of acute liver disease

apart from jaundice and an enlarged liver. In chronic liver disease there are many possible clinical features.

- Spider naevi may be present on the chest and upper body. These are red spots with a spidery appearance that blanch on pressure.
- The hands may show palmar erythema.
- Clubbing occasionally occurs.
- The liver may be enlarged at first but becomes small and hard later.
- Gynaecomastia and testicular atrophy may occur in males.
- Clotting factor deficiencies lead to bruising and bleeding tendencies.
- The liver breaks down drugs so these will be metabolized more slowly.
- Jaundice.
- Ascites (fluid in the peritoneal cavity) – abdominal swelling may accumulate over many weeks or over a few days. If ascites is very severe, respiratory distress may occur.
- Mild abdominal discomfort may be present.
- Peripheral oedema sometimes.
- The patient will feel tired.

Complications include portal hypertension and oesophageal varices.

- Seventy percent of patients with cirrhosis will develop varices but only about one-third will bleed from them.
- Bleeding is likely from large varices and in severe liver disease.
- Severe life-threatening haematemesis may occur from varices.

- The patient will need prompt correction of hypovolaemia with plasma expanders or a blood transfusion if possible.
- Vasoconstrictor therapy may be used in an emergency to try and control bleeding.
- Vasopressin or glypressin may be used.
- Balloon tamponade may be needed to control bleeding. A Sengstaken–Blakemore tube is usually used. The inflated balloon presses on the bleeding veins.

Portosystemic encephalopathy is a chronic neuropsychiatric condition secondary to chronic liver disease. It is not fully understood but is due to the effects of toxic metabolites on the brain.

- May occur in cirrhosis.
- Ammonia seems to play a major role and is produced by the breakdown of protein by intestinal bacteria.
- In chronic cases there is a disorder of mood, personality and intellect. Sleep patterns are affected. The patient may be irritable, may become confused and have slurred speech. Convulsions and coma occur as severity increases.
- Treatment includes a low-protein diet, lactulose three times daily to limit ammonia absorption, avoiding too much diuretic therapy which may cause electrolyte imbalance and avoiding constipation.
- Renal failure may occur as the hepatorenal syndrome in advanced cirrhosis. Diuretic therapy should be stopped and the prognosis is poor.

Cirrhosis of the liver

The liver structure becomes irreversibly destroyed by fibrosis and regeneration of liver cells. Cirrhosis is a cause of chronic liver disease.

Causes

- Alcohol – the most common cause in the Western world
- Post hepatitis
- Primary biliary cirrhosis – genetic autoimmune condition, 90% female
- Haemachromatosis (increased iron absorption)
- Wilson's disease – inherited disorder of copper metabolism

Treatment is that for chronic liver disease but the alcoholic must be advised to abstain from alcohol for life. If this is done, the 5-year survival is 90%.

Delirium tremens (withdrawal symptoms) may be treated with clomethiazole or diazepam.

Follow-up shows that the majority of patients continue to abuse alcohol.

Neoplasms of the liver

- These are usually metastases, commonly from breast, colon, stomach, uterus and lung.
- The patient will have lost weight, have pain over the liver and an enlarged abdomen.
- Jaundice occurs late and is a very poor prognostic sign.
- Chemotherapy or hormonal therapy (breast) may be tried.
- When tumours originate from the gastrointestinal tract, palliative care may be all that is available.

Jaundice

This is a yellow coloration of the skin and the whites of the eyes. It indicates an excess of bilirubin in the blood.

- Obstructive jaundice occurs when the bile made in the liver does not reach the intestine due to an obstruction of the bile ducts which may be due to gall stones or cancer of the head of the pancreas.
- The urine is dark and the stools are pale.
- The patient may have pruritus (itching).

Conditions causing obstructive jaundice

- Stones in the common bile duct (see p. 213) – will have pain and perhaps a history of gall stones. The jaundice may be progressive or fluctuating as the stone moves.
- Carcinoma of the head of the pancreas – the jaundice is progressive and painless.
- Other tumours such as secondaries in the porta hepatis or carcinoma of the gall bladder (rare).
- Intrahepatic bile duct obstruction caused by liver secondaries or cirrhosis.
- As a reaction to certain drugs such as chlorpromazine.

> ⚠️ Biliary obstruction leads to poor fat absorption and so poor absorption of vitamin K (fat soluble). This vitamin is needed for the synthesis of prothrombin and the result is deficient blood clotting. Intramuscular vitamin K is given several days preoperatively and this is usually sufficient to improve the prothrombin level.

Hepatocellular jaundice is due to liver disease such as hepatitis or cirrhosis and the liver is unable to deal with all the bilirubin. In acute and chronic hepatitis the stools may be pale and the urine dark. *Haemolytic jaundice* is due to excessive production of bilirubin when there is excessive destruction of red blood cells. The urine and faeces are a normal colour.

> ⚠️ Patients with jaundice should always be assumed to represent a high risk for transmission of hepatitis.

Acute viral hepatitis

May be due to several different viruses. The general features are similar but there is a difference in occurrence and prognosis between the various types.

Hepatitis A (HAV)

- Transmitted by the faecal–oral route.
- Incubation is about one month and carriers have not been detected.
- It is usually a mild illness and flu-like symptoms with myalgia (pain in the muscles) occur. Jaundice occurs later.
- Progression to chronic liver disease does not occur.
- No specific treatment and admission to hospital is not usually necessary.

Hepatitis B (HBV)

- The virus is present worldwide with a low prevalence in the UK.

- Spread is by the IV route, e.g. transfusion of infected blood or blood products, contaminated needles with drug addicts, tattooists or acupuncturists, sexual intercourse particularly in male homosexuals. Transmission from mother to child during parturition can occur.
- Symptoms similar to hepatitis A but the illness may be more severe and there may be an immunological syndrome with a rash and painful joints. Fever is unusual.
- The majority of patients make a full recovery but fulminant hepatitis occurs in 1% and some go on to develop chronic hepatitis or hepatocellular carcinoma or become asymptomatic carriers.
- There is no specific treatment.
- Prevention is by avoiding risk factors.
- Vaccination is available and should be given to all healthcare personnel in the UK.
- Carriers may be treated with interferon-alpha.

Hepatitis D (HDV)
- Especially seen in IV drug abusers.
- Unable to replicate on its own and is activated by HBV.
- Chronic HDV is a severe form of liver disease and 60–70% of patients will develop cirrhosis in the long term.
- Interferon-alpha produces remission but relapse is common.

Hepatitis C (HCV)
- Identified in 1988 and causes 70–90% of post-transfusion hepatitis. Now screening of HCV in donor blood occurs but it is estimated that 76% of haemophiliacs in the UK may have been infected.
- Transmitted intravenously, including by sexual intercourse.
- Flu-like symptoms.
- Less than 20% develop jaundice.
- Most not diagnosed until they present years later with chronic liver disease.

Hepatitis E
- Enteral hepatitis and usually water borne.
- Epidemics have occurred in many developing countries.
- Mortality 1–2% and no carrier state.

Fulminant hepatic failure (FHF)
Severe hepatic failure with encephalopathy developing in less than 8 weeks in a patient with a previously normal liver. It is rare but life threatening and may complicate acute hepatitis due to any cause. There is massive necrosis of the liver tissue.

> ⚠ **Paracetamol overdose is the most common cause of FHF in Britain.**

- The patient is jaundiced.
- Mental state varies from slight drowsiness to total disorientation or unresponsive coma with convulsions.
- Signs of chronic liver failure such as ascites are absent.
- Fever, vomiting, hypertension and hyperglycaemia occur.

- Complications include bacterial infections, gastrointestinal bleeding, respiratory arrest, renal failure and pancreatitis.
- A very high prothrombin (PT) level gives a poor prognosis.
- The patient needs to be managed in an intensive care unit.
- Cerebral oedema is the major cause of death and mannitol may be given by intravenous infusion.
- In special units 70% of cases due to paracetamol poisoning survive even if coma and convulsions have occurred. The survival of those with viral hepatitis is poorer.
- Liver transplantation has been a major advance and specialist centres have developed guidelines dependent on prognosis.

Ascites

This is an accumulation of fluid within the abdominal cavity and has many causes.

Malignant causes

- Tumours of the ovary or colon may lead to the peritoneum becoming 'seeded' with tumour deposits. The malignant cells produce a protein-rich fluid that contains malignant cells and may reach a volume of several litres.
- Severe congestive cardiac failure.
- Severe hypoalbuminuria.
- Cirrhosis when there is obstruction to the venous drainage of the liver.
- Liver metastases when there is obstruction to the venous drainage of the liver.

THE PANCREAS

The head of the pancreas is encircled by the duodenum and the tail lies in contact with the spleen. The pancreas is a fleshy gland with both endocrine and exocrine functions. The endocrine function is described in on p. 260.

Pancreatitis

Inflammation of the pancreas.

Acute pancreatitis

- Associated with gall stone disease, possibly alcohol and some other rare causes.
- Full recovery of the gland usually.
- Mortality varies from 1% in mild cases to 50% in severe cases.

Clinical features

- Vary according to severity of the attack.
- Abdominal pain that may radiate to the back.
- Varies from mild to excruciating pain.
- Nausea and vomiting usually accompany the pain.
- Diagnosis depends on the serum amylase. If this is raised more than five times the normal, acute pancreatitis is very likely.

Care and managemnt

- Nasogastric suction to reduce vomiting and abdominal distension.
- All feeding is stopped and in severe cases nothing at all is given by mouth.
- Analgesia with an opiate other than morphine.

- Intravenous infusion to replace fluid and electrolytes.

Chronic pancreatitis
- Results in permanent damage.
- Majority of cases are due to high alcohol consumption.
- The disease may arrest if the patient stops drinking.
- Abdominal pain is the main symptom and may be almost as severe as acute pancreatitis.
- Some acute episodes appear to be precipitated by alcohol.
- Severe weight loss due to anorexia.
- Steatorrhoea (fatty stools) when lipase is reduced by 90%.
- Development of diabetes is common.

Treatment
- Stop drinking alcohol.
- Pain control, often with narcotics.
- Surgery is occasionally used in specialized units for intractable pain.

Carcinoma of the pancreas
- Incidence is increasing in Western countries.
- Fourth most common cause of cancer death in USA and UK.
- Incidence increases with age and most are over 60 years old.
- Mostly adenocarcinomas from the ductal epithelium.
- Sixty percent are in the head of the pancreas.
- Tumour spreads locally to involve the lymph nodes and the liver.

Clinical features
- Painless jaundice due to obstruction of the common bile duct.
- Most patients will have pain as the disease progresses.
- Weight loss.

Diagnosis
- Ultrasound is used.
- CT scan and fine needle biopsy may be done.
- In almost all cases the tumour is discovered too late for resection to be done.

Care and management
- Five-year survival is extremely low at 1%.
- Resection with total pancreatectomy is not usually possible and itself carries a mortality of 20%.
- Jaundice is usually relieved by a bypass procedure, done endoscopically with the placement of a stent through the narrowest part of the common bile duct to allow drainage.
- Analgesia with long-acting morphine should be used.

Cystic fibrosis
- The most common cause of pancreatic disease in childhood.
- Inherited as an autosomal recessive condition.
- Basic defect in all exocrine glands and thick viscoid secretions are produced.
- Diagnosis is by sweat testing.
- Pancreatic supplements are given and a low-fat diet.

- Chest disease and bronchiectasis also occur but many patients are now surviving into adulthood because of improved therapy.

4.5 THE RENAL SYSTEM

The kidneys' main role is the elimination of waste material and the regulation of fluid and electrolyte balance by the formation of urine.

The functioning unit of the kidney is the nephron and there are approximately one million nephrons in each kidney.

Functions of the kidney

- *Excretory* – elimination of waste products
- *Regulatory* – control of body fluid volume and composition
- *Endocrine* – production of erythropoietin, renin and prostaglandins
- *Metabolic* – metabolism of vitamin D

Renal disease may be suspected from the following:

- symptoms in the urinary tract
- hypertension
- elevated blood urea (from protein breakdown – usually excreted in the urine)
- abnormalities in urinalysis (see p. 57).

Haematuria is blood in the urine. It may be caused by:

- infection of the urinary tract
- stones (calculi)
- glomerulonephritis

- neoplasms anywhere in the renal system
- polycystic disease
- trauma
- warfarin excess.

Discoloured urine may be seen with:

- porphyria (a disturbance in the metabolism of the breakdown products of haemoglobin, the porphyrins, which are excreted in the urine, discoloring it)
- beetroot ingestion
- certain drugs (e.g. rifampicin).

Glycosuria is glucose in the urine. It may be caused by:

- diabetes mellitus
- sepsis
- renal tubular damage
- corticosteroids.

Proteinuria is protein in the urine. It may be caused by:

- urinary tract infection
- vaginal mucus contaminating the sample
- diabetes with nephropathy
- glomerulonephritis
- nephrotic syndrome
- CCF
- hypertension
- systemic lupus erythmatosus (SLE) – a chronic inflammatory condition of connective tissue, affecting the skin and some internal organs
- myeloma.

Anuria is failure of the kidneys to produce urine.

- The urine output is less than 50 ml in 24 hours.
- Lack of production of urine has to be differentiated from an

obstruction in the renal tract preventing the flow of urine.
- Can occur in a variety of conditions that result in a sustained drop in blood pressure.
- It is associated with increasing levels of urea in the blood.
- Haemodialysis may be required.

Oliguria is the production of an abnormally small volume of urine – less than 400 ml in 24 hours. It may be due to:

- kidney disease
- profuse sweating associated with physical activity and /or hot weather
- loss of blood or other body fluids
- diarrhoea.

Uraemia is the presence of excessive amounts of urea and other nitrogenous waste in the blood. These waste products are normally excreted by the kidney in the urine and their accumulation in renal failure results in:

- nausea
- vomiting
- headache
- lethargy
- hiccups
- drowsiness
- convulsions
- coma and death if not treated.

The normal range for blood urea is 2.8–7.0 mmol/l.

URINARY TRACT INFECTION (UTI)

This is an infection of any part of the urinary tract as shown by the growth of microorganisms from a midstream specimen of urine (MSU).

A urinary tract infection (UTI) is usually defined as the presence of >100 000 organisms per ml of urine and symptoms of genitourinary (GU) inflammation.
Pyelonephritis means the kidneys are involved. *Cystitis* means the bladder is involved. The principal danger is that a lower UTI can travel up towards the kidneys.

UTI is much commoner in women as their urethra is so much shorter and is nearer the anus.

Predisposing factors
- Urinary stasis which could be due to:
  —obstruction to urine flow (enlarged prostate, renal calculi)
  —poor fluid intake and/or excessive sweating
  —infrequent voiding
- Trauma
- Instrumentation (catheterization, cystoscopy)
- Malformations of the urinary tract
- Diabetes mellitus
- Pregnancy

Causative organisms
The most common is *E. coli* which causes >70% of UTIs outside hospital but <41% in hospital. *Staphylococcus, Pseudomonas, Strep. faecalis* and *Proteus* are other examples.

Clinical features of lower UTI
- Frequency of micturition
- Pain on micturition – 'burning'
- Suprapubic pain
- Pyrexia
- Unpleasant-smelling urine – *E. coli* infection smells of raw fish

- Frank haematuria (visible to the naked eye) sometimes

Clinical features of upper UTI and pyelonephritis

- Clinical features of lower UTI (sometimes)
- Loin pain and tenderness
- Headache, anorexia, malaise
- Pyrexia and rigors sometimes
- Raised pulse rate
- Nausea and vomiting
- Retention of urine sometimes

Management and nursing care

- Urinalysis – contains blood and protein.
- Obtain MSU before commencement of antibiotics to identify the causative organisms.
- Commence antibiotic therapy – amoxicillin or trimethoprim (see p. 319) usually but may need to be changed if the report shows a lack of sensitivity to the antibiotic.
- Drink plenty – two cups an hour (>3 l daily).
- Intravenous fluids may be needed if cannot tolerate oral fluids.
- Monitor urine output.
- Urinate frequently and not 'hold on' because of pain.
- Care of pyrexial patient (see p. 94).
- Analgesia if needed – pyelonephritis can be very painful.
- Repeated infections must be investigated to detect the cause.

Urethral syndrome or abacterial cystitis

This occurs only in women and is the presence of urgency, frequency and dysuria (painful micturition) in the absence of readily identifiable bacteria in the urine. It is induced by cold, stress, intercourse and nylon underwear. The cause is unknown.

RENAL STONES AND RENAL COLIC

Stones may be made of uric acid, cystine, xanthine, calcium oxalate or calcium phosphate and magnesium ammonium phosphate. The latter follow UTIs, especially those caused by Proteus.

Clinical features

- Some large stones may be symptomless if in the kidney whilst some very small stones can cause intense spasm and pain if in the ureter.
- Stones in the kidney cause loin pain.
- Stones in the ureter cause renal colic, which is a very severe pain that often radiates from the loin to the groin.
- Nausea and vomiting often occur with renal colic.
- The patient cannot lie still and tends to be writhing around or walking about.
- There will be haematuria.

Management and nursing care

- Analgesia – pethidine may be used or a NSAID such as diclofenac.
- Sieve all urine to 'catch' the stone.
- High fluid intake.
- Test urine for blood.
- Send an MSU for culture.
- Investigations – IV urogram.

A small stone will pass spontaneously. Larger stones will need to be extracted or dissolved using ultrasound.

Measures to prevent recurrence may need to be taken. These will depend partly on the type of stone but the patient should be encouraged to raise his fluid intake, especially in summer.

ACUTE RENAL FAILURE

This is an acute failure of renal excretory function due to depression of the glomerular filtration rate lasting for days or weeks, accompanied by a rapidly rising serum urea, creatinine and potassium (K^+).

> ⚠️ Acute renal failure can cause sudden, life-threatening disturbances in the biochemistry of the blood and is a medical emergency.

Causes

Prerenal
May be prerenal when there is a failure of blood supply to the kidneys. Occurs with hypovolaemia and hypotension

- Haemorrhage
- Burns
- Diarrhoea
- Diuretics

Decreased cardiac output and hypotension

- Myocardial infarction
- Massive pulmonary embolism
- Congestive cardiac failure

Renal vasoconstriction

- Sepsis
- Non-steroidal antiinflammatory drugs

Systemic vasodilatation

- Liver disease
- Sepsis
- Drugs

The kidney is structurally normal but functionally compromised and function will return to normal rapidly if a good blood supply is restored. However, if severe or prolonged, these factors may lead to acute tubular necrosis.

Renal
May be renal when there are established structural abnormalities in the kidney.

- Acute tubular necrosis (ATN), which is due to ischaemia of the medulla of the kidney and is secondary to poor renal circulation.
- All the prerenal causes above can lead to ATN.
- The outcome of the condition depends on the severity and duration of the ischaemia.
- Even relatively mild cases may last for up to 6 weeks.
- Glomerulonephritis.
- Drug-induced nephrotoxicity.
- Interstitial nephritis.
- Malignant hypertension.
- Blood transfusion.

Postrenal
Although this is more likely to be chronic renal failure.

- Bilateral ureteric obstruction.

- Bladder outflow obstruction, e.g. prostatic enlargement, stones, pelvic mass.

Clinical features

- Oliguria (production of an abnormally small amount of urine: <400 ml in 24 hours).
- Early stages may be asymptomatic despite the accumulation of metabolites in the blood.
- Symptoms are commonly present when the blood urea rises above 40 mmol/l but may occur before this.
- Nausea and vomiting.
- Confusion.
- Loss of appetite.

Clinical progression of acute renal failure with recovery is in three phases.

- *Oliguria* – usually lasts 1–3 weeks but may regress in hours or may be extended to several weeks, dependent on renal damage.
- *Diuresis* – as renal function improves, diuresis is progressive. In the early phase the renal tubules are still damaged and there is danger of hypokalaemia. Fluid losses may be up to 3–4 l daily and volume depletion may occur. Fluid and electrolyte balance needs to be carefully monitored.
- *Recovery*.

Management and nursing care

Fluid balance

- In the hypovolaemic patient fluid replacement is essential (see p. 125).
- In acute renal failure of any cause, the fluid intake must be adjusted

so that the patient is neither hypovolaemic nor overloaded.
- Urine output must be accurately measured hourly and the patient will be catheterized.
- Any other fluid losses such as diarrhoea, sweat and vomit must be charted.
- The patient may be weighed daily to monitor fluid balance.
- If the patient is overloaded diuretics may be used and fluid intake limited.

Hyperkalaemia

Potassium levels rise in renal failure (hyperkalaemia) and patients will need to restrict their fluid intake.

Fruit and fruit juices are high in potassium.

Hyperkalaemia can lead to cardiac arrhythmias and the patient will be attached to a cardiac monitor.

Measures may need to be taken to reduce the serum potassium. Calcium resonium is an ion exchange resin that may be used either orally or rectally. In acute renal failure insulin and glucose bring down serum potassium levels faster and may be administered according to a standard regime.

Acidosis

The pH of the blood is normally kept within the narrow range of 7.35–7.45. If there are excess hydrogen ions that are not being eliminated, the pH will fall and acidosis occurs. This happens in renal failure (see p. 68).

Sodium bicarbonate (an alkali) may be used to counteract this but can cause oedema and hypertension.

Dialysis

Uraemic toxins can be removed by dialysis and this is indicated if the plasma potassium remains high, acidosis occurs, pulmonary oedema is present or there is a symptomatic uraemia.

CHRONIC RENAL FAILURE (CRF)

This is a permanent reduction in glomerular filtration rate caused by loss of nephrons. In the early stages the plasma urea and creatinine will not be raised but there is impaired concentrating ability in the kidneys and this leads to polyuria and thirst. As the condition worsens there will be sodium and water retention.

Causes
- Glomerulonephritis
- Diabetes mellitus
- Chronic pyelonephritis
- Polycystic kidneys
- Hypertension

Clinical features

The early stages may be asymptomatic. Most symptoms appear when the glomerular filtration rate (GFR) is reduced to 10–15 ml/min (normal GFR is 120 ml/min).

Eventually the metabolism of the body becomes very disordered in chronic renal failure, uraemia results and most body systems are affected.

Gastrointestinal tract
- anorexia
- nausea
- vomiting
- hiccups

Skin
- Itching
- Uraemic frost – if the urea is very high it may crystallize in the sweat: rare

Blood
- Anaemia due to reduced erythropoietin and depression of the bone marrow by uraemic toxins
- Tendency to bleed due to abnormal platelet function – mainly capillaries

Cardiovascular system
- Hypertension, anaemia and fluid retention may lead to heart failure
- Increased incidence of coronary artery disease due to abnormal fat metabolism

Bones

Renal osteodystrophy is caused by:

- increased bone resorption
- inadequate vitamin D production

and may cause:

- bone pain
- occasionally pathological fractures

Nervous system
- Accumulation of toxic metabolites leads eventually to uraemic neuropathy.

- Poor concentration, apathy, insomnia and irritation occur at first.
- Slurring of speech, tremors and seizures may occur eventually if untreated.
- Peripheral neuropathy may occur in the late stages of renal failure.
- In children failure to grow is an important complication.

Management and nursing care

The aim is to prevent any further decline in renal function.

- Treatment of underlying factors – hypertension, infection.
- Control of blood pressure with antihypertensive agents reduces the rate of progress of CRF.
- Removal of nephrotoxic drugs from medication.
- The client will be under the care of the dietitian. There is much ongoing research into the amount of protein that should be recommended in CRF. There can be both deficiency and toxicity present. Protein restriction is not usually commenced until GFR falls to 25 ml/min; there is some evidence that earlier restriction may delay the onset of symptomatic uraemia but this is controversial.
- Patients may have a negative salt and water balance which needs correcting. High fluid intake allows excretion of metabolites despite inability to concentrate the urine.
- Fluid restriction may be needed in patients with oedema.
- Potassium intake is restricted to reduce hyperkalaemia.

- Occasionally calcium resonium may be prescribed.
- Anaemia can be treated with synthetic (recombinant) human erythropoietin.
- Patient education and involvement in care help to prepare for the future and the possibility of dialysis or transplantation.
- Job prospects and finances need to be discussed.

END-STAGE RENAL FAILURE (ESRF)

This is terminal renal failure and occurs when the kidney function is so poor that the patient requires dialysis or renal transplantation to survive.

Renal replacement therapy

The aim is to mimic the excretory functions of the normal kidney, including the excretion of nitrogenous waste such as urea and the maintenance of fluid and electrolyte balance (see p. 125).

Haemodialysis

The blood from the patient is pumped through a dialyser which is a collection of semipermeable membranes ('artificial kidney'). These bring the blood into close contact with the dialysing fluid and the biochemistry of the blood changes towards that of the dialysate due to diffusion of molecules down their concentration gradient. The concentration gradient is maintained by replacing used dialysis fluid with fresh solutions.

An adult of average size usually requires 4–5 hours of haemodialysis three times a week, which may be performed in hospital or by home dialysis.

All patients are anticoagulated, usually with heparin, as contact with foreign surfaces activates clotting mechanisms.

Haemofiltration

This removes plasma water and its dissolved constituents such as K^+, Na^+, urea and phosphate by convective flow across a high-flux semipermeable membrane and replaces it with a solution of desired biochemical composition. It can be used for acute or chronic renal failure. High volumes need to be exchanged to achieve adequate removal and in acute renal failure 1000 ml/hour is exchanged. It is often performed on very sick patients in intensive care units.

Peritoneal dialysis

This is used for less severe renal failure.

The dialysate is fed into the peritoneal cavity via a flexible tube and the peritoneum itself acts as the semipermeable membrane.

Continuous ambulatory peritoneal dialysis is now used (CAPD). Two litre exchanges are performed three or four times a day. This technique is easy to learn and in chronic renal failure the patient can use it at home.

Bacterial peritonitis is the commonest severe complication of peritoneal dialysis. Infection with *Staph. epidermidis* is responsible for about 50% of cases. Treatment is with peritoneal antibiotics.

Transplantation

The only complete rehabilitation in ESRF is successful renal transplantation. In very successful units, graft survival is 80% at 10 years. The kidney can be obtained from cadavers or, more frequently nowadays, close relatives with ABO compatibility and close HLA matching.

Graft rejection is reduced by giving long-term immunosuppressive therapy with corticosteroids, azathioprine and cyclosporin.

GLOMERULONEPHRITIS

This is an inflammatory response (see p. 19) within the kidney due to the deposition of immune complexes in the glomerulus. The cause is often unknown but antigens derived from certain viruses or bacteria are sometimes involved.

Some causes of glomerulonephritis

- Beta-haemolytic streptococcus
- *Streptococcus viridans* (infective endocarditis)
- Mumps virus
- Hepatitis B virus
- Tropical infections, e.g. schistosomiasis
- Systemic lupus erythematosus (SLE)
- Malignant tumours
- Drugs, e.g. penicillamine

Clinical features

Glomerular nephritis presents in one of four ways:

- asymptomatic proteinuria/haematuria

- acute nephrotic syndrome (acute glomerular nephritis)
- nephrotic syndrome
- renal failure.

Acute glomerular nephritis

This is often a poststreptococcal nephritis. It typically develops in a child, 1–3 weeks after a streptococcal sore throat. The antigens from the bacteria become trapped in the glomerulus, leading to acute glomerulonephritis.

There is an abrupt onset.

Clinical features

- Haematuria (macroscopic or microscopic)
- Proteinuria
- Hypertension
- Oedema – around eyes but may also be feet and ankles
- Oliguria
- Uraemia

Treatment

- Antibiotics to clear up any remaining infection.
- Good prognosis and spontaneous recovery usually takes place.
- Hypertension is treated with salt restriction, diuretics and vasodilators.
- Fluid balance is monitored by daily weighing and a fluid chart.
- Fluid restriction may be necessary if oliguria is present.
- In some cases due to SLE, steroids, e.g. prednisilone, may be given as immunosuppressants.

NEPHROTIC SYNDROME

This is not a disease but a triad of symptoms:

- heavy proteinuria (> 3.5 g/24 hours)
- hypoalbuminaemia
- oedema – severe and affects the eyes, face, ankles and genitals.

Blood lipids are usually raised.

All types of glomerulonephritis can cause the nephrotic syndrome. Other damage to the basement membrane in the glomerulus can also be responsible, e.g. advanced diabetic nephropathy.

When present as a secondary complication of renal disease, the prognosis is usually more severe.

Of those who have a remission, approximately 30% relapse within 3 years.

Treatment

- In children a renal biopsy may not be necessary as most cases are secondary to acute glomerular nephritis. In an adult, a renal biopsy is often undertaken to establish the cause.
- Oedema is treated with rest, salt restriction and diuretics.
- Diuresis must not be too vigorous or it may precipitate circulatory collapse.
- Steroids are usually given, especially in children.
- The diet is normal protein, low salt and low fat.
- Occasionally albumin replacement may be necessary.
- The underlying cause, if known, should be treated.

UROLOGICAL TUMOURS

Renal cell carcinoma

Clinical features
- Classic triad of frank haematuria, loin pain and a loin mass.
- Intravenous urogram confirms the diagnosis.
- Renal ultrasound will be done.

Treatment
- Surgery – a radical nephrectomy for a unilateral tumour.
- Lung metastases are common.

Transitional cell carcinoma of the renal pelvis and ureter
- Haematuria and renal colic are the presenting signs.
- Treatment is a nephroureterectomy.
- Postoperative radiotherapy may be given.
- Check cystoscopies as can recur around the ureteric orifice.

Carcinoma of the bladder
- Male:female is 3:1.
- 5000 deaths per year.
- Non-invasive papillary tumour – bladder warts.
- May be single or multiple.
- 5–10% progress to become invasive.

Carcinoma in situ
- Thirty to fifty percent progress to invasive. Most recurrences are in the first 2 years.
- Can be multifocal.

Invasive carcinoma
- Sixty percent have no previous history of bladder tumours.
- Lymphatic involvement and spread via the lymphatics.

Risk factors
Associated with smoking and exposure to aniline dyes as well as urinary stasis.

Treatment
Cystoscopic resection and regular cystoscopic follow-up for superficial tumours.

For invasive tumours, options will depend on the tumour and include:

- radiotherapy
- cystectomy (removal of the bladder)
- partial cystectomy.

4.6 THE NERVOUS SYSTEM

The nervous system consists of:

- the central nervous system – the brain and spinal cord (Fig. 4.9)
- the peripheral nervous system – somatic and autonomic nervous systems.

THE BRAIN

Divided into the forebrain, midbrain and hindbrain. The forebrain is called the cerebrum and is the largest part. It receives and interprets sensory input and is responsible for motor output.

There are two cerebral hemispheres. A lesion of one hemisphere shows its effects on the opposite side of the body. The left is the dominant hemisphere in all right-handed people and also in 70%

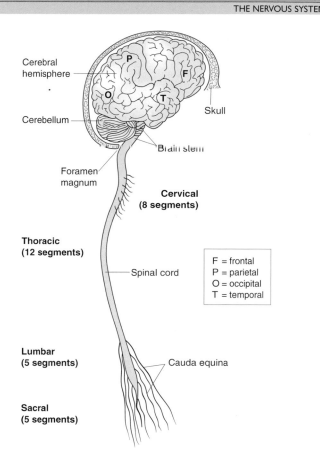

Fig. 4.9 The central nervous system. From Bickerstaff/Neurology for Nurses, reproduced with permission of Arnold

of those apparently left-handed. The speech area is in the dominant hemisphere.

Clinical features of lesions of the cerebral hemispheres depend on the focus of a cerebral lesion. Abnormalities depend upon:

• the lobe affected by the lesion
• how large the lesion is

• how deeply it extends into the brain.

Destruction of the motor area in the frontal lobe produces a *hemiplegia* – paralysis down one side of the body. A lesion in the occipital lobe will affect vision. A parietal lobe lesion will affect sensation on the opposite side of the body.

- *Aphasia* is loss of or defect in language and is caused by lesions that affect the speech area (usually the left frontoparietal region).
- *Dysphasia* is difficulty in speaking and is very common following a stroke if the damage is to the left side of the brain.
- *Dysarthria* is disordered articulation that could occur due to problems with facial muscles or weakness and is common in Parkinson's disease, for instance.

An irritative lesion of the cerebral cortex can produce convulsions of the opposite side of the body.

The cerebellum is responsible for maintaining posture and balance. A lesion may produce the following on the same side of the body:

- decreased muscle tone
- reduced tendon reflexes
- flexor plantar reflexes
- intention tremor
- marked ataxia

There are 12 cranial nerves that originate in the brain. Neurological disease can affect any of these. The cranial nerves are detailed in Table 4.5.

Papilloedema is swelling of the optic disc seen through the ophthalmoscope. It may be an early sign of a tumour in the brain but is also seen in oedema of the brain, accelerated hypertension, optic neuritis and subarachnoid haemorrhage.

Clinical signs of damage to nervous tissue
- Destruction leads to paralysis or loss of sensation.

- If there is damage to the motor system, weakness or wasting of the muscles will result. If damage is to the sensory system, tingling or pain may result.

Motor neurons
Lesions may affect the upper motor neuron, between the brain and spinal cord, or the lower motor neuron, between the spinal cord and the muscle. Clinical features of upper and lower motor neuron disease are shown in Figure 4.10 and Table 4.6.

LESIONS OF THE PERIPHERAL NERVES

These are mostly mixed nerves that carry both motor and sensory fibres. Each supplies a specific muscle group and has an area of skin from which sensation is carried. Damage to the nerve will lead to weakness in a group of muscles and a patch of analgesia and anaesthesia.

Sometimes many nerve endings may be diseased together and symptoms will be present in the periphery of all four limbs. This occurs in diabetic neuropathy, polyneuritis and other causes of peripheral neuropathy.

LESIONS OF THE SPINAL CORD

Complete destruction at any point causes paralysis and loss of sensation to all parts of the body supplied by nerves leaving or entering the cord below the level of the lesion. A lesion in the cervical spine will paralyse the arms, legs

Table 4.5 Cranial nerves – some lesions affecting their functions

Nerve number	Name	Controls	Lesion causes	Caused by
I	Olfactory	Smell	Loss of smell	Head injury Tumour of optic groove
II	Optic	Vision	Visual field defect or loss of sight	Compression in pituitary tumour or aneurysm Papilloedema Optic neuritis
III	Oculomotor	Eye movements	Unilateral complete ptosis, eye facing down and out, fixed and dilated pupil	Aneurysm, coning of the temporal lobe, tumour
IV	Trochlear	Eye movements	Diplopia	Isolated lesion rare
V	Trigeminal	Sensory for light and touch. Motor for mastication	Sensory loss in face, reduced corneal reflex Pain in trigeminal neuralgia	MS, brainstem glioma and other tumours, aneurysm Trigeminal neuralgia – unknown cause
VI	Abducens	Eye movements	Convergent squint with diplopia	MS, compressed in raised ICP May be infiltrated by nasopharyngeal cancer
VII	Facial	Muscles of facial expression	Unilateral facial weakness	Bell's palsy, trauma, infection of middle ear, tumours, herpes zoster
VIII	Vestibulo-cochlear	Hearing, balance and posture	Deafness and tinnitus Vertigo Nystagmus	Ménière's disease Middle ear infection Noise Vestibular neuritis
IX	Glosso-pharyngeal	Sensation to throat and taste	Usually IX and X together	Glossopharyngeal neuritis – painful throat on swallowing – rare
X	Vagus	Muscle of pharynx (gag), larynx and oesophagus Parasympathetic supply to heart and gut	Loss of gag reflex Depression of cough reflex Paralysis of vocal cords Difficulty in swallowing, choking and hoarseness	Motor neuron disease Cancer of nasopharynx Polyneuropathy Brainstem infarct
XI	Accessory	Motor to trapezius and sternomastoid	Weakness of rotation of head and neck	Motor neurondisease Cancer of nasopharynx Polyneuropathy Brainstem infarct
XII	Hypoglossal	Motor to tongue	Unilateral weakness, wasting and fasciculation of the tongue	Motor neuron disease Cancer of nasopharynx Trauma to the neck

ICP – intracranial pressure, MS – multiple sclerosis

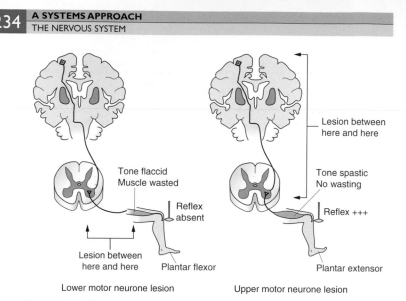

Fig. 4.10 Clinical features of upper and lower motor neuron disease. From Bickerstaff/ Neurology for Nurses, reproduced with permission of Arnold

Table 4.6   Some signs of upper and lower motor neuron disease

	Upper motor neuron	Lower motor neuron
Wasting	Slight	Very marked
Weakness	Could be any degree	Usually marked
Muscle tone	Increased (spastic)	Decreased (flaccid)
Tendon reflexes	Exaggerated	Absent
Plantar reflexes	Extensor	Flexor
Flexor spasms	Common	Do not occur
Fasciculation	Absent	Common if cells involved

and the respiratory muscles if high enough.

If there is partial damage to the cord a variety of clinical features are present affecting both movement and sensation.

TRAUMA

The skull provides very good protection but may be fractured by a severe blow. The fracture may be:

- simple
- compound
- comminuted
- depressed (Fig. 4.11).

The type of fracture is of little consequence as it is the damage to the brain below that is important.

Extradural haematoma

Follows trauma and is usually due to rupture of the middle meningeal artery. Bleeding occurs between the

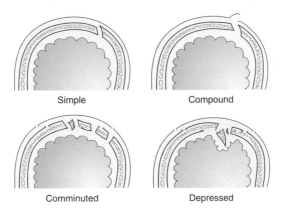

Fig. 4.11 Different types of skull fracture. From Bickerstaff/Neurology for Nurses, reproduced with permission of Arnold

bone and the dura. Usually collects and enlarges fairly quickly (Fig. 4.12).

The patient may be knocked unconscious and recover consciousness rapidly but within a few hours:

- start to feel drowsy
- develop paralysis down one side of the body
- one pupil dilates due to pressure of the expanding haematoma
- requires emergency surgery to remove the clot.

If left untreated, the patient will die.

Subdural haematoma

- Due to head injury that may be minor.

- Fine arteries between the arachnoid and the dura mater are damaged.
- Blood collects slowly and signs may be delayed over a period of days or weeks.
- Patient may have variations in drowsiness and fits as the cerebral cortex is irritated.
- Complains of increasing headache.
- Usually involves a fractured skull in the young but in the elderly may occur without.
- Treatment is by surgical evacuation of the clot.

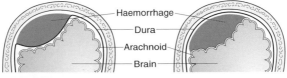

Fig. 4.12 Extradural and subdural haematomas. From Bickerstaff/Neurology for Nurses, reproduced with permission of Arnold

Traumatic subarachnoid bleeding

- The vessels between the arachnoid and pia maters may be torn and bleeding into the subarachnoid space occurs.
- On recovering consciousness the patient will have severe headache and stiffness of the neck that gradually improve.

SUBARACHNOID HAEMORRHAGE (SAH)

This is a spontaneous intracranial haemorrhage where the bleeding occurs into the subarachnoid space between the arachnoid and pia maters. It accounts for about 10% of cerebrovascular disease.

It is usually due to a weakness in the vessel wall. An aneurysm or bulge may be present in one of the cerebral arteries and is called a *berry aneurysm* because of its shape. SAH is due to berry aneurysms in 70% of cases, 10% are due to arteriovenous malformation and in 20% no lesion is found.

Clinical features

- The patient may be young and have a history of headaches or may rapidly develop a devastating occipital headache that spreads down the back of the neck.
- Vomiting occurs.
- *Photophobia* (dislike of the light) is present.
- Neck stiffness.
- Restlessness and irritability occur.
- There is often loss of consciousness.

- If small, the blood will be reabsorbed but if large, paralysis and death can follow.

Investigations

- CT scan.
- Cerebrospinal fluid (CSF) is pink because of the blood it contains.
- Carotid and vertebral angiography to establish the site of bleeding prior to surgery.
- Needs to be differentiated from severe migraine and meningitis.

Care and management

- Nearly half the cases die before they reach hospital.
- A further 10–20% die in the following few weeks due to a second bleed.
- Patients unconscious or with severe neurological deficits have a poor prognosis.
- Neurosurgery may be performed to clip the neck of the aneurysm and prevent further bleeding.
- Immediate treatment is bedrest and supportive measures.
- Hypertension should be controlled.
- Nimodipine is a calcium channel blocker that has been shown to reduce morbidity.

EPILEPSY

People who have epilepsy show a tendency to have recurrent seizures (also known as fits) with little or no provocation. Epilepsy is not a disease, it is a disorder or condition. A seizure is an altered chemical state of the brain leading to bursts of excessive electrical activity within it.

Some causes of epilepsy

- Head injury
- Brain infection, e.g. meningitis
- Stroke
- Brain damage – could be birth trauma or hypoxia
- Drugs and alcohol
- Biochemical imbalance
- Hormonal changes
- Cerebral palsy
- Brain tumour
- 50% no known cause

Causes of individual seizures

- Forgotten or incorrect medication
- Lack of sleep
- Stress
- Excitement
- Boredom
- Alcohol
- Flashing lights (only 3–5% of people with epilepsy are photosensitive)
- Drugs

Common types of seizure

Generalized
- Tonic-clonic
- Absence
- Tonic
- Atonic
- Myoclonic

Partial (focal)
- Simple partial – no impairment of consciousness
- Complex partial – with impairment of consciousness
- Secondary generalized – start as partial but evolve to tonic-clonic

There are also *febrile convulsions* in children with a high temperature.

Pseudoseizures are of behavioural or psychological origin.

Care and management

Emergency treatment of a seizure is to ensure that the patient does himself no harm and that the airway is patent.

Wooden mouth gags, tongue forceps and physical restraint should not be used as they cause more harm than good (see p. 22).

Anticonvulsant drugs are used for long-term treatment. Examples are phenytoin, sodium valproate and carbamazepine. Ideally the epilepsy should be controlled with one drug (see p. 20).

Status epilepticus

This is when seizures follow each other without recovery of consciousness. It is a medical emergency and there is a risk of death from cardiorespiratory failure.

It is necessary to stop the fitting and intravenous diazepam may be given. Some patients may need to be anaesthetized and ventilated.

PARKINSON'S DISEASE

This is the most common cause of progressive neurological disorder in older patients. It is increasing in incidence alongside longevity.

It is due to a loss of nerves in an area of the brain called the substantia nigra. These cells are in the basal ganglia, an area of the brain that has a role in regulating motor function. The cells here use a neurotransmitter called *dopamine* and in Parkinson's disease there is a reduced ability of the cells in the substantia nigra to manufacture dopamine.

Dopamine is one of two transmitters produced and usually they are in balance. The other one is *acetylcholine* (ACH). When there is a reduction in dopamine this means that the ACh has excessive action. The symptoms of Parkinson's disease are due to a decline in dopamine and a relative excess of ACh. Parkinson's disease is progressive but with the treatments now available, life expectancy is near normal.

The loss of cells from the substantia nigra and the progress of the disease occur at variable rates and to a variable extent. Some patients may become rapidly disabled in a few years and others may have a mild, slowly progressive disorder that does not need treatment for several years. The majority of cases fall in between these two extremes and the condition slowly becomes more incapacitating over a period of about 10 years.

Aetiology

Parkinson's disease is common worldwide but the aetiology is not completely understood. In Britain it affects 1:1000 of the population and has a prevalence rate of about 1 in 200 over the age of 70. Males and females are equally affected. In two-thirds of cases the first symptoms occur between the ages of 50 and 60 years.

Most cases are idiopathic, i.e. the cause is not understood, but there are likely to be some environmental elements alongside a genetic risk of developing the disease.

Some known causal factors include the following.

- Postinfective – survivors of a disease called encephalitis lethargica (sleeping sickness), an epidemic between 1916 and 1926.

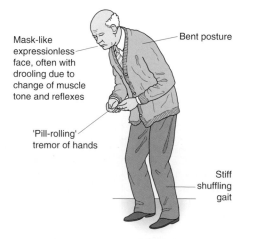

Fig. 4.13 Some features of Parkinson's disease. From Mallett J, Bailey C/Manual of Clinical Nursing Procedures 4e, reproduced with permission.

- Intracranial tumours.
- Ischaemia (lack of blood supply) in that part of the brain due perhaps to atherosclerosis.
- Cerebral atrophy.
- Trauma – often over a long period, e.g. boxing.
- Toxic substances:
  —drugs of the phenothiazine group that are used in schizophrenia: these work by blocking dopamine and so can lead to drug-induced symptoms of Parkinson's disease
  —copper: Wilson's disease
  —manganese and mercury also when used in industrial processes
  —carbon monoxide
  —MPTP: an impurity formed when opioids are manufactured illegally. In the 1970s in California there was an epidemic of young people with rapidly progressive Parkinson's disease following administration of illegal heroin.

Clinical features

It is believed that there is a long presymptomatic phase in Parkinson's disease and the dopamine produced by the brain is reduced by 70–80% before any symptoms appear.

Tremor

- Present at rest at first and reduced or eliminated by movement. It usually starts in one hand or arm and takes 2–3 years to spread to the other hand and arm.
- The tremor is rhythmic in nature and may be described as a 'pill-rolling movement'. It is less marked when the patient is involved in activity and is absent in sleep but is increased by stress, fatigue and cold. It eventually spreads to include the lips, face, tongue and lower limbs.
- Although the tremor is rarely disabling it is very upsetting for the patient and a cause of embarrassment and anxiety. It may limit the amount of socializing the patient feels able to do and such activities as eating out may be curtailed.

Rigidity

- This may occur in virtually all skeletal muscle and throughout the full range of movement of the joints. Rigidity may be present in the limbs, trunk and neck.
- In the limbs it has a 'cogwheel' effect and also affects such actions as turning in bed. Satin-type sheets may help here.
- Fine movements such as fastening buttons become difficult.
- As the disease progresses there is a stooped posture and the body and head are flexed forward. The acceleration present in the steps when walking may now lead to falls.

Bradykinesia (slowness or poverty of movement) and akinesia (lack of spontaneous movement)

- At first this leads to a difficulty with fine movements such as fastening buttons.
- The writing becomes smaller.
- When the legs are affected this leads to a 'shuffling gait'. The patient starts walking slowly but then speed builds up – *festinating gait*.

- Hesitation at doorways and difficulty in entering.
- Need to make a deliberate effort to initiate all movement.
- As spontaneous movement declines there is a mask-like expression.
- The hands no longer swing on walking.
- The eyes do not blink and there is a staring expression.
- The speech becomes a monotone and dysarthria occurs. Speech is weak and slurred.
- There is difficulty in eating and increased salivation. This is embarrassing and tends to lead to a desire to eat alone.
- There are slow reaction times.
- Later the cough reflex may be lost and chest infections occur.
- Fatiguability of repeated movements.
- Difficulty in performing two movements at once, e.g. rising from a chair and shaking hands.

Postural instability

This makes turning difficult and there is poor balance on standing and moving. This may result in frequent falls.

Common problems

Constipation

- Due to lack of exercise and problems with chewing and swallowing as well as actual problems in defaecation, sometimes due to spasm of the sphincter.
- Mental capacity is not usually affected although there is a 20% risk of some dementia occurring.

- The diagnosis may be made by the GP and the patient treated at home but you will meet many patients with Parkinson's disease on care of the elderly wards.

Eating

- It becomes difficult to cut up food and eating a meal takes a long time.
- As there is loss of control of hand movement, it may be difficult to prevent spillage.
- Excessive salivation adds to the embarrassment of the patient.
- Due to muscular rigidity and paucity of movement, there are problems with chewing and swallowing so the patient needs encouragement to eat and a diet that can be easily managed.

Communication

- The same person is still there inside a body that feels as though it will no longer do what is asked of it.
- This means there is still a strong desire to communicate and show facial expressions such as smiling.
- The presence of a mask-like expression and the inability to respond rapidly to conversation, together with a monotonous slow voice, mean that the patient may become introverted and avoid company.
- Education of those around the client will enable them to understand the condition and so promote better communication.

Depression

This may accompany the disease and may be partly due to the chronic nature of the illness and its effect on social activity. Doctors may treat this with antidepressant drugs with reasonable success in some patients.

> ⚠ **Always remember that the client with Parkinson's disease usually has an active mind locked inside a body that will not allow communications such as facial expression and talking clearly.**

Drug treatment of Parkinson's disease

Selegeline
Prevents the breakdown of dopamine in the brain and is often used as the first-line treatment.

Levodopa
The introduction of levodopa in the 1960s revolutionized the treatment of Parkinson's disease. Although it is dopamine that the brain is lacking, it cannot be given as treatment as it does not pass the blood–brain barrier and remains in the peripheral circulation. Levodopa is the precursor of dopamine and it does get into the brain. It is converted into dopamine by an enzyme in the brain tissue. It is given as Madopar or Sinemet and treatment starts with low doses. There are problems with long-term treatment and this means the drug should not be used until necessary.

MULTIPLE SCLEROSIS (MS)

Multiple sclerosis (MS) is a common disease of unknown cause whereby areas of discrete demyelination develop at many sites in the brain and the spinal cord. It is one of the commonest causes of neurological disability amongst people under the age of 50. The disease usually presents between 20 and 40 years of age. It affects 1 in 2000 of the population in this country but less than 1 in 100 000 in equatorial regions. The highest incidence in the world is in Orkney and Shetland.

Lesions develop at different sites at different times, usually with some capacity for regeneration and restoration of function. Remyelination is never complete and the new myelin is thinner than the old.

The sizes of the plaques vary and ongoing disability is variable. Nerve conduction in the affected axon is slow and inefficient.

The disease usually takes the form of relapses and remissions but in some cases a slowly progressive deficit occurs.

Aetiology
- Cause is not known.
- Believed to be an autoimmune disorder.
- Commoner in females than males – ratio 1.5:1.
- Increased incidence in close relatives – about 10-fold.
- More common in temperate than equatorial regions. Those who move to a low-risk area before puberty acquire low risk. If they move after puberty, they do not.
- Higher consumption of animal fat in high-risk areas.
- Some antibodies, e.g. to the measles virus, are higher in those with MS.

Clinical features

- The onset may be acute or insidious and because of the highly variable distribution of the plaques, signs and symptoms are varied.
- A common first symptom is blurring of vision due to a lesion affecting the optic nerve. Colour vision may be affected. Recovery usually occurs in 4–8 weeks and 5 years later, the patient often has difficulty remembering which eye was affected.
- Twenty-five percent of patients present with visual symptoms.
- Thirty percent of those with optic neuritis have no other evidence of MS and do not go on to develop the disease.
- Brainstem demyelination may cause diplopia, vertigo, facial numbness and dysphagia.

If a lesion affects the spinal cord it most often interferes with the legs and may cause:

- heaviness, dragging or weakness of arms or legs
- loss of pain and temperature sensation
- tingling, numbness, sense of coldness, sense of skin wetness in arms or legs
- bladder or bowel dysfunction:
  —spastic bladder: frequency, urgency, precipitance of micturition, ultimately incontinence
  —spastic bowel: constipation.

Remissions may last for many years and their length is unpredictable
Fatigue and depression both may be problems as the disease progresses. Intellectual function is usually preserved.

Features are often worse in hot weather, after a hot bath, during fever and after exertion.

Prognosis

- Seventy-five percent relapse and remit.
- Twenty percent have no significant disability after 5 years.
- Average life expectancy is 20–30 years.
- Five percent of cases are rapidly progressive and fatal within 5 years.
- Poor prognostic factors are late age of onset, development of dementia and early ataxia.
- There is relative protection from the disease in pregnancy but an increase in the proportion of attacks in the postnatal period.

Investigations

There is no single diagnostic test for MS.

- CSF examination has been used to support the diagnosis. White cells and protein are often raised.
- Magnetic resonance imaging (MRI) identifies the plaques readily and may be useful when diagnosis is unsure.

Treatment

- A potentially disabling disease with no curative treatment. Wide variations in severity and course of the disease.
- Corticosteroids may promote remissions and probably relieve oedema and inflammation in the plaques. They have no effect on the outcome of a relapse and do not protect against a further relapse.

- Long-term immunosuppression has been tried but is not proven to help.
- Treatment is symptomatic and supportive.
- Muscle relaxants, e.g. baclofen, benzodiazepines and dantrolene reduce the pain and discomfort of spasticity.
- There are four disease-modifying drugs licensed in the UK for use in MS. About 2–3% of those with MS receive these drugs compared to 13–15% in other European countries. The National Institute for Clinical Excellence (NICE) is determining whether these drugs should be prescribed.
- Interferon is a naturally occurring protein in the body which protects us against viruses. It has been manufactured in several forms using genetic engineering. Interferon beta–1a (Avonex) is given as a weekly injection and has been shown to reduce disability progression and exacerbations in some patients. Side-effects include flu-like symptoms and the injection should be given at bedtime.

MOTOR NEURON DISEASE

This is a progressive degenerative disease of unknown cause which affects the upper and lower motor neurons in the brain and spinal cord.

- It is of entirely unknown cause and affects 6 in 100 000 of the British population.
- Onset is uncommon before the age of 40.
- The mean survival is 3 years; 20% may live 5 years or more but it is doubtful if this is the same disease.
- The sensory system is not involved.
- There is degeneration of the anterior horn cells of the spinal cord and the lower motor neurons in the cranial nerves.
- Upper cranial nerves controlling eye movements and motor nerves to the bladder and bowel sphincters are spared.
- Family history in only a very small number of cases.
- Pathology is not inflammatory.
- No evidence to indicate an immune mechanism.
- Searches for toxic factors have been fruitless.
- The disease has a focal onset but becomes more generalized with time.

There are three main patterns of presentation.

Progressive muscular atrophy
- This usually gives lower motor neuron symptoms first.
- Wasting may begin in the small muscles of one hand and then spread through the arm. May begin unilaterally but soon spreads to both sides.
- Fasciculation is common and fibrillary twitching occurs.
- Cramps may occur.

Amyotrophic lateral sclerosis
- This is a disease of the lateral corticospinal tracts and produces a spastic paralysis.
- Amyotrophy means atrophy of muscle which would be unusual in other forms of spastic paralysis.

Progressive bulbar palsy

- Bulbar – relating to the medulla oblongata. Palsy – paralysis.
- Lower motor neuron degeneration only may occur here. More usually both upper and lower motor neuron degeneration occurs.
- Results in dysarthria, dysphagia, choking and regurgitation of fluids as common symptoms.
- This form is commoner in women than men for an unknown reason.

Course

- Remission is unknown.
- The disease progresses, spreading gradually and causes death.
- Survival for more than 3 years is most unusual.
- Awareness is preserved and dementia is unusual.
- Sphincter disturbances do not usually occur. If they do, it is very late in the disease.
- There is progressive respiratory paralysis and, together with aspiration pneumonia, this is the usual cause of death.
- Intermittent positive pressure ventilation only increases the length of suffering.

Treatment

- No treatment has been shown to alter the progression of the disease.
- Patients remain alert and drug treatment to alleviate distress is indicated.

DELIRIUM

This is a toxic confusional state where impaired consciousness is associated with abnormalities of perception or mood. Impairment of consciousness is variable and often fluctuates.

Confusion is often worse at night and there may also be hallucinations and delusions. Restlessness and aggression may be present.

Causes include:

- liver or renal failure
- disorders of electrolyte balance
- hypoxia
- hypoglycaemia
- vitamin B_{12} deficiency
- vitamin B_1 deficiency usually in alcoholics
- brain damage as in trauma, abscess, tumour or subarachnoid haemorrhage
- drug intoxication with anticonvulsants, opioids, anxiolytics or hypnotics.

Management is that of the underlying disease.

DEMENTIA

This is a chronic or persistent disorder of mental processes and is due to organic brain disease. It is marked by memory loss and disorders, personality changes, impaired ability to reason and disorientation. Consciousness is not affected.

It affects 10% of those aged 65 or over and 20% of those over 80 years of age.

There are many causes but the commonest is Alzheimer's disease, accounting for 70% of cases. Other causes include cerebral infarctions, alcoholism and hypothyroidism.

Alzheimer's disease

This is a degenerative condition of the brain, the cause of which is still not clear. There is a gradual reduction in neurons in parts of the brain and the deposition of amyloid plaques.

Clinical features
- Insidious onset (slow) that progresses over several years.
- Memory loss is usually the first sign.
- Slow disintegration of personality and intellect occurs.
- Difficulty with performing familiar tasks such as preparing a meal.
- Problems with language and word use.
- Disorientation to time and place.
- Poor and decreased judgement, e.g. may wear lots of jumpers on a hot day.
- Problems with abstract thinking.
- Misplacing things – putting things in unusual places.
- Changes in mood and behaviour – can show rapid mood swings.
- Changes in personality – may become very dependent on one person.
- Loss of initiative and desire to do things – may sit for hours in front of the television.
- All aspects of cortical function are eventually affected.

Investigations
- CT scanning will demonstrate cerebral atrophy and will exclude some other possible causes that could be curable, e.g. depression, adverse drug reactions and metabolic changes or nutritional deficiencies.
- There is no single diagnostic test. The patient needs a comprehensive assessment.

- Examination of the brain at autopsy will confirm.

Care and management
- This is extremely difficult as the disease is degenerative in nature.
- Although there is no cure for the disease, medical and social management can help all concerned.
- For those close to the patient it is hard to see their relative changing into perhaps an unrecognizable person with a different personality and weak intellectual ability.
- Management should be in the community if at all possible and support should be given to carers.
- There are four drugs currently approved for the treatment of Alzheimer's – tacrine (Cognex), donepezil (Aricept), rivastigmine (Exelon) and galantamine (Reminyl).

INFECTIVE AND INFLAMMATORY DISEASE

Meningitis
This is inflammation of the meninges which may be caused by bacteria, viruses, fungi, drugs and contrast media or blood (following SAH). Usually refers to infection by microorganisms, which reach the meninges by direct spread from the ears or nasopharynx, via a cranial injury or by spread in the bloodstream.
Bacteria causing meningitis include:

- *Neisseria meningitidis* (meningococcus)

- *Haemophilus influenzae*
- *Streptococcus pneumoniae*
- *Myobacterium tuberculosis*.

Clinical features
- Acute bacterial meningitis has a sudden onset with rigors and a high fever.
- A petechial rash is evidence of meningococcal meningitis.
- Severe headache, photophobia and vomiting are often present.
- Should be considered for all patients that have a headache and fever.
- Consciousness is not usually impaired although the patient may be delirious.
- Drowsiness and loss of consciousness signal complications such as venous sinus thrombosis, severe cerebral oedema or cerebral abscess.
- Mortality is about 15% even with treatment. The earlier the antibiotics are started, the better the prognosis.
- In fulminant meningococcal septicaemia there are often large ecchymoses (bruises) and gangrenous skin lesions may occur.

Diagnosis
- Confirmed by lumbar puncture.
- The CSF is cloudy due to the presence of pus. It is also sent for protein and glucose levels as well as microscopy. White cells in the CSF will be raised, protein will be raised and glucose may be low in the presence of bacteria.
- Blood cultures.

Care and management
- If the diagnosis is suspected intravenous antibiotics must be started immediately.
- Treatment is started with cefotaxime or penicillin. Those allergic to penicillin are given chloramphenicol.
- Subsequent antibiotic treatment depends on the CSF microscopy which tells us what the bacteria are sensitive to.
- All cases of meningitis must be notified to the local public health authority.

Meningococcal prophylaxis
Oral rifampicin is given to very close contacts to eradicate nasopharyngeal carriage of the meningococcus.

Viral meningitis
Usually a benign and self-limiting disease that lasts 4–10 days. Headache may continue for several weeks but there is no long-term damage.

Encephalitis
This is inflammation of the brain itself which may be caused by viruses or bacteria. In HIV infection, opportunistic organisms (e.g. *Toxoplasma gondii*) are important.

Acute viral encephalitis
Echo, coxsackie, mumps and herpes simplex are the most common causative viruses in Britain.

Clinical features
- Mostly a mild, self-limiting illness.
- Headaches and drowsiness.

- Sometimes severe with hemiparesis and dysphasia, seizures and coma.
- Usually due to herpes simplex when severe – mortality of about 20% with treatment.
- Prognosis is poor if the patient is in a coma.

Investigations
- Viral serology
- CT scan – shows oedema
- EEG may show slow wave activity.

Treatment
Herpes simplex, if suspected, is immediately treated with intravenous aciclovir.

Cerebral abscess
The causes are shown in Box 4.6 but often no direct cause is found.
   Common bacteria are *streptococci, staphylococci* and *enterobacter*. Sometimes a chronic abscess may be due to tuberculosis.

Clinical features
- Fever
- Seizures
- Focal neurological signs
- Raised intracranial pressure

Care and management
- Intravenous antibiotics
- Surgical drainage

INTRACRANIAL TUMOURS
These make up 2–7% of all tumours and 20% of childhood cancers. Primary brain tumours do not usually metastasize outside the brain but spread by local infiltration and may seed into the subarachnoid space or ventricles. Many brain tumours are secondaries from other primary tumours.

Primary tumours
Malignant (40%):

- gliomas
- astrocytoma – commonest
- oligodendroglioma

Benign (30%):

- meningioma – commonest
- neurofibroma

Secondary tumours (30%)
- Bronchus
- Breast
- Prostate

Clinical features
- Headache
- Altered mental function
- Convulsions
- Focal neurological deficit
- Raised intracranial pressure (ICP) may produce:
   —early morning headache
   —vomiting
   —papilloedema

Box 4.6 Causes of a cerebral abscess	
Direct spread of microorganisms	**Spread in bloodstream**
Skull fracture	Lung in bronchiectasis
Focus of infection in paranasal sinuses	Heart in endocarditis
Focus in middle ear	Bone in osteomyelitis

—hypertension
—bradycardia
—decreased conscious level

Investigations
- CT or MRI scanning
- Biopsy or CSF examination for histology
- If cerebral metastases are suspected then investigations for the primary tumour, e.g. chest X-ray

Care and management
This will depend on the tumour and the prognosis. Dexamethasone is a steroid that reduces cerebral oedema and is given to all patients with raised ICP or focal signs. It can produce outstanding improvements, with the unconscious patient often recovering consciousness.

Astrocytoma
- Differ in histological grade –a low-grade tumour has a 5-year survival of about 50%, high grade is 5%
- Surgery – may be repeated in low-grade tumours
- Radiotherapy mostly in unresectable low-grade tumours
- Chemotherapy – CCNU, a fat-soluble drug that crosses the blood–brain barrier, is the basis of treatment

Meningioma
- Tumour of the meninges of the brain.
- Very slow-growing and usually benign.
- Interval to recurrence following surgical excision is about 4 years.

- Surgery is usually the mainstay of treatment and radiotherapy is limited to those patients in whom surgical excision was incomplete or recurrence occurs.
- Prognosis is usually very good.

HYDROCEPHALUS

An excessive amount of CSF in the cranium. May occur when there is obstruction to the flow of CSF and is very rarely due to an increased production of CSF. In children it is due to a congenital malformation of the brain, meningitis or haemorrhage. In adults it may be due to:

- late presentation of a congenital defect
- cerebral tumour
- subarachnoid haemorrhage
- meningitis
- head injury.

Clinical features
- Headache
- Vomiting
- Papilloedema
- All caused by raised ICP
- May also be nystagmus

Treatment is usually surgical with the insertion of a shunt to drain the CSF.

DISEASES OF VOLUNTARY MUSCLE

These are the myopathies. Weakness is the dominant feature. Some may be congenital, e.g. muscular dystrophy, some are inflammatory and some may be associated with drugs, toxins and endocrine weakness.

Potassium deficiency (hypokalaemia) may cause a generalized flaccid weakness if severe.

Myasthenia gravis

An autoimmune disease where antibodies attack and destroy the acetylcholine receptors at the muscle endplate. The thymus gland is enlarged in about 70% of those under 40 and a thymic tumour is found in about 10%.

Clinical features

- Fatiguability.
- Proximal limb muscles, eye muscles and muscles of mastication and facial expression are those most commonly involved.
- In 65% of cases the eye muscles are the first to be involved.

Investigations

Tensilon test – injection of an anticholinesterase that prevents the destruction of acetylcholine results in rapid temporary improvement in the weakness.

Care and management

- Anticholinesterase drugs such as neostigmine are used.
- The dose is determined by the patient's response.
- In those under 45 years with severe disease, thymectomy may be performed.
- Immunosuppressive treatment may also be considered.

4.7 THE ENDOCRINE SYSTEM

The endocrine system, alongside the nervous system, is responsible for control and communication within the body. The glands are ductless and release their secretions directly into the bloodstream to act upon a target organ that may be far away from the gland itself.

THE PITUITARY GLAND

Although normally only the size of a pea, the pituitary gland secretes many vital hormones, the majority of which are important in the control of other endocrine glands. It is often known as 'the leader of the orchestra' or the master endocrine gland and is attached beneath the hypothalamus in a bony cavity (sella turcica) at the base of the skull. Pituitary hormones are shown in Table 4.7.

Diseases of the posterior pituitary gland

These are rare and are usually related to antidiuretic hormone (ADH) secretion.

Diabetes insipidus

- This is due to insufficient ADH.
- Leads to poyluria and polydipsia.
- It is most often due to a lesion in the hypothalamus or posterior pituitary gland. This would include tumours, aneurysms, thrombosis and infections.
- The person has either partial or total inability to concentrate the urine.

Table 4.7 Pituitary hormones

Hormone	Function
Anterior pituitary	
Growth hormone (GH or somatotrophin)	Stimulates the growth of long bones Increases protein synthesis
Adrenocorticotrophic hormone (ACTH)	Controls secretion of corticosteroid hormones from the adrenal cortex
Melanocyte-stimulating hormone (MSH)	Stimulates the production of melanin
Thyroid-stimulating hormone (TSH)	Stimulates the production of thyroid hormones by the thyroid gland
Gonadotrophins 1. Luteinizing hormone (LH)	Stimulates ovulation, corpus luteum formation and the production of progesterone Stimulates androgen synthesis in the testes
2. Follicle-stimulating hormone (FSH)	Stimulates the ripening of follicles in the ovary Stimulates the formation of sperm in the testes
Prolactin	Stimulates milk production after childbirth
Posterior pituitary	Hormones are synthesized in the hypothalamus but stored and released from the pituitary
Vasopressin (antidiuretic hormone – ADH)	Increases the reabsorption of water by the kidneys and so prevents excessive water loss from the body Also constricts the blood vessels
Oxytocin	Causes contraction of the uterus in labour Stimulates the flow of milk from the breast

- Total urine output varies between 4 l and 12 l per day.
- Usually there is an acute onset and dehydration may develop rapidly if fluids are not replaced.

Clinical presentation
- Polyuria
- Nocturia
- Thirst – especially a desire for cold drinks
- Low urine osmolality
- High plasma osmolality

Treatment
- Replacement therapy with a synthetic vasopressin analogue –

desmopressin (DDAVP) – may be needed.
- Oral hydration is often sufficient.

Pituitary tumours
These are usually benign, slow-growing adenomas. Symptoms may arise due to:

- over- or under-secretion of the hormones secreted by the pituitary gland
- pressure on the surrounding tissues
- infiltration of the tumour.

Overproduction
The tumour secretes the hormone of the cell type from which it arose.

This is no longer beneficial to the body and is not under control of normal feedback mechanisms.

- Growth hormone excess results in acromegaly or gigantism
- Prolactin excess
- Cushing's disease from excess ACTH

Underproduction

- This is due to pressure on the cells by the growing tumour.
- Leads to hypopituitarism.
- Progressive loss of hormones.
- Luteinizing hormone and follide-stimulating hormone are usually affected first, resulting in menstrual irregularity and amenorrhoea.
- Growth hormone (GH) loss may be silent except in children.
- TSH and ACTH are usually last affected, resulting in hypothyroidism and Addison's disease.
- ADH secretion is affected if the tumour extends to the hypothalamus.

Local effects

- Headaches.
- Visual loss with field defects. This is caused by pressure on the optic chiasma (where the optic nerves from the eye cross over in the brain). It can lead to blindness.
- Obesity and altered appetite and thirst due to involvement of the hypothalamus.
- Seizures.
- Early puberty may occur in children due to hypothalamic involvement.
- Hydrocephalus may result from an interruption in the flow of CSF.

Diagnosis

- Radiographic examination of the skull and CT scan in conjunction with contrast material.
- Laboratory evaluations.

Treatment

Surgery and radiation therapy are used.

Hypersecretion of growth hormone

- In a child this leads to gigantism. In an adult it leads to acromegaly.
- Relatively rare disorder.
- Fifteen percent of pituitary tumours do secrete growth hormone and the commonest cause of acromegaly is a pituitary adenoma.
- Occurs more frequently in women than men.
- Slow progressive disease which, if untreated, results in a decreased life expectancy.
- There is an increased risk of hypertension, left ventricular failure and diabetes mellitus.
- Headache and other symptoms of a space-occupying lesion may be present.

Diagnosis

- Measurement of serum GH
- Treatment
- Removal of the tumour or treatment with radiation therapy

THYROID GLAND

The activity of the thyroid gland affects the whole body. It is involved in the control of body metabolism and its hormones govern cellular oxygen consumption and thus all heat and energy production.

Produces the hormones thyroxine (T_4) and triiodothyronine (T_3). Thyroxine is the hormone produced in the greatest quantity and its release is stimulated by TSH from the pituitary gland.

Goitre

A goitre is an enlargement of the thyroid gland and may be due to either increased or decreased activity of the thyroid or a lack of iodine needed to synthesize thyroid hormones. It is commoner in women than men.

The thyroid may enlarge at puberty and in pregnancy but this is often associated with normal activity (*euthyroidism*) and does not warrant treatment.

It is often first noticed as a cosmetic defect and is usually painless. Large goitres can cause dysphagia (difficulty in swallowing) and difficulty in breathing when they compress the oesophagus or trachea.

Endemic goitre was common in areas where iodine content in the soil was low. It was so common in Derbyshire that it became known as 'Derbyshire neck'. Iodine is now added to foods, e.g. table salt, and endemic goitre is virtually unknown.

Thyrotoxicosis

This is due to increased activity of thyroid hormones, whatever the cause. It leads to:

- an increased metabolic rate
- heat intolerance
- increased tissue sensitivity to stimulation by the sympathetic nervous system.

Causes
- Hyperthyroidism – excess thyroid hormones are produced by the thyroid gland:
  —Graves' disease – autoimmune and familial
  —toxic nodular goitre
  —thyroid cancer:
  —increased TSH secretion
  —drugs – amiodarone
  —acute thyroiditis
- Ectopic thyroid tissue (outside the thyroid gland)
- Ingestion of excessive thyroid hormone

Clinical features
All forms of thyrotoxicosis share some common characteristics. These are shown in Figure 4.14.

Endocrine
- Enlarged thyroid gland (97–99% of cases)
- Increased breakdown of cortisol
- Hypercalcaemia (see p. 121) and decreased parathyroid hormone levels
- Decreased sensitivity to insulin due to increased degradation of insulin

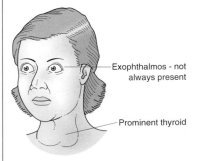

Fig. 4.14 Some features of thyrotoxicosis. From Govan/Pathology Illustrated, reproduced with permission.

Exophthalmos - not always present

Prominent thyroid

Gastrointestinal
- Weight loss and increased appetite
- More frequent passage of less formed stools due to increased peristalsis
- Decreased blood lipid levels due to malabsorption of fat

Skin – due to the hyperdynamic circulation
- Excessive flushing and warm skin
- Heat intolerance
- Sweating
- Fine, soft hair and sometimes temporary hair loss

Cardiovascular
- Tachycardia at rest (raised sleeping pulse rate)
- Increased cardiac output
- Palpitations and atrial fibrillation, especially in the elderly

Respiratory
- Breathlessness

Nervous system
- Hyperactivity and restlessness
- Insomnia
- Short attention span
- Tiredness
- Fine tremor

Eyes
- In Graves' disease there is exophthalmos – protrusion of the eye balls

- Elevated upper eyelid – leads to lack of blinking and staring expression
- Oedema of the conjunctiva
- Retroorbital inflammation and oedema, probably caused by antibodies, lead to protrusion of the eyes

Graves' disease
This is the commonest form of hyperthyroidism and is an autoimmune disorder where antibodies bind to the TSH receptor and stimulate the production of thyroxine. It is associated with other autoimmune disorders such as myasthenia gravis and pernicious anaemia. It affects more women than men, mostly between the ages of 20 and 40 years.

The thyroid is enlarged (goitre) and there is exophthalmos. The condition may relapse and remit.

Diagnosis of thyrotoxicosis
Clinically, a mild case may be difficult to differentiate from an anxiety state. Diagnosis may be obvious but treatment will never be started without biochemical tests, some of which are shown in Table 4.8. TSH is suppressed, T_3 and T_4 are raised.

Ultrasound may be used to determine the size and shape of the

Table 4.8 Thyroid function tests	
Test	Results
Total thyroxine (T_4)	Low in hypothyroidism Raised in thyrotoxicosis
Total T_3	Raised in thyrotoxicosis
TSH (immunoradiometric assay)	Suppressed in thyrotoxicosis Hypothyroidism Hypothalamic-pituitary disease

gland and whether there is any tracheal compression present.

Treatment of hyperthyroidism
Three possible treatments are available:

- antithyroid drugs – most cases initially
- radioactive iodine
- surgery.

Antithyroid drugs
Carbimazole 10–20 mg 8 hourly inhibits the formation of thyroid hormones. It is also an immunosuppressive agent. Improvement may not be seen for 10–20 days as although synthesis is reduced rapidly, thyroxine has a long half-life of 7 days (this means it is only eliminated slowly from the body).

Beta-blockers are used for more immediate symptomatic control as many of the symptoms are mediated via the sympathetic nervous system. Propranolol 40–80 mg 6–8 hourly may be used but should be avoided in asthma. The beta-blockers are stopped when a euthyroid state is obtained.

The production of thyroxine may be blocked totally by carbimazole and a replacement regime of thyroxine tablets, 0.1 mg daily, given. This is continued for 18 months and then reviewed.

> ⚠ The major side-effect of carbimazole is a potentially fatal, but reversible, agranulocytosis (1 in 1000 patients within 3 months of commencement of treatment) Regular white cell counts (every 3 months) must be done during drug therapy.

As an alternative, the dose of carbimazole may be reduced after 4–6 weeks, according to the levels of thyroid hormones. Review in 2–3 months and reduce again. Gradually over 12–18 months the dose is reduced to 5 mg daily and then when the patient is euthyroid on this, it is discontinued.

About 50% of patients will relapse and a repeat course of carbimazole or other forms of treatment, including surgery, will be considered.

Radioactive iodine therapy
- Administered orally in doses 100 times higher than those used for scanning.
- Usually used in middle-aged or elderly patients.
- The radioactive iodine is rapidly taken up by the gland and emission of radiation then destroys it.
- Very simple but results are slow to take effect and unpredictable.
- Late underactivity of the gland may occur, requiring thyroxine.
- Small theoretical risk of inducing malignancy.
- Absolutely contraindicated in pregnancy due to damage to the fetus.

Surgery

Subtotal thyroidectomy

Indications for surgery
- When quick and effective cure is required, especially in the young with Graves' disease.
- When antithyroid drugs have been unsatisfactory due to

persistent side-effects or non-compliance.

- More effective in some types of nodules and goitres.

Preoperative care

- Vocal cord function is assessed by indirect laryngoscopy. This looks at the function of the recurrent laryngeal nerve, which can occasionally be damaged in the operation.
- There may be a change in voice quality after any thyroidectomy and the patient should be warned of this.
- Whenever possible, patients should be rendered euthyroid prior to surgery.
- If they are thyrotoxic there are anaesthetic risks such as cardiac arrhythmias.
- Also, when the gland is manipulated in the operation, there can be a massive release of thyroid hormone into the bloodstream. This precipitates a thyroid crisis, which may be lethal.
- Thyroid activity is reduced by antithyroid drugs such as carbimazole in the weeks before surgery. Beta- blockers may also be used if control is difficult.
- Antithyroid drugs increase the blood flow to the thyroid and so are stopped 10–14 days before surgery. Potassium iodide (Lugol's iodine), 60 mg three times daily, is given by some surgeons to reduce the vascularity of the gland, although its efficacy is unproven.

Partial thyroidectomy

The aim is to remove enough of the gland to render the patient euthyroid whilst leaving enough of the gland to prevent hypothyroidism.

Complications of thyroid surgery

- In theatre uncontrolled haemorrhage is possible, but rare.
- Unilateral or bilateral damage to the recurrent laryngeal nerve in the operation presents as a laryngeal obstruction after tracheal extubation. It necessitates the performance of an immediate tracheostomy.

Immediate postoperative complications

- Major haemorrhage may cause severe blood loss and tracheal compression. This presents as a rapid swelling of the neck and a large volume of blood loss via the wound drain.
- To avoid suffocation from bleeding, a clip or suture-removing pack must always be at the patient's bed-side for emergency reopening of the wound.
- Emergency surgical exploration is essential to find the bleeding point.
- Laryngeal oedema – presents as stridor and may necessitate intubation.
- Thyrotoxic crisis – abrupt onset of extreme agitation and confusion, hyperpyrexia, profuse sweating and rapid tachycardia or arrhythmia. Requires emergency treatment with beta-blockers, intravenous hydrocortisone and potassium iodide.

- The mortality is 10% from coma, pulmonary oedema or circulatory collapse.

Late postoperative complications
- Hypoparathyroidism due to erroneous removal of the parathyroids, normally embedded in the four poles of the thyroid. This presents with muscle cramps, paraesthesia and tetany within 36 hours of operation.
- Unilateral recurrent laryngeal nerve damage – presents as hoarseness and defective cough.
- Superior laryngeal nerve damage leads to a change in quality of the voice.

Long-term complications
Hypothyroidism. May be overlooked as it develops slowly and insidiously. Loss of energy, weight gain, depression and an intolerance of cold weather are symptoms. Treatment is with thyroxine for life.

Thyroid cancer
- Relatively uncommon (<1% of all malignancies) and responsible for about 400 deaths each year in the UK. Types of thyroid cancer are shown in Table 4.9.
- Thyroidectomy is usually the treatment and this may be followed by radioactive iodine, which will be taken up by any remaining cancer cells and metastases.
- Replacement thyroxine will be needed.

Hypothyroidism
This is a reduced level of thyroid hormone and is sometimes called myxoedema because of swelling under the skin. It is the commonest disorder of the thyroid gland.

Aetiology
- Autoimmune thyroiditis. Antithyroid antibodies are produced and result in defective secretion of thyroid hormones. This leads to an increased production of TSH and often, a goitre. It is then called Hashimoto's disease. Sometimes the gland atrophies without producing a goitre. There may be

Table 4.9	Types of thyroid cancer			
Cell type	Frequency	Characteristics	Spread	Prognosis
Papillary	70%	Young people Slow growing	Local Sometimes lung and bone metastases (secondaries)	Good, especially in young
Follicular	20%	Commoner in females	Metastases to lung and bone	Good if resected
Anaplastic	<5%	Aggressive	Locally invasive	Very poor
Lymphoma	<2%	Variable		Sometimes responds to radiotherapy
Medullary cell	5%	Often familial	Local and metastases	Poor

a history of autoimmune disorders and 10% of patients also have pernicious anaemia.
- Loss of tissue following partial thyroidectomy.
- Disorders of the pituitary gland may cause a lack of TSH and so low secretion of thyroid hormones.
- Peripheral resistance to thyroid hormone may be the cause.

Clinical features
- Onset is insidious and the disease may be advanced before it is recognized. It may be confused with depression.
- Diminished energy and also physical tiredness.
- Intolerance to the cold. Cold skin.
- Diminished sweating.
- Increase in weight with decrease in appetite.
- Constipation.
- Hoarseness of the voice.
- Dry and rough skin; dry, brittle hair. Reduced nail growth.
- Slow thought processes and confusion; memory loss.
- Slow pulse rate.
- Slow respirations may lead to hypoventilation and carbon dioxide retention.

Investigations
- All suspected cases should be investigated.
- Thyroid hormone levels. There is a low level of thyroxine, which stimulates pituitary secretion of TSH.
- Anaemia may be present.
- ECG shows a slow rate and flattened or inverted T waves.
- Rise in titre of thyroid antibodies.

Treatment
Thyroxine is given in doses of 25–50 µg a day, starting with a low dose and raising it every 14 days until normal levels of TSH are achieved. The average daily maintenance dose is 250 µg. The patient should be warned that treatment is for life.

PARATHYROID GLANDS

Parathormone (PTH) from the parathyroid glands controls the concentration of calcium and inorganic phosphorus in the blood. It raises the plasma calcium by removal of calcium from bone, by increasing intestinal absorption of calcium and reducing renal excretion. It increases the synthesis of vitamin D and lowers serum phosphate by enhancing its excretion.

In health, parathormone levels rise as plasma calcium levels fall.

Hyperparathyroidism

Causes
- Parathyroid adenoma
- Conditions causing hypocalcaemia, e.g. chronic renal failure

Clinical features
- If mild, may be asymptomatic.
- Symptoms are related to hypercalcaemia. They include malaise, anorexia, nausea and vomiting. Drowsiness or confusion may occur.
- Peptic ulceration and acute pancreatitis.

- Kidney involvement may present with renal colic from stones, haematuria or polyuria from tubular damage.
- Bone pain suggests involvement of the bones and backache is common.

Investigations
- Plasma calcium is high and plasma phosphate is low.
- Alkaline phosphatase is raised, reflecting increased osteoblastic activity.
- Radiological changes may include demineralization.

Treatment
Surgical removal of the tumour.

Hypoparathyroidism
- This is a failure of secretion and is rare.
- Major causes are postnatal and postsurgical following thyroidectomy.
- Idiopathic hypoparathyroidism may be associated with autoimmune disorders such as Addison's disease.
- Clinical features are caused by hypocalcaemia.
- Tetany occurs, which is characterized by carpopedal spasm. This is Trousseau's sign and may be provoked by inflating a sphygmomanometer cuff to just above systolic pressure for at least 2 minutes.
- Treatment of tetany is with intravenous calcium and long-term oral calcium and an active metabolite of vitamin D are needed.

ADRENAL GLANDS
The adrenal glands are small, triangular in shape and situated on the superior poles of each kidney. They have an outer cortex and an inner medulla.

The adrenal medulla secretes adrenaline (epinephrine) and noradrenaline (norepinephrine).

The cortex secretes steroid hormones – glucocorticoids (cortisol), mineralocorticoids (aldosterone) and some sex hormones (mostly androgens).

The secretion of aldosterone is under the control of the renin–angiotensin system. The secretion of glucocorticoids is controlled by ACTH from the anterior pituitary gland, controlled in turn by cortisol release factor (CRF) from the hypothalamus. Cortisol is secreted in response to circadian rhythm, stress and other factors.

Glucocorticoid hormones
Cortisol is the main hormone.

- Essential to life although it is not known why.
- Secreted more in stress.
- Influence metabolism of most body cells.
- Concerned with the metabolism of carbohydrates, fats and proteins.
- Glucocorticoids have an antiinflammatory and immunosuppressive action and it is for these actions that they are used therapeutically. All their other actions then become unwanted side-effects.

- There are a number of synthetic compounds with similar action, e.g. prednisolone.

Addison's disease – primary hypoadrenalism

An uncommon condition, in which there is destruction of the adrenal cortex resulting in a deficiency of corticosteroid production.

Aetiology

- Eighty percent result from antibodies being produced against adrenal cortex antigens.
- Associated with other autoimmune conditions such as Hashimoto's thyroiditis, Graves' disease and type 2 diabetes mellitus.
- Rarer causes include tuberculosis, surgical removal, haemorrhage (in meningococcal septicaemia) and malignant infiltration.

Clinical features

- Insidious onset with lethargy, depression, anorexia, muscular weakness and weight loss.
- May also present as an emergency with vomiting, abdominal pain and hypovolaemic shock.
- Important signs are hypotension caused by salt and water loss and hyperpigmentation caused by increased secretion of ACTH, stimulating melanocytes to produce melanin, which is responsible for skin pigmentation.
- There may be hypoglycaemia.

Investigations

- Serum urea and electrolytes.

- Adrenal antibodies are detected in most cases of autoimmune adrenalitis.
- Chest radiography will show TB.
- Diagnosis may be made by using the tetracosatrin (synthetic ACTH) test.
- Treatment should not wait for any results if it is an emergency. Hydrocortisone 100 mg should be given immediately after taking a sample of blood for measurement of plasma cortisol (will be low) and ACTH (will be high due to loss of negative feedback).

Treatment

- Lifelong replacement with steroid tablets.
- In normal individuals, steroids are released in stress of any type, e.g. infection, trauma and surgical operations. In Addison's disease, the dose of steroid must be increased in any of these situations.
- The patient must carry a steroid card and wear a MedicAlert bracelet in case of accidents.

Cushing's syndrome

Caused by persistently and inappropriately raised levels of glucocorticoids.

Aetiology

- Most cases result from the administration of steroids for the treatment of medical conditions, e.g. asthma.
- Spontaneous Cushing's syndrome is rare but may result from a pituitary adenoma, ectopic

ACTH-producing tumours (e.g. small cell lung cancer), adrenal adenoma and very rarely adrenal hyperplasia.

Clinical features
- Obese with central fat distribution affecting the trunk, abdomen and neck (buffalo hump).
- Moon face and plethoric complexion.
- Protein catabolism causes the skin to be thin and to bruise easily.
- Purple striae on the abdomen, breasts and thighs.

Investigations
- Raised plasma cortisol level is confirmed by the low-dose dexamethasone suppression test. Dexamethasone, a potent synthetic glucocorticoid, is given in a low dose, 0.5 g 6 hourly, orally for 48 hours. This will suppress the serum cortisol in normal individuals by 48 hours.
- Raised 24-hour urine level of free cortisol.

Treatment
- Surgical removal of any tumours, if possible.
- Metyrapone is an inhibitor of cortisol synthesis and may be useful if removal is not possible.
- Reduction of steroid dose in iatrogenic cases.

Phaeochromocytoma
A rare, benign (usually) tumour of the adrenal medulla in which one or both of the catecholamines are secreted in excess.

Hypertension (may be paroxysmal) is the commonest sign, along with headache, pallor, sweating, palpitations and apprehension.

The treatment is surgery where possible under alpha and beta blockade using phenoxybenzamine and propranolol, started before the operation. These drugs can be used in long-term treatment where surgery is not possible.

DIABETES MELLITUS AND THE PANCREAS

This is a syndrome characterized by a persistently raised blood glucose level associated with a deficiency or lack of effectiveness of insulin. An estimated 1.4 million people in the UK have diabetes (Diabetes UK 2002).

Box 4.7 shows the classification of diabetes by the WHO.

Action of insulin
- Insulin is a hormone secreted by the beta cells of the islets of Langerhans in the pancreas.
- Its secretion is dependent upon the level of glucose in the blood.
- After a meal when glucose levels rise, insulin is secreted.
- Insulin is necessary to allow glucose to enter the body cells and be used for energy. If there is excess glucose, insulin encourages its storage as glycogen in the liver and muscles and triglycerides in the adipose tissue.
- If there is insufficient insulin the body cannot utilize its glucose which will then accumulate in the blood and spill over into the urine.

Box 4.7   Classification of diabetes mellitus (WHO)

Type I diabetes – beta cell destruction and eventually insulin dependent
(IDDM)
Type 2 diabetes – usually non-insulin dependent (NIDDM); may be
predominantly insulin resistant or predominantly secretory deficit
Other specific types of diabetes:

- secondary to pancreatic disease, e.g. chronic pancreatitis, pancreatectomy
- secondary to endocrine disease, e.g. Cushing's syndrome, acromegaly
- drug induced, e.g. steroids, thiazide diuretics
- associated with genetic syndromes

Gestational diabetes

Diagnosis

- Urine test positive for glucose – insufficient on its own.
- Random blood glucose measurement above 11 mmol/l.
- Fasting blood glucose level above 7.8 mmol/l.
- Oral glucose tolerance test (GTT) if borderline.

Oral glucose tolerance test

Normal blood glucose ranges from 3.5 mmol/l when fasting to 7.8 mmol/l after food. The subject should have fasted for at least 10 hours but no longer than 16 hours. Blood glucose is measured before and 2 hours after the ingestion of 75 g glucose. A fasting blood glucose level above 6.7 mmol/l rising to above 11.1 mmol/l after glucose is diagnostic of diabetes mellitus. Impaired glucose tolerance is when the fasting level is below 6.7 mmol/l and the venous level 2 hours after the glucose load is 6.7–10.0 mmol/l.

Type I diabetes mellitus

Used to be called insulin-dependent diabetes mellitus (IDDM).

- Dependent upon insulin and without it the patient would eventually die. Less than 25% of those with diabetes are insulin dependent.
- Autoimmune disorder, the causes of which are not entirely understood. The beta cells in the pancreas are attacked by antibodies and eventually totally destroyed.
- Certain individuals have a genetic predisposition towards the disease but an environmental trigger factor is needed. This may be a virus.
- The onset of the disease has its highest incidence around 11–12 years of age and although it can occur at any age, it is uncommon over the age of about 40 years.

Clinical features

- Polyuria (passing lots of urine)
- Thirst
- Polydipsia (drinking lots)
- Weight loss
- Lack of energy

Without treatment the body has to utilize fat for energy and as it cannot use any glucose without insulin, the fat breakdown forms ketones, which are acidic and accumulate in the blood. Ketones will also be present in the urine.

On diagnosis the patient will require treatment with insulin, which will be lifelong. Ideally the patient will not need admission to hospital.

Insulin therapy

The normal production of insulin by the pancreas has to be mimicked as closely as possible by the administration of insulin by injection.

Insulin cannot be given orally as it is inactivated by gastrointestinal enzymes. It is usually given subcutaneously and the injection site is rotated on a systematic basis, using the thighs and the abdominal wall. Some clients also use the upper arms or buttocks.

The patient may have to inject himself up to four times daily and for some, this is the worst aspect of their illness. New, very fine insulin needles have now made the process practically painless.

Types of insulin

- Insulin used to be extracted mainly from the pancreas of pigs (porcine) and also from cows (bovine) but human insulin is made by genetic engineering.
- In Britain, insulin is presented in one strength of 100 iu (international units) per ml. There are special insulin syringes that are marked in units.
- Insulin syringes now come disguised in other forms, such as pens that children can take to school. For information on the devices available contact the diabetes specialist nurse linked to your hospital.
- Soluble (fast-acting) insulin is the type that would be used in an emergency and at the time of surgical operations on those with diabetes. This is a clear fluid. It may also be given intravenously in an emergency.
- There are also modified insulins available that are longer acting and so need to be administered less frequently.
- New insulin analogues such as Lispro are faster acting than soluble insulin and may be injected at the start of a meal.

Table 4.10 Types of insulin

Approx. length of action	Type	Examples
Short		
Onset within 0.5–1 hour	Soluble	Actrapid
Peak about 3–4 hours		Humulin S
Last no more than 8 hours		
Intermediate	Isophane	Insulatard
Onset 1–2 hours		Humulin I
Peak 4–12 hours		
Duration 12–24 hours	Insulin zinc suspension	Human Monotard
Long acting	Insulin zinc suspension	Human Ultratard

Biphasic insulins are a mixture of soluble and isophane insulins in various quantities. Mixtard 30/70 is 30% soluble and 70% isophane, suitable for twice-daily injecting.

Administration of insulin
- Vary the injection site.
- Always use a special insulin syringe.
- Insert needle at 45° if no pinch-up is to be used.
- If a pinch-up is used the needle may be inserted at 45° or 90°.
- Skin should be clean and dry but an alcohol swab is not needed.

Fingerprick glucose monitoring
- This is done using a test strip and a special meter of which there are many different types now available.
- It is essential that those involved in this procedure have been trained.
- Great care has to be taken when obtaining blood from the finger of a diabetic person.
- Accuracy is vital and reading the glucometer needs practice – most hospitals offer training by specialist staff in this area and often supply a certificate of competence afterwards.
- Those with type 1 diabetes will be used to monitoring their own blood glucose using these simple machines and may well have been taught to adjust their insulin accordingly.

Type 2 diabetes mellitus
Used to be called non-insulin dependent diabetes mellitus (NIDDM).

- Either insufficient production of insulin or an inability of the body to use the insulin adequately (insulin resistance).
- Patients not dependent on insulin for their survival. May be receiving some insulin to help control their diabetes, but can live without it.
- This is a different disorder to type 1 and does not usually happen in the young.
- The symptoms develop much more insidiously and patients may even be diagnosed on having a routine urine test. They may have had the disorder for years and not known about it.
- It is still very important to treat this condition as the complications of diabetes, especially heart disease, still occur.
- Incidence increases with age and as people are living longer, so the disease is getting more common.
- The disorder is also linked to obesity and runs in families but the exact cause is not known.
- This type of diabetes may be controlled by diet alone or the patient may be on medication, oral hypoglycaemic agents, to bring down the blood glucose.

Aims for type 1 and type 2 diabetes are similar.

- To maintain a blood glucose that is within the normal range if possible and thus prevent or reduce the complications of diabetes.
- Through communication and education, to encourage patients to have control of their own disorder.

- To help the client to lead as normal and active a life as possible.

Results of the Diabetes Control and Complications Trial (DCCT) in type 1 diabetes and the United Kingdom Prospective Diabetes Survey (UKPDS) for type 2 diabetes have shown that the higher the glucose levels in diabetes, the more likely it is that complications will occur. They have also shown that blood pressure control is extremely important in the prevention and control of complications.

The diet in diabetes

On diagnosis, the client will see a dietitian.

Contrary to popular thinking, the diet in diabetes is one that can be eaten by the whole family. It is a 'healthy eating' diet. The diet should:

- meet the patient's overall daily energy requirements; these depend partly on age, sex and level of activity
- be low in fat, especially saturated or animal fat
- give about 50% of calories in the form of carbohydrate, aiming to increase the complex carbohydrate in the diet (this is found in such foods as pasta, potatoes and bread) and reduce the fast sugars such as sucrose
- contain at least five portions of fruit and vegetables daily.

If you wish to know more about the diet in diabetes you should contact your hospital dietitian or diabetes specialist nurse.

Diabetic emergencies

Hypoglycaemia

This occurs when the blood glucose falls below about 3.5 mmol/l. It does not occur in the diabetic who is diet controlled but may occur if someone with type 2 diabetes is on oral hypoglycaemics of the sulphonylurea group, such as tolbutamide or gliclazide. It is most common in those receiving insulin.

Causes

- Too much insulin (either accidental or deliberate)
- Missing or delaying a meal or snack
- Excessive exercise with no reduction in insulin
- Alcohol

Clinical features

- Pallor
- Trembling
- Sweating
- Feeling 'lightheaded'
- Blurred vision
- Tachycardia
- Increasing confusion – sometimes aggression
- Incoherent speech

An attack of hypoglycaemia may occur very rapidly and if the nurse notices a change in behaviour of a client with diabetes and he becomes irritable or lethargic, she should seek help immediately. Prompt action may mean oral instead of intravenous glucose may be given.

Treatment

- Glucose may be given orally if the client is awake and fully conscious.

- If he is unconscious the doctor will give intravenous dextrose 50% 50 ml.
- Glucagon 0.5–1 unit may be given intramuscularly if intravenous dextrose is not available. This is a hormone produced by the pancreas that causes the release of glucose from stores in the body.

Diabetic ketoacidosis

- This happens when there is insufficient insulin in the body. The cells cannot utilize glucose, which accumulates in the bloodstream. Fat stores have to be used for energy with the production of ketones.
- Compared to hypoglycaemia, deterioration is slow.
- Hyperglycaemia is present and ketones are heavily present both in the urine and on the breath.
- Polyuria is present and at first polydipsia but as the acidosis increases, nausea and vomiting may occur, making drinking impossible.
- Dehydration will now increase, leading to a lowering of blood pressure and a rapid, thready pulse.
- The respirations become deep and the ketones can be smelt on the breath (they smell of acetone, which is nail varnish remover, or pear drops).
- Without treatment drowsiness and coma will follow.

> **Diabetic ketoacidosis is a medical emergency and urgent intervention is needed.**

Causes
- Untreated diabetes, i.e. undiagnosed patient.
- Illness, e.g. urinary tract infection or throat infection. Infection increases the body's insulin requirement but the patient may actually omit his insulin as he has no appetite for food.
- Vomiting followed by the total omission of insulin. It is of vital importance that insulin is never totally stopped when the patient is ill.

Treatment
- Assessment of the patient's conscious level half hourly
- Have a suction machine by the bed in case of vomiting.
- Half hourly monitoring of vital signs – blood pressure, pulse and respirations.
- An intravenous infusion of normal (0.9%) saline will probably be commenced by the medical staff to help combat the dehydration. It is possible that the patient may be depleted of up to 8 l of fluid. Fluids given may be prescribed with added potassium.
- Bloods will be taken for blood glucose measurement and urea and electrolytes. An arterial sample may be taken for blood gases to assess the amount of acidosis present.
- The patient will be attached to a cardiac monitor as there is likely to be a potassium deficiency in the body which may lead to cardiac arrhythmias.
- Insulin therapy will be commenced with a short-acting

insulin such as Actrapid or Humulin S.

- Insulin will be given according to the blood glucose measurements which may be taken hourly at first.
- If acidosis is severe, sodium bicarbonate may be given but this is rarely needed.
- Once the blood glucose has fallen to 11 mmol/l the normal saline infusion is likely to be replaced by dextrose 5%.

Long-term complications of diabetes

These may be divided into small vessel and large vessel diseases.

Small vessel disease (microvascular)
This type of disorder only happens in diabetes. It is much more common when the blood glucose levels are maintained above 11 mmol/l. The incidence of complications also rises with the length of time the patient has had diabetes.

Retinopathy. The small vessels at the back of the eye are affected and if untreated, eventually this can lead to blindness. All diabetics need an annual eye check. Treatment with photocoagulation can prevent blindness.

Nephropathy. This is damage to the kidney. There will be albumin in the urine and usually a raised blood pressure. If the damage continues chronic renal failure can follow.

Neuropathy. This is damage to the peripheral nerves, which may lead to sensory loss and is one of the reasons why extreme caution is

needed when dealing with the feet of those with diabetes. The chiropodist should be consulted on a regular basis and the nurse should never attempt to cut the toe nails of the client with diabetes.

Damage to the skin of the feet in the presence of both neuropathy and poor circulation is one of the reasons why amputations are so common in patients with diabetes.

Large vessel disease (macrovascular)
- Cardiovascular disease – may lead to angina and heart attacks
- Cerebrovascular disease – may lead to stroke
- Peripheral vascular disease – may lead to severe pain on walking and contribute to poor healing of any injuries to the foot

All of these occur in the non-diabetic population but are much more common in those with diabetes due to their more rapid development of atherosclerosis.

4.8 DISEASES OF BONES AND JOINTS

Bone is a collagen-based matrix with mineral laid upon it. Its strength depends upon both these components. The minerals are calcium, phosphorus and magnesium. Vitamin D, parathormone and calcitonin (produced by the thyroid gland) are important in bone mineralization. The new bone is deposited by the osteoblast cells and old bone is resorbed by the osteoclast cells. Bone is not static and is constantly remodelling throughout life.

OSTEOPOROSIS

The most common metabolic bone disease in which there is a loss of bone mass per unit volume. Bone composition remains normal. This leads to reduced strength and the weakened bone fractures easily. Damage is particularly likely to occur to the femoral neck, the dorsal vertebrae and the distal radius. The trauma precipitating this damage may be very minor.

Aetiology

Most examples are the result of progressive decrease in bone mass with age.

- Bone formation and resorption are balanced in adulthood. With ageing, the balance swings towards bone resorption and whether this reaches a critical point or not depends largely on the bone mass achieved as an adult. This is greater in men than women and also greater in blacks than whites.
- Changes in body oestrogen levels also cause more bone resorption in women after the menopause as oestrogen prevents bone resorption. As women also live longer, on average, than men they have more problems with osteoporosis.
- Exercise throughout life helps to maintain bone mass and immobility for any reason may precipitate premature osteoporosis.
- Occasionally direct causes can be found such as Cushing's syndrome, diabetes, thyrotoxicosis, chronic renal failure and use of drugs such as glucocorticoids and long-term heparin.

Clinical features

- Asymptomatic osteoporosis is common.
- Backache is common.
- The vertebrae may collapse due to typical crush fractures and there may be an exaggeration of the curvature of the thoracic spine.
- Collapse of vertebrae may lead to loss of height.

Investigations

- X-ray will demonstrate decreased bone density and thinning of the cortex.
- Lumbar and thoracic vertebrae become biconcave in shape.
- Blood levels of calcium, phosphate and alkaline phosphatase are normal.

Treatment and prevention

- Once osteoporosis occurs, treatment is unsatisfactory. The loss of bone mass has already occurred and fractures should be treated as and when they happen.
- Prophylaxis is preferred and a good diet, with plenty of calcium and low alcohol in take, will help.
- Early oestrogen replacement during the menopause (HRT) will prevent osteoporosis in most women and may even increase the bone mass.
- Adequate intake of calcium and vitamin D is needed but calcium supplements after the

menopause have not been proven to be beneficial. Research is conflicting but as they do not usually cause harm they can be taken.

- Regular exercise against gravity is recommended.

VITAMIN D DEFICIENCY

- Results in rickets in children and osteomalacia in adults. It is uncommon in the UK but may occur in Asian immigrants and the elderly as a result of dietary lack and failure to be exposed to sunlight.
- May also occur in malabsorption from any cause including previous gastric surgery and coeliac disease.
- Rare causes include long-term use of anticonvulsants, liver and renal failure.
- The main function of vitamin D is to ensure an adequate concentration of calcium for bone formation. Deficiency leads to a failure of calcification. Soft bones lacking in tensile strength result but there is no interference with bone bulk.

Childhood rickets

The bones become distorted and there may be pain and weakness. It leads to the stunting of growth and bowing of the lower limbs. There may be a pigeon deformity of the chest and delay in closure of the anterior fontanelle.

Distortion of the pelvis in females may lead to difficulties with childbirth.

Osteomalacia in adults

May produce pain and tenderness as well as spontaneous fractures. Muscle weakness is also present. Plasma calcium may be low and tetany may ensue.

Treatment

- Prevention is better than cure!
- Education and living standards are important and susceptible populations should be targeted.
- A good diet with vitamin D and calcium supplements should be given.
- Exposure to sunlight is also important.
- Patients on long-term anticonvulsants should receive supplements.

PAGET'S DISEASE OF THE BONE

- This is known as osteitis deformans and is common in the elderly (up to 10%).
- There is a familial tendency to develop the disease although its aetiology is not known.
- British cases are clustered in the northern part of the country.
- There is an increase in osteoclast activity that leads to an increase in osteoblast activity. This results in abnormal architecture of the bones, with the legs and axial skeleton (including the skull) most commonly affected.
- Often the patient is asymptomatic but constant localized bone pain may occur and this is unrelieved by rest.

- The features may be distorted and the affected areas may feel warm.
- Complications are due to compression by the bony overgrowths and include blindness and deafness.
- Simple analgesics and physiotherapy are used.
- Etidronate disodium (Didronel), calcitonin, corticosteroids or cytotoxic drugs may be used when symptoms or complications are present.

OSTEOMYELITIS

This is infection in the bone. It may be bloodborne or occur from direct spread of microorganisms. Predisposing conditions are shown in Box 4.8. It is difficult to treat and may result in extensive physical disability.

Acute osteomyelitis is usually caused by *Staphylococcus aureus* but other organisms include *Pseudomonas aeruginosa*, *Salmonella*, *Streptococci*, Candida and mixed aerobic and anaerobic organisms.

There is fever, pain and tenderness over the affected bone. Blood culture or needle biopsy is done for diagnosis but treatment may be possible from the clinical picture alone.

Chronic osteomyelitis usually results from untreated or undertreated acute osteomyelitis. There is bone erosion and areas of cystic degeneration. Necrosis of bone follows and there may be intermittent flare-up of the disease over a period of years with fever, local pain and sinus formation.

Treatment
- Antibiotics and drainage of inflammatory exudates.
- Evaluation is by bone scanning and MRI.
- Chronic osteomyelitis may require a combination of surgery and antibiotic therapy.
- Hyperbaric oxygen is sometimes used.

BONE TUMOURS

Many different types of tumour involve the skeleton but primary bone tumours are rare and occur mainly in the young.

Secondary metastases in bone are common, especially from malignancies of the breast, bronchi, prostate, thyroid and kidney.

The rate is low below 15 years (3% of all malignancies), adolescents have the highest rate and the lowest rate of all is between 30 and 35 years. Over 35 years, the incidence slowly rises due to metastases in bone.

Box 4.8 Acute osteomyelitis – predisposing conditions	
Direct spread	**Bloodborne**
Open fractures	Skin sepsis and ulcers
Penetrating trauma, e.g. animal bite	Intravenous drug abuse
Replacement joints	Chronic urinary tract infection
Penetrating ulcer, e.g. in diabetic neuropathy	Sickle cell disease
	Chronic diverticulitis

Osteosarcomas

These malignant bone-forming tumours account for about 38% of bone tumours. Occurrence is 3:2 times more common in males. Sixty percent occur in the under-20s and a secondary peak occurs in the 50–60 age range, mostly in those with Paget's disease.

Ninety percent of these tumours are located in the metaphyses of long bones, especially the femur. Fifty percent occur around the knee joint.

Clinical features
- Pain and swelling.
- Pain slight and intermittent at first but becomes more intense and of longer duration. It is often severe at night and analgesia becomes necessary.
- Usually there is a coincidental history of trauma.
- Sometimes may present with a fracture.

Diagnosis

Early recognition is essential for a reasonable prognosis. Many could be diagnosed early but often the individual does not seek medical attention. There may be vague symptoms that could be related to minor trauma or inflammatory conditions.

Radiologic studies including plain X-ray, CT scan and an MRI enable diagnosis and often staging to be done. MRI may also be used to follow the progress of the tumour with treatment.

Treatment
- Surgery is the treatment of choice. Amputation used to be the rule but now chemotherapy may be given first and limb salvage made possible by removal of the tumour whilst preserving the limb.
- Chemotherapy is usually given both pre- and postoperatively using combinations of drugs.

Ewing's sarcoma
- Originates from cells within the bone marrow space.
- Most frequently diagnosed between 5 and 15 years of age. Rare after 30 years of age.
- Most common in the mid-shaft of long bones or in flat bones.
- Most common complaint is pain and swelling but fever may be present with malaise and anorexia.
- The tumour breaks through the bone and may form a soft tissue mass. It is most common in the femur and pelvis but can occur in any bone.
- It metastasizes early to nearly every part of the body and metastases are usually present at diagnosis or within one year. Common sites are the lungs and other bones.
- Bone scan, chest X-ray and chest CT are used to detect metastases.
- Biopsy is used to establish the diagnosis.
- Preoperative chemotherapy is used prior to surgery or radiotherapy or a combination of both. Chemotherapy is then continued for 12–18 months afterwards.
- Prognosis is poor with a 5-year survival of 5–10%. Survival for localized tumours with aggressive

treatment, however, may reach 60%.

Other tumours

Tumours may arise from any tissue and there are rare tumours occurring in cartilage and collagen. These may be benign or malignant.

INFLAMMATORY JOINT DISEASE

Commonly termed arthritis, this is characterized by inflammatory damage and destruction of the synovial membrane or articular cartilage in the joints. There are also systemic signs of inflammation including fever, malaise, anorexia and a raised white cell count.

Rheumatoid arthritis

This is a classic autoimmune disorder with self-perpetuating inflammation occurring in the joints and resulting from immune reactions. It can be described as a non-suppurative, non-infectious, proliferative synovitis.

The first tissue to be affected in the joint is the synovial membrane that lines the joint cavity. Eventually it may lead to the progressive destruction of articular cartilage. The result is a progressively disabling arthritis with pain, joint deformity and loss of movement.

Over 70% of patients present with a bilateral and symmetrical polyarthritis, usually of insidious onset. All synovial joints may be affected but some are more commonly affected than others (Fig. 4.15). There may be extra-articular involvement of other tissues and in

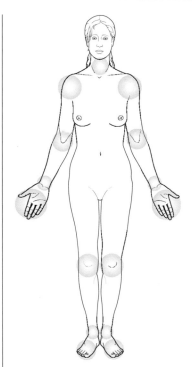

Fig. 4.15 Joints affected by rheumatoid arthritis.

this way the disorder resembles systemic lupus erythematosus and other multiorgan autoimmune disorders. These patients tend to have a poorer prognosis.

The trigger factor is unknown and various agents have been suggested including some of the enteric bacteria and the Epstein–Barr virus. The precise triggering may vary from person to person.

Incidence
- Predominantly female – 3:1.
- Occurs in 2% of the population worldwide.

- Just as common in tropical countries as in cold, damp Britain.
- Does not appear to have occurred in ancient times.
- May commence at any age from 10 to 70 years.
- Commonest time of onset is 30–40 years.
- Genetic factors seem to be vitally important in determining a predisposition.
- Hormonal factors may have an influence as the disease is commoner in women and tends to become quiescent in pregnancy.

Aetiology

> ⚠ The joint damage of rheumatoid arthritis is autoimmune in nature, appearing in genetically predisposed individuals, after exposure to an unknown trigger.

Normally the immune system does not attack 'self'; any part of self is tolerated. In autoimmune disorders something has gone wrong with this mechanism and the body starts to make antibodies to certain body proteins. In diabetes it is to the islets of Langerhans and so this is organ specific. In rheumatoid arthritis there is a more generalized reaction, which may cause systemic problems as well as those in the joints. Quiescent episodes may cause a reduction in the inflammation and pain but there will always be some lymphocytes in the synovium (i.e. some inflammation).

Those with rheumatoid factor present are seropositive. In 20% of cases the client may be seronegative and not have the rheumatoid factor. The rheumatoid factor does not always mean rheumatoid arthritis. It is present in some other diseases, e.g. SLE, TB and in some elderly clients whose relatives have RA but who have no evidence of the disease.

There are changes in the synovial fluid. An increase in volume occurs, the turbidity increases, mucin decreases and the numbers of white cells in it are increased.

Clinical features
- Pain and swelling in symmetrical small joints (e.g. fingers and toes).
- Morning stiffness in affected joints.
- May be additional general symptoms, especially tiredness, irritability and depression.
- Usually of insidious onset but in the minority of patients, it may begin with acute fever, weight loss and excessive fatigue.
- Gradually the disease spreads: fingers to hands and wrists, toes to feet and ankles, elbows, shoulders and knees can be affected.
- The joints take on a characteristic deformed appearance. There is difficulty holding cutlery and problems with walking and even dressing.
- There are periods of exacerbation and remission throughout the course of the disease.

Because rheumatoid arthritis is a systemic disorder there may be other changes throughout the body.

Subcutaneous nodules in 25% of cases. Usually in those positive for rheumatoid factor. Most common in the elbows adjacent to the olecranon process, but also at the back of the skull and the Achilles tendon. May occur at any subcutaneous site that is exposed to contact or pressure. Nodules are rounded, firm masses in the subcutaneous tissue varying in diameter from less than 0.5 cm to several centimetres. There is an outer layer of granulation tissue containing lymphocytes and an inner zone of fibrinoid necrosis.

Vasculitis. This occurs at many sites and can involve any major organ. Usually in patients with high titres of rheumatoid factor. Small vessel vasculitis involves arterioles, venules and capillaries and leads to localized purpura and petechiae. Severe digital vasculitis is rare. Presents with pallor, cyanosis and coldness of the distal digits. Pain and ischaemic ulcerations with necrosis of the finger ends occur. Dry gangrene will result unless treated. Amputation may be indicated.

Fibrinous pleurisy and fibrosis of the lungs. At autopsy 50% of all RA patients have had pleural involvement. Less than 20% will actually experience symptoms and less than 5% will have pleural effusions. Chronic bronchitis may be secondary to RA but this is controversial. Those with RA who smoke appear 2–3 times more likely to develop chronic bronchitis.

Cardiac involvement. Pericarditis is the most frequent manifestation. At autopsy about 40% show some evidence of previous pericardial involvement. Very few experience any symptoms. If they do, it is likely to be chest pain.

Neuropathy. Usually relatively mild distal sensory neuropathy showing as paraesthesia. Decreased touch sensation in the feet.

Carpal tunnel syndrome. This may occur due to compression of the median nerve by proliferative tenosynovitis of the wrist. The symptoms may precede the onset of RA by years in some cases.

Eye changes. Keratoconjunctivitis (dry eyes) and scleritis commonly. Those with scleritis will get severe pain, photophobia and impairment of vision. Ten percent will develop keratoconjunctivitis from decreased tear secretion.

Splenomegaly. This is often associated with leucopenia and known as Felty's syndrome. There are often high titres of rheumatoid factor. Skin ulceration and recurrent infections are likely to occur.

Anaemia. Mild normocytic, hypochromic anaemia. Due to poor erythropoiesis and the type that commonly occurs in chronic illness. May be aggravated by blood loss from NSAIDs.

Fatigue, malaise and depression. Fatigue is a common symptom and can precede the onset of joint synovitis by many months.

Investigations
- Immunological investigations show a positive rheumatoid factor in about 80% of patients.
- Anaemia may be present (see above).
- Platelet and white cell count may be raised.

- The ESR may be raised.
- Radiological changes – may not be present very early in the disease.

Treatment and nursing management
- Main objective is to reduce pain and enable the patient to lead as normal a life as possible.
- Many patients notice a reduction in symptoms following the application of heat in the form of wax, heating pads or whirlpool-type baths. Care should be taken to explain to the patient that the heat should not be too intense and that it is not 'the hotter, the better'. Some of the joint symptoms may also be helped by ice packs, ultrasound and weak electrical stimulation.
- Physiotherapy forms an important part of the care, with exercises to try and maintain joint movement and strengthen weak muscles.
- Occupational therapists are involved and provide splints for joint protection as well as aids and appliances to increase independence.

Drug treatment
Several classes of drug are utilized, including analgesics to control the pain, NSAIDs, corticosteroids, immunosuppressive drugs and disease-modifying antirheumatic drugs (DMARDs).

NSAIDs are the mainstay of treatment and are usually well tolerated by the patient. They decrease pain and also inflammation but may produce gastrointestinal side-effects. They have little or no effect on the underlying disease process and do not prevent joint destruction.

Juvenile chronic arthritis (Still's disease)
- This is persistent synovitis in one or more joints for at least 3 months.
- Treatment is with NSAIDs.
- Steroids should be avoided as they suppress growth.
- Physiotherapy and joint protection are important.

Osteoarthritis (OA)
This is a common degenerative disease of the joints and affects 10% of all adults, both men and women. The prevalence increases with age and it is commoner in men under 45 years and women over 55 years. By the age of 75, 85% of people have some osteoarthritis. It occurs worldwide in all climates.

It most commonly affects the weight-bearing joints, especially the knees, and interphalangeal joints of the hands. It is also common in the hip joint.

It may be:

- primary – a degenerative disease and the result of wear and tear on the joint
- secondary – attributable to other causes, e.g. joint injury in athletics or trauma.

Excessive joint loading may be a contributing factor.

- Obesity
- Postural defect
- Malformed joint
- Long-term occupational or athletic stress on a joint

Clinical features
- Joint aches and stiffness arising gradually in middle age.
- Increase with activity and decrease with rest.
- No systemic signs or symptoms.
- As the degeneration increases, the pain becomes more persistent and stiffness increases.
- Limitation of movement in the affected joint.
- Most serious loss of mobility is from hip and knee involvement.

Management and nursing care
- No prevention or arrest of the process.
- Analgesia is helpful, usually in the form of NSAIDs.
- Physiotherapy and the use of activities that reduce strain can help.
- Joint replacement often becomes necessary.

FRACTURES

A fracture may be a complete break in the continuity of a bone or it may be an incomplete break or crack.

Clinical features

The clinical manifestations vary according to the type of fracture and the site.

- When a fracture occurs there will be soft tissue injury as well and blood vessels and nerves may be damaged. Neurovascular assessment is needed. There may be impaired sensation and numbness.
- Typically fractures are painful and there is loss of function. The pain is due to muscle spasm and is worse on movement.
- Deformity (unnatural alignment) occurs at the fracture site.
- Swelling is caused by the fracture haematoma and soft tissue oedema.
- Tenderness, muscle spasm and pain are usually present.
- There may be angulation at the fracture site with shortening of the limb and rotational deformities.
- Crepitus may occur. This is abnormal movement at the fracture site. The broken bone ends grind against each other.
- Shortening may occur due to overlapping of fragments and muscle spasm.
- Sometimes reasonable function may be retained as in a stress fracture or an impacted fracture. This may lead to the doctor missing the fracture.

It may be the case that the fractures sustained by a patient are only a small part of the damage and in cases of multiple injuries, other trauma is more important. Maintaining the airway is always the first priority. There may be spinal injuries or head injuries also.

Diagnosis

X-ray of the whole length of the bone, including the adjacent joints, should be done.

Causes

Trauma
Sudden injury is the cause of the majority of fractures. They occur in previously healthy bone.

- May be direct trauma, e.g. hitting the ulna with a stick. The fracture occurs at the site of the injury.
- May be indirect trauma, e.g. a fall on the hand may fracture the clavicle. Force was applied at a site remote from the injury.

Stress

The bone is fatigued by repeated stress, e.g. a fractured tibia in an athlete, ballet dancer or military recruit. This type of fracture is often due to new strenuous and repetitive activity when gains in muscle strength occur more rapidly than gains in bone strength.

Pathological

This occurs when a bone is already weakened by disease. The trauma needed may be quite trivial or the fracture may occur spontaneously. Examples of diseases are osteoporosis, cancer metastases in bone, bone cysts and Paget's disease.

Classification of fractures
(Fig. 4.16)

Closed or simple fractures

There is no communication between the site of the fracture and the exterior of the body.

Open or compound fractures

The overlying skin is broken and the wound leads down to the site of the fracture. This means infection may enter the bone. The skin break may be a small puncture or the bone may protrude right through the skin. Infection in the bone is called *osteomyelitis* (see p. 269) and may be difficult to eliminate.

All fractures are either open or closed.

A fracture is comminuted when there are more than two fragments to the bone. This type of fracture may be difficult to align.

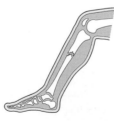

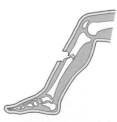

A. Closed or simple fracture
There is no communication between the fractured bone and the body surface.

B. Open or compound fracture
There is a wound leading down to the site of fracture. Organisms may gain access through the wound and infect the bone.

Fig. 4.16 Open and closed fractures. From Crawford/Outline of Fractures, reproduced with permission.

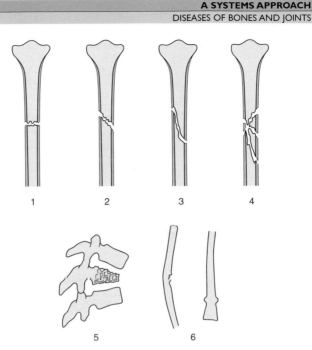

Fig. 4.17 Common patterns of fracture. I Transverse. 2 Oblique. 3 Spiral. 4 Comminuted. 5 Compression. 6 Greenstick. From Crawford/Outline of Fractures, reproduced with permission.

Patterns of fracture

Complete fracture
The bone is completely divided into two separate fragments. Different fractures are shown in Figure 4.17.

The fracture is often described in terms of the pattern seen on the X-ray as:

- transverse – occurs straight across the bone and is usually caused by an angulation, not twisting, force. Unlikely to become displaced after reduction
- oblique – occurs at a 45° angle to the shaft of the bone and is more difficult to stabilize at reduction
- spiral – encircles the bone and is usually caused by a twisting

force and prone to redisplacement following reduction.

Incomplete fracture
Occurs more frequently in the more flexible, growing bones of children. The bone is not completely broken into two parts.

A *greenstick* fracture occurs in children, especially under the age of 10. Their bones have elasticity and buckle. If the force applied is strong enough, a complete fracture will occur in a child.

A *hairline* fracture occurs when little force has been applied.

An *impacted* fracture may occur in adults. The bone fragments are jammed into each other. This is common in a fractured neck of femur.

A *crush* or *compression* fracture may occur in cancellous bone when it has been compressed beyond the limits of tolerance, e.g. heels (calcaneum), as a result of falling from a height, or vertebrae.

Complicated fracture

There is accompanying damage to neighbouring structures such as nerves, blood vessels or tendons, e.g. a fractured humerus may damage the brachial artery.

Depressed fracture

A segment of bone is depressed below the level of the bone. This is usually due to a sharply localized blow and is common in skull fractures.

Displacement

This is present if the bone ends have moved from each other. Reduction of a fracture is realignment of the bone ends. It is only necessary if there is some displacement.

Dislocation

A dislocation is loss of congruity between the articular surfaces of a joint. Sometimes a fracture dislocation occurs when the joint is dislocated and at least one of the bones involved is fractured.

A Pott's fracture is dislocation of the ankle joint with fracture of the tibia or fibula.

Treatment

This depends very much on the type and site of the fracture.

First aid

Immobilization by the use of a sling, a splint or traction will lessen the pain. Great care must be taken with spinal injuries.

Uncomplicated fractures

There are three fundamentals of treatment for fractures:

- reduction
- immobilization
- preservation of function.

Reduction. This is realignment of the bone fragments. It is not always necessary either because there is no displacement or because the displacement is immaterial to the final result. Reduction may be carried out in three ways.

Manipulative reduction. Closed manipulative reduction is usually carried out under general anaesthesia but local or regional anaesthesia may sometimes be used. Most fractures can be realigned by this method. The skin is not opened and the bones are moved back into place.

Mechanical traction. This is necessary when there are strong muscles exerting a displacement force, as in a fractured femur. It aims to draw the bone fragments back to their normal length. It may be done rapidly under general anaesthesia or more slowly by prolonged traction without anaesthesia.

Operative reduction. Reduction takes place with direct vision of the bones at an open operation. This is done when an acceptable reduction cannot be maintained by closed methods and is common when there is nerve or articular surface involvement. The fragments will be fixed internally to ensure maintenance of their position.

Immobilization. Some fractures require rigid splinting to maintain their position until union of the bone can occur but others do not and immobilization can do more harm than good in some cases.

Immobilization is done to:

- prevent displacement of the bone fragments
- prevent movement that may interfere with union
- relieve pain.

A fracture that has required reduction will always require immobilization to prevent redisplacement.

Prevention of movement is virtually always needed in fractures of the scaphoid, ulna and femur whereas a fractured clavicle, scapula, stable fracture of the pelvis and fractured ribs will all heal well without immobilization.

Methods of immobilization include:

- plaster of Paris or other external splint
- continuous traction
- external fixation
- internal fixation.

Plaster of Paris. The plaster cast is the standard method of immobilization for most fractures. Plaster of Paris is calcium sulphate, which reacts with water to become hydrated. Plaster bandages come ready prepared and must be soaked in cold water before application. When the wet plaster is applied, the reaction takes place and the plaster feels warmer as it sets. A thin lining of stockinet is used close to the skin, for comfort and to prevent the plaster sticking, and a layer of cotton wool bandage is applied before the plaster. This allows for some swelling of the limb to take place.

There used to be no alternatives to plaster of Paris but now there are many synthetic substitutes with such advantages as lightness, radiolucency (do not interfere with radiographical procedures) and imperviousness to water.

The plaster may be applied as a normal bandage, round and round the limb, but if a lot of swelling is expected, a backslab may be applied and a full plaster used when the swelling has subsided.

Plaster is removed by the use of an electric plaster saw and plaster-cutting shears.

Observation of a plaster. When a plaster cast has been applied to a new fracture or following a manipulation there are precautions that need to be observed. There is a danger of restricting the circulation, should the limb swell. This may be sufficient to impede the arterial flow to the fingers or toes and is most likely to occur between 12 and 36 hours after application of the plaster.

The clinical features of a restricted circulation are:

- pain
- swelling of the fingers or toes
- numbness of the digits or pins and needles
- change in colour – should be pink; any blue, grey or white colour should be reported

- cold digits – this may not be a sign, especially if no other sign is present, but warm digits are more reassuring.

Cast bracing. This is the application of a supportive device that allows continued function of the part. It is especially used in fractures of long bones such as the tibia and femur and allows some use of the limb. As the support is less with this type of splint, it is not usually applied until the fifth or sixth week when healing is well under way.

Traction. Sustained traction is used when it is not possible to hold the bones in place with a plaster cast, usually due to muscle contraction. It is more common in fractures of the femur, distal shaft of humerus and some fractures of the tibial shaft. The pull of the muscles is balanced by sustained traction on the distal fragment of the fracture, usually by weights. Traction is usually combined with splintage to give support to the limb and prevent angular deformity, e.g. a Thomas splint for fractured femur and a Braun splint for fractured tibia.

External fixation. The bone fragments are anchored to an external device, such as a metal bar, by pins inserted into the distal and proximal fragments of a long bone fracture. It is used especially when infection is a danger, as in an open fracture, as internal fixation would carry a greater risk of spreading infection.

Internal fixation. This involves an operation and the insertion of some form of metallic plate, intramedullary nail, screwplate or nailplate. It carries a much higher risk of introducing infection into the bone and the surgeon often has to balance this risk with the advantage of early mobilization. The age of the patient, his occupation and the site of the fracture have all to be taken into account. With the advent of improved antibiotic cover and the use of closed-suction drainage the dangers are becoming less.

Internal fixation is used:

- when the fracture cannot be maintained in an acceptable position by splintage and/or traction
- following an open reduction when it is usually necessary to internally fix the fragments to prevent displacement
- to provide rapid control of limb fractures when there are other severe injuries
- to rigidly fix the fracture for early mobility, e.g. neck of femur.

Open (compound) fractures

The big risk here is infection and the wound should be kept covered with a sterile dressing and not disturbed until the patient can urgently go to theatre. Here, the wound can be cleaned, dead tissue removed, leaving only healthy and well-vascularized tissue able to fight off infection by microorganisms.

Most wounds will not be immediately sutured unless very recent and obviously clean and uncontaminated. Other wounds are sutured when it is certain that any infection has been prevented, often in 4 or 5 days.

The fracture itself is better treated by closed methods. Internal fixation runs the risk of spreading any infection. Antibiotics are always administered. These will be broad spectrum such as a cephalosporin (see p. 320). Tetanus prophylaxis must be given if not up to date.

The patient should be closely observed for signs of infection, especially a sustained rise in temperature.

Healing of fractures

This starts as soon as the bone is broken and usually proceeds through several stages until the break is healed. These stages include haematoma formation around the fracture, cellular proliferation by the osteoblasts, laying down of calcium to form callus and finally consolidation into mature bone.

Restoration of function

Rehabilitation is always necessary and should begin as soon as the fracture is treated. Patients can help themselves with the aid of the physiotherapist as active use is much better than passive movement. The physiotherapist will explain the exercises that are needed to help retain or restore function and these need to be commenced as soon as possible.

> ⚠ If rehabilitation is ignored and a limb is kept immobile for long periods the muscles will waste and the joints will stiffen.
>
> There may be permanent impairment of function.

Complications of fractures

These may be associated with the fracture itself or with the surrounding soft tissues.

Infection

Usually occurs in an open fracture but may also occur when a closed fracture is converted into an open one by operative reduction. Osteomyelitis (see p. 269) is infection of the bone and is difficult to treat, often leading to long-term problems. The acute infection often becomes a chronic one and part of the bone may die due to lack of blood supply. This leads to a chronic discharge of pus through a sinus and the infection often prevents or delays union of the fracture.

Prevention is by early cleaning of the wound in theatre and removal of all dead tissue. The wound should not be sutured immediately. Antibiotics are always administered.

If infection is present then free drainage is allowed and antibiotics administered. A combination of flucloxacillin and fusidic acid may be appropriate but does depend on the sensitivity of the invading organisms.

Delayed union

The fracture does not unite as quickly as expected and is freely mobile after a period of 3 or 4 months. If it persists, it will become non-union. If healing does not occur after about 6 months, bone grafting may be considered. If callus has formed then internal fixation may be used.

Non-union

This is a failure of the bone ends to grow together and can be diagnosed by X-ray. Healing is not going to occur and the bone ends are dense and rounded. The gap between the bones is filled with fibrous tissue and not callus.

Non-union may be due to infection, inadequate blood supply to one or both fragments, loss of apposition between fragments, interposition of soft tissue between fragments, movement between fragments or destruction of bone by a tumour in pathological fractures.

The treatment depends partly on the site of the fracture, as in some cases it may not affect mobility too greatly and may be left, e.g. scaphoid fracture. Bone grafting is often used. The graft is usually obtained from the patient and may come from the ilium when cancellous bone is required or from the tibia if a stronger bone is needed.

Electromagnetic stimulation may be used to encourage bone healing.

Malunion

The bone is healed but in an imperfect position. It may result in shortening or there may be some rotation or overlap of the fragments. Often occurs to a small degree but can need correcting in some instances.

Shortening

May be due to malunion, crushing or actual loss of bone as in a comminuted fracture or in children when there is interference with the growing ends of long bones (epiphyses). It is only really important in the legs and may require raising of the shoe if more than 2 cm or an operation to correct it or shorten the other leg. It can cause backache due to tilting of the pelvis and osteoarthritis of the hip in later life.

Avascular necrosis

This is death of bone due to interference with its blood supply and may have serious consequences. It can lead to non-union and severe osteoarthritis. It is only a problem usually when a joint is involved. The avascular bone loses its structure and eventually collapses. This may occur within a year of the injury but may take 3 or 4 years. The affected joint is likely to be arthritic whether or not union eventually occurs.

Common sites are the head of the femur following a fractured neck of femur and the scaphoid. On diagnosis, early operation may be attempted.

Blood vessel injuries

There is always some damage to soft tissues when a bone is broken but usually healing occurs without a problem. If an important artery is damaged, however, this can occasionally lead to loss of a limb. It is more likely to result in ischaemic damage such as a Volkmann's ischaemic contracture of muscle, especially common following injury to the brachial artery in a supracondylar fracture of the humerus (at the elbow), commonly seen in children.

It is vital that observation of the peripheral circulation occurs following a fracture of a long bone.

The radial pulse should be checked at regular intervals following a supracondylar fracture. There may be numbness of the digits and pain due to ischaemia.

Compartment syndrome

Within a muscle compartment swelling occurs and the pressure rises. This can lead to ischaemia as a result of small vessel occlusion and the operation of fasciotomy is urgently necessary as permanent loss of function can occur in 6–8 hours.

Injury to nerves

This is more common than damage to major arteries. If there is slight damage, recovery is spontaneous in a few weeks. In more severe damage recovery takes many months and may not occur without excision of the damaged section.

The nerve is often contused (bruised) by a sharp bone fragment and recovery is complete.

Injury to viscera

Examples include lung complications following fractured ribs and bladder injury following a fractured pelvis.

Tendon injuries

Tendons attach muscle to bone and if they are severed, movement is prevented. The treatment here is surgical reconstruction.

Injuries to joints

There may be dislocation, subluxation (partial displacement) or strain of the ligaments. The long-term result is often joint stiffness and osteoarthritis, from any fracture involving the joint. Adhesions may occur and the best preventive measure is early mobilization and exercise. The knee, elbow, shoulder and finger joints stiffen easily whereas the wrist usually regains its mobility. Exercises are always necessary and physiotherapy may continue long after the fracture has healed.

Osteoarthritis is likely to develop in any joint that has been involved in a displaced fracture. The risk varies according to the joint involvement at the time and the residual damage to the joint. The arthritis may occur within 6–9 months after a severe injury but may not become apparent for 15 or 20 years if the damage is slight.

Fat embolism

Uncommon but often fatal. Globules of fat enter the venous circulation and pass through the lungs to the systemic circulation. Small blood vessels may be blocked by the fat globules and this usually occurs in the lungs (resulting in difficulty in breathing and hypoxaemia) or the brain. Fat embolism most often follows a fractured shaft of femur.

Recovery occurs if the patient can be supported over the dangerous period of hypoxia. Oxygen is given and heparin may be administered to aid capillary flow.

4.9 THE IMMUNE SYSTEM

Immunology is the study of the way in which organisms fight off disease. It includes the study of how they differentiate between self and non-self. The immune system is a defence system that will identify and destroy all substances, dead or alive, not recognized as self. It is a remarkably adaptive defence system that has evolved in vertebrates to protect them from invading pathogenic microorganisms and cancer.

- The complexity of the network rivals that of the nervous system.
- It is able to differentiate between what is foreign and what are the body's own cells and proteins.
- Once a foreign organism is recognized there are a variety of cells and molecules which will effect an appropriate response.
- Later exposure to the same foreign organism will initiate a memory response, which is characterized by heightened immune activity to eliminate the pathogen and prevent disease.

Immunity has both specific and non-specific components.

- *Innate* immunity is non-specific and refers to the basic resistance to disease that an individual is born with.
- *Acquired* immunity is specific and involves white blood cells called lymphocytes and antibodies.

Innate immunity can be seen to be composed of four types of barriers.

Anatomic barriers
- Skin
- Mucous membranes

Physiological barriers
- Temperature – body temperature inhibits the growth of some

pathogens, e.g. chickens have a high body temperature which makes them immune to anthrax
- Low pH
- Chemical mediators – lysozyme, interferon, complement

Phagocytic barriers – white blood cells
- Neutrophils
- Macrophages

Inflammatory barriers
- Tissue damage and infection induce leakage of vascular fluid, which contains serum proteins, and an influx of phagocytic cells occurs into the affected area.
- Inflammatory response includes vasodilatation, increase in capillary permeability and an influx of phagocytes.

ACQUIRED IMMUNITY

This needs the presence of a functional immune system that is capable of recognizing and selectively eliminating organisms. Acquired immune responses are adaptive and display antigenic specificity and immunological memory.

Acquired immunity involves two major populations of white blood cells:

- B lymphocytes – produce antibodies
- T lymphocytes – produce chemicals to 'help' the B lymphocyte in antibody production.

AGEING AND THE IMMUNE SYSTEM

- Immune function decreases with age.
- Diminished T cell function and antibody responses to antigenic challenge.
- However, circulating autoantibodies and immune complexes increase.
- Those over 60 have decreased delayed hypersensitivity reactions, decreased T cell responses to infection and decreased T cell activity.

HYPERSENSITIVITIES

The immune system is a finely tuned network that protects the host against foreign antigens, particularly infectious agents. Sometimes this network breaks down and the immune system reacts inappropriately.

Type 1 hypersensitivity is an immediate allergic response due to the production of IgE antibodies to an allergen. It is an exaggerated response to an environmental antigen – called an *allergy*. It is responsible for the severe response in anaphylaxis and for hay fever, asthma and eczema.

Hypersensitivity reactions are immediate or delayed depending on the time required for the reaction to appear after re-exposure to an antigen. *Immediate* hypersensitivity reactions occur in a few minutes to hours. *Delayed* hypersensitivity reactions may take several hours and are at maximum severity several days after reexposure to the antigen.

Anaphylaxis is the immediate hypersensitivity reaction (see p. 15).

- It is a rapid and severe response occurring within minutes of re-exposure to the antigen.
- It can be systemic or localized.
- Symptoms include itching, erythema, urticaria (hives), vomiting, abdominal cramps, diarrhoea and breathing difficulties.
- In severe cases, laryngeal oedema and vascular collapse may occur and result in respiratory distress,

---

Box 4.9   Common antigens associated with type 1 hypersensitivity

Proteins
Foreign serum
Vaccines

Plant pollens
Rye grass
Ragweed
Timothy grass
Birch trees

Drugs
Penicillin
Sulphonamides
Salicylates

Foods
Nuts
Seafood
Eggs
Peas, beans

Insect products
Bee venom
Ant venom
Cockroach calyx

Mould spores

Animal hair and dander

decreased blood pressure, shock and death.

- Severe anaphylaxis, when there is difficulty in breathing or collapse, is treated with adrenaline 1 in 1000, 0.5 ml, intramuscularly.
- Chlorphenamine (Piriton) and hydrocortisone are also given to reduce symptoms.

General predisposition

- Certain individuals are prone to allergies and are *atopic*.
- Atopic individuals tend to produce higher quantities of IgE.
- The airways and skin of atopic individuals are also more responsive to all types of stimuli.
- In families where one parent has an allergy, allergies develop in about 40% of the offspring.
- If both parents have allergies, the incidence in offspring is about 80%.
- Atopic individuals are more susceptible to asthma, hay fever and eczema.

Skin testing is available to determine allergies against which individuals are sensitized but can be dangerous. The allergen is injected intradermally or put onto the skin in a scratch test. A local anaphylactic response occurs within 30 minutes in sensitized individuals.

Localized anaphylaxis (atopy)

The reaction is limited to a particular tissue or organ, often involving the epithelial surfaces at the site of entry of the allergen.

Atopic allergies affect at least 20% of individuals in developed countries and include hay fever (allergic rhinitis), asthma, eczema and food allergies.

ECZEMA

This is a form of dermatitis that is non-specific and may be acute, subacute or chronic.

Dermatitis is the name given to inflammatory conditions of the skin. They may involve the dermis or epidermis but usually involve both.

- The skin becomes red and itchy. The epidermis and superficial dermis are involved.
- There may be oedema in the acute stages.
- Tiny blisters called vesicles develop in the epidermis: fluid accumulates between the epidermal cells (*spongiosis*), eventually forming small fluid-filled collections. These burst, causing weeping and oozing of clear yellow fluid, and then crust over.
- In chronic phases, scaling and fissuring occur.
- Excoriation may lead to secondary infection.
- Intense itching and scratching cause secondary changes due to trauma to occur. This leads to chronic dermatitis.
- The skin is thickened and cracked and often covered with a thick opaque scale.
- The skin looks a bit like the bark of a tree due to its increased thickness and the underlying oedema. This is called *lichenification*.
- The dermis shows increased fibrosis.

Dermatitis may be due to many causes but one of the most common in childhood is atopic eczema, which usually starts in infancy. Where the disorder starts early in life, there is a good chance that it will clear in adolescence; 90% of those with infantile eczema will be clear in adulthood. A few may be able to correlate the onset of itching with dietary factors and removal of the food item, e.g. eggs, milk, from the diet will improve the condition.

There is a tendency to dry, flaky skin (*xeroderma*) even when the eczema is not present.

Exacerbating factors

- Heat
- Humidity
- Drying of the skin
- Contact with woolly clothing may cause a flare-up

Staphylococcus aureus is found on the skin in a higher percentage of these individuals than normal and may be present in 90% of lesions.

Eczema is never present at birth but it may develop after a few weeks. Atopic eczema affects 3% of all infants.

Patterns of disease

- *Infantile eczema* – usually first appears on the facial skin at a few months of age.
- With time there is spread to other flexures.
- *Flexural or childhood dermatitis* – in toddlers or children; the skinfolds are usually involved. Some facial involvement may persist.
- *Adult dermatitis* – flexures at the neck, elbow, wrist, ankle, knee

and the limbs are usually involved. Chronic eczematous changes are common on the face.
- *Seborrhoeic dermatitis* – a coarse, yellowish crust scale is seen on the scalp. May be called cradle cap or milk crust. Disappears by the age of a year.
- *Napkin dermatitis* – this is a form of contact dermatitis; 50% of babies may be affected at some time. Bright erythema is present.

AUTOIMMUNITY

In autoimmune diseases the immune system reacts against self antigens and destroys host tissues. Antibodies against self are called *autoantibodies* and are produced by healthy individuals, especially the elderly, without overt autoimmune disease.

Autoimmune diseases affect 5–7% of the population and may be:

- organ specific
- systemic.

Systemic autoimmune diseases

- The response is directed towards a large number of target antigens and involves a number of organs and tissues.
- They reflect a generalized defect in immune regulation.
- Tissue damage is widespread from both cell-mediated immune responses and direct cellular damage caused by autoantibodies.
- Includes systemic lupus erythematosus (SLE) and rheumatoid arthritis.

Table 4.11 Some organ-specific autoimmune diseases in humans

Disease	Organ
Addison's disease	Adrenal glands
Haemolytic anaemia (autoimmune)	RBC membrane protein
Graves' disease	Thyroid
Hashimoto's thyroiditis	Thyroid cells
Idiopathic thrombocytopenic purpura	Platelets
Type I diabetes mellitus (IDDM)	Pancreatic beta cells
Myasthenia gravis	ACh receptor
Pernicious anaemia	Gastric parietal cells

Treatment of autoimmune disease

- Ideally the treatment should be aimed at reducing the autoimmune response while leaving the rest of the immune system intact. To date, this ideal has not been reached.
- Current therapies are not cures but palliatives.
- Aim to reduce symptoms to give the patient a reasonable quality of life.
- Most provide non-specific suppression of the immune system and do not differentiate between a pathogenic immune response and a protective one.
- Immunosuppressive drugs such as corticosteroids, azathioprine and cyclophosphamide are given to slow the proliferation of lymphocytes. However, the patient is then at a much greater risk of infection and cancer.
- Removal of the thymus has been used in myasthenia where it is often abnormal.
- Plasmapheresis has been shown to help some patients. Plasma is removed from the patient's body by continuous flow centrifugation. The red blood cells are resuspended in a suitable medium and returned to the patient. This removes antigen–antibody complexes for a short period.

ALLOIMMUNITY

Alloimmune disease occurs when the immune system of one individual produces an immunological reaction against the tissues of another individual. It may be observed in reactions against transfusions, grafted tissues or the fetus in pregnancy.

Preventing graft rejection

The severity of rejection is determined by certain genetic differences and whether an organ is a good match or not can be determined by *tissue typing*. Closely related individuals are likely to have similar tissue types and grafts between identical twins are completely accepted.

Immunosuppressant drugs are given to try and suppress the

immune response and graft rejection.

IMMUNODEFICIENCY DISEASES

A diverse spectrum of illnesses that stem from various abnormalities of the immune system. Basic manifestations are frequent, prolonged, severe infections, which are often caused by organisms with normally low pathogenicity.

An immunodeficiency disease may result from:

- a primary congenital defect
- a secondary cause, such as viral or bacterial infection, malnutrition or a drug treatment.

Acquired immune deficiency syndrome (AIDS) is the most significant immunodeficiency arising from secondary causes. AIDS is an epidemic of a retroviral disease characterized by profound immunosuppression. It is caused by the human immunodeficiency virus HIV-1 and is associated with opportunistic infections, secondary neoplasms and neurological manifestations. HIV-1 infects humans, chimpanzees, pigtailed macaques and SCID-human mice but causes immune suppression only in humans.

AIDS renders its victims susceptible to opportunistic infections and certain rare forms of cancer, which are the immediate cause of death. Transmission is possible via:

- sexual intercourse
- contaminated blood products and organ donation – very rare since screening was introduced in 1985
- contaminated needles in IV drug users or in needlestick injuries
- passage of virus from infected mothers to their newborns.

Infected mothers transmit AIDS by three routes:

- transplacental, in utero
- during delivery
- via breast milk – not usual.

Vertical transmission by these routes occurs in 12–30% of infants at risk.

Although originally more common in homosexual males, the rate of increase of heterosexual transmission has outpaced transmission by all other means. The number of women with AIDS is increasing rapidly. The presence of any other sexually transmitted disease such as *Treponema pallidum* or herpes simplex virus increases the likelihood of transmission because of genital ulceration.

There is an extremely small but definite risk to healthcare workers and seroconversion has been reported following an accidental needlestick injury. The risk is believed to be 0.3%. By comparison the risk for hepatitis B would be 30%.

Genetic variation in HIV
- HIV is capable of tremendous genetic variation with mutation occurring at rates millions of times faster than observed in human DNA.
- The influenza virus also has a high mutation rate and this has hampered the production of an effective flu vaccine.
- The rate of mutation in HIV is 65 times that of the influenza virus.

- No two AIDS patients carry an identical virus.
- HIV isolates taken from the same individual at different times can differ substantially.

Diagnosis of infection

- Most individuals develop symptoms of HIV 8–10 years after infection but approximately 25% of infected individuals have remained symptom free for some 10–12 years.
- Soon after infection with HIV the virus replicates and can be detected in the serum but is only there for a few weeks and then disappears as the antibody response (seroconversion) develops.
- In most cases the time between infection and seroconversion is 6 weeks but in some it has lasted for 3 years.
- At seroconversion antibodies to HIV can be detected in the blood (serum).
- Within a few weeks these decline and IgG appears.
- As long as the antibody to core protein remains high, an individual remains asymptomatic.
- When the antibody declines this is associated with progression from latency to infection.

The CD4 cell (T helper) in AIDS

- Uninfected persons have about 1100 CD4 cells per microlitre of blood.
- In AIDS this drops dramatically and may be as low as 200.
- About 40% of AIDS patients manifesting opportunistic

infections have no detectable CD4 cells at all.
- The CD4 count drops very slowly over 8–10 years and then rapidly in most cases.

Clinical features

The spectrum of illnesses associated with AIDS is very broad.
The following classification is that of the Centers for Disease Control (CDC).

Group I Acute seroconversion illness
Occurs 4–8 weeks after exposure in some patients. It is a self-limiting and non-specific illness with fever, myalgia (muscle aching), oral ulceration, generalized lymphadenopathy (enlarged lymph glands) and a maculopapular rash (small red spots).

Group II Asymptomatic infection
A period when the number of HIV-infected lymphocytes is gradually increasing. Individuals may remain well but they are infectious. This stage may last up to 10 years.

Group III Persistent generalized lymphadenopathy
The presence of enlarged lymph nodes of more than 1 cm in diameter at two or more sites for more than 3 months.

Group IV symptomatic HIV infection
Divided into subgroups A–E.

- A – continuous symptoms of fever, weight loss and diarrhoea
- B – neurological disease: dementia, peripheral neuropathy, myelopathy
- C – opportunistic infections
- D – secondary cancers
- E – other conditions – thrombocytopenia

Management

Zidovudine inhibits the reverse transcriptase of the virus and so prevents replication in the host cells. It reduces mortality and opportunistic infections in patients with symptomatic HIV infection.

Prevention and control

- Screening of blood products
- Use of condoms in sexual intercourse
- Advice to drug addicts not to share needles or the provision of free sterile needles

4.10 CANCER

Known since the time of the ancient Egyptians, cancer occurs in most plants as well as animals. *Neoplasia* means new growth. *Neoplasms* are often referred to as tumours and the study of tumours is called *oncology*.

Malignant tumours are collectively referred to as cancers, from the Latin for 'crab'. The lesion can invade and destroy adjacent structures and spread to distant sites (*metastasise*) to cause death.

Benign tumours

May affect any tissue

- Grow locally but do not spread or invade
- Damage tissues by pressure
- Resemble the tissue of origin and, if endocrine, are likely to produce hormones
- Usually have a capsule of connective tissue

Malignant tumours

- Cellular abnormalities are present and there may be invasion of the surrounding tissues
- Local increase in cell number and increased mitotic activity
- Loss of normal regular arrangement
- Variation in cell size and shape
- Increase in nuclear size and density of staining
- No well-defined capsule
  C = M = epidose

Carcinoma in situ is a small tumour that remains localized in the epithelial layer, usually on the cervix or skin but can be the bladder and other organs. There is no invasion of underlying tissue, the cancer remains where it began – in situ.

The only definite evidence of malignancy is invasion of the underlying tissues and metastases.

NAMING TUMOURS

The generic name, which describes the tissue of origin and whether the tumour is benign or malignant, is qualified by the specific tissue of origin and this may be further qualified by further terms describing the cell of origin and the pattern of growth. Benign tumours tend to be named by adding *-oma* to the cell type from which the tumour arises.

Tumours of the epithelium

- Benign tumours
- May be papillary (warty) or solid
- Glandular tissue – adenomas and may be solid or papillary

- Malignant tumours
- Generic name is carcinoma
- Can qualify as squamous cell or basal cell if the skin is involved
- Glands – adenocarcinoma but can also describe the cell type, e.g. columnar cell

Tumours of the mesenchyme

- Benign tumours – named from the cellular tissue from which they arise: fibroma (fibrous tissue), osteoma (bone), angioma (blood vessels), etc.
- Malignant tumours – generic name is sarcoma and as with carcinoma, this is qualified by the cell of origin and growth type, e.g. osteosarcoma – tumour of bone, osteogenic sarcoma – tumour of bone-forming cells.
- Most sarcomas grow rapidly.

Tumours of the reticuloendothelial system

This is a complicated field. Benign tumours do exist but are difficult to distinguish. There are two main types:

- those arising from blood-producing cells – leukaemias
- solid tumours – lymphomas

Tumours of the nervous system

- Benign and malignant but malignant very rarely spread outside the nervous system.
- Tumours of nerve cells proper – neurons – only arise in the embryo or shortly after birth – neuroblastomas and retinoblastomas.

- Almost all tumours are either gliomas, that arise from the supporting connective tissues within the brain, or meningiomas, that arise from the membranes surrounding the brain.

Tumours of mixed tissues

Very rarely tumours which contain a whole range of different tissues may be found – teratomas. They are thought to arise from primitive cells of embryonic type and are usually found in the testes or ovary. Sometimes they are benign but often malignant changes occur.

- Sometimes the tissue of origin can be identified and the tumour is *differentiated*.
- Other tumours may follow a very undifferentiated growth pattern and be classed as *poorly differentiated*.
- Malignant neoplasms composed of undifferentiated cells are said to be *anaplastic*. This is the most extreme disturbance in cell growth and structure of the tissue is lost.
- The rate of growth of malignant tumours correlates in general with their level of differentiation.
- *Dysplasia* is a term used to describe disorderly but non-neoplastic proliferation which exhibits loss of uniformity and architectural orientation. This is seen in epithelial tissue and if marked and involving the entire thickness of the epithelium, the lesion is known as *carcinoma in situ*.

CARCINOGENESIS

This is a multistage process that is still not completely understood. There is an evolving process causing changes to the genetic material (DNA) within the nucleus of the cell. The tumour appears to be derived from a single stem cell.

Theories suggest that there is an initiation stage, such as contact with a carcinogen, which does not lead to the immediate development of a tumour but is rapid and essential for development to occur. The initiated cells may be dormant for very long periods or even the whole lifespan of the individual and several further independent accidents may have to occur to the same cell for tumour development to continue. This would explain why most forms of cancer increase in incidence as we get older, i.e. the chances of cumulative accidents to the cell increase with time. Examples of carcinogens include cigarette smoke, viruses, radiation and certain chemicals in foods named *xenobiotics*.

Cancers in humans can be divided into three groups dependent on age and incidence.

- Embryonic
  —Neuroblastoma (tumours of embryonic nerve cells)
  —Wilms' tumours (embryonal tumours of the kidney)
  —Retinoblastomas
- Those occurring predominantly in the young
  —Some leukaemias
  —Tumours of the bone and testes
- Those with an increasing incidence with age

—Prostate, colon, breast, skin, salivary glands, etc.

There are at least three possible explanations for age-related tumour incidence.

- Continuous exposure throughout life to low levels of carcinogens.
- Hormonal changes occur with age and these allow neoplastic changes to occur.
- Age-associated changes in some cells increase susceptibility to neoplastic transformation.

TUMOUR SPREAD

- Local
- Via the lymphatic system
- Via the bloodstream
- Seeding within body cavities

Cancers grow by progressive infiltration, invasion, destruction and penetration of surrounding tissue.

Basal cell carcinomas of the skin and primary tumours of the central nervous system are highly invasive in their primary sites but only rarely metastasize. At the other extreme are osteogenic sarcomas that have usually metastasized to the lungs before discovery.

Approximately 30% of newly diagnosed patients with solid tumours present with metastases. An additional 20% have occult metastases at the time of diagnoses.

- When local invasion occurs, tumours may penetrate the lymphatics and be carried to the regional lymph nodes where they may be arrested.
- Some are destroyed but some grow.

LN = C
X S

- If tumour cells get into the bloodstream they can be carried to any organ in the body.
- Many are destroyed but others grow into secondary tumours.
- Arteries are less readily penetrated than veins.
- All portal drainage flows to the liver and all caval blood flows to the lungs.
- Carcinomas often involve the lymph nodes, sarcomas do not.
- Metastases are common in the lungs, liver and bone but rare in muscle and spleen.

BREAST CANCER

This has now taken over from lung cancer as the most common cancer in Britain. Approximately 1 in 8 women in England may develop breast cancer during their lifetime and 3.5% of all women die of this disease.

The risk increases with advancing age and the peak incidence is between 45 and 64 years. In this age group breast cancer is the leading cause of death.

Risk factors

- Reproductive – the younger a woman has her first full-term pregnancy, the lower the risk of breast cancer.
- Hormonal – late menarche and early menopause reduce the risk. Removal of the ovaries is protective. Increasing oestrogen levels may be a risk.
- Hormone replacement therapy (HRT) has been linked to an increased incidence of breast cancer but this is with prolonged use of HRT (over 8 years) and the risk is lost as soon as the HRT is discontinued.
- Environmental – high-dose radiation.
- Diet perhaps – results of research are mixed but there may be a higher risk with a high-fat diet. There is a low incidence in Japan that could be related to diet.
- Some studies show that there may be a correlation between alcohol consumption and breast cancer.
- Viral factors have been suspected following research with mice.
- Trauma is not thought to have any effect.
- Familial – 7% of breast cancers are familial. Autosomal dominant gene with 90% penetration by the age of 50.

Screening

In the UK screening is commenced at the age of 50 years and is offered every 3 years until the age of 64. Regular screening can reduce breast cancer mortality by up to 25%. Mammography has a 90% accuracy but is less accurate premenopausally due to the density of breast tissue.

Screening should begin earlier for those at high risk and regular breast self-examination should be practised by all women.

Diagnosis

The patient may present with a breast lump, nipple retraction, breast pain, a discharge from the nipple, inflammation or an axillary lump. Mammography, ultrasound, examination and cytology or needle biopsy may all be involved in the diagnosis.

BC = CS (BN)(NI)
= Ic (I)

- Needle biopsy – 95% accuracy.
- Frozen section – 99.4% accuracy.

Pathogenesis

Most cancers arise from the ductal epithelium. There are two classes of breast cancer.

Carcinoma in situ – non-invasive

- Growth is confined to the basement membrane of the duct or gland.
- Difficult to detect because there may be no fibrous lump; the cancer does metastasize, (extend) though.
- The usual treatment consists of complete local excision with radiotherapy and/or tamoxifen.
- Paget's disease of the nipple is an intraduct carcinoma, which presents as a red scaly lesion of the nipple.

Infiltrating carcinoma – invasive

- Most breast cancers are of this type.
- Infiltrating ductal carcinomas account for 75% of all tumours.
- Invasive lobular carcinoma – 10%.
- Other types include tubular, medullary and mucinous; these carry a better prognosis usually.
- Sixty percent of tumours occur in the upper, outer aspect of the breast because most glandular tissue is found here.

Presentation

- Early signs are insidious.
- A non-tender lump, most often in the upper, outer quadrant of the breast.

- At first the lump is mobile and pain is usually absent until the later stages.
- Dimpling or retraction of the skin over the lump – peau d'orange appearance. This is due to oedema caused by blockage of the small lymphatic ducts.
- Retraction of the nipple, due to a shortening of the ducts.
- Asymmetry of the breasts may be noted on mirror examination. The affected breast appears more elevated.
- The lump appears fixed to the chest wall at a later stage.
- Nodular axillary lumps may be present. These are enlarged lymph nodes.
- In the late stages ulceration may occur.

Treatment of invasive breast cancer

- In early operable breast cancer, a mastectomy (removal of the breast) may be done.
- Axillary clearance or sampling of the axillary lymph nodes is necessary as histology of the lymph nodes is vital to determine if the cancer has spread.
- Cytotoxic chemotherapy in premenopausal women and tamoxifen in postmenopausal women reduce the death rate at 10 years by about 25%.

Routes of spread

Locally

- Involving a progressive amount of breast tissue.
- Eventually results in skin involvement and ulceration or

attachment to the muscle and chest wall.

BC(T)

Via the lymphatic system

- To axillary nodes at an early stage; 50–60% of those with operable cancer have axillary nodes.
- To internal mammary lymphatics.
- Skin lymphatics – leads to multiple tumour nodules. The skin becomes stiff and board-like.
- Mediastinal and abdominal nodes later in the disease.

Via the blood

- Very common and present in virtually all fatal cases.
- Most frequent metastases occur in the lungs, liver, bones and brain.
- The patient may first present with a pathological fracture or bony pain.

Staging

It is not easy to be totally accurate in this. The T (tumour) N(nodes) M(metastases) classification is also used.

Stage I

- Tumour confined within the breast
- Less than 2 cm in size
- Not fixed to skin or fascia
- Axillary and internal mammary glands not involved
- Eighty-six percent survival rate at 5 years

Stage 2

- Larger growth but less than 5 cm
- Some local involvement
- Lymph nodes may be involved but mobile
- Forty-five percent survival at 5 years

Stage 3

- More advanced
- Skin involvement and may be fixed to the chest wall
- Twelve percent survival at 5 years

Stage 4

- Evidence of distant metastasis
- Twelve percent survival at 5 years

All grades with uninvolved lymph nodes – 75% survival at 5 years. All grades with involved lymph nodes – 30%.

CANCER OF THE PROSTATE GLAND

This is a disease of older men and the third most common male cancer.

The prostate gland is situated around the upper end of the urethra just below the bladder. It is involved in the secretion of prostatic fluid that nourishes sperm.

At postmortem 30% of men over 75 years have prostate cancer.

Risk factors

- Associated with circulating testosterone – does not occur in castrated men.
- Reports of increased risk following vasectomy.

Clinical features

- May be asymptomatic and found following operation for benign prostatic hyperplasia (BPH).
- Routine screening may show raised serum prostate specific antigen (PSA).

- Difficulty in passing urine is usually the first symptom – poor stream, hesitancy, terminal dribbling, frequency and nocturia.
- Perineal pain may be present in advanced disease.
- Often metastasizes to bone and pathological fracture may be the first sign.

Investigations
- Rectal examination usually reveals a hard irregular prostate.
- FBC and biochemical profile.
- Serum PSA (prostatic specific antigen) and acid phosphatase.
- Transrectal ultrasound.
- Cystourethroscopy with examination under anaesthetic (EUA) and biopsy or transrectal biopsy.
- Bone scan – looking for metastases.

Treatment
- Localized tumour that is well differentiated may sometimes be left untreated in an elderly man.
- Localized tumours can be treated with radical prostatectomy or local radiotherapy.
- Transurethral resection of the prostate (TURP) relieves obstruction and allows histology of the tumour.
- Radical prostatectomy involves removal of the seminal vesicles and prostatic urethra.
- These operations used to be associated with a high incidence of impotence but nerve-sparing procedures have reduced this.
- Radiotherapy.
- External beam therapy using CT scan planning.

- Hormone therapy to reduce circulating testosterone levels. Cyproterone acetate is a testosterone antagonist. GRH (gonadotrophic hormone) agonists shut down stimulation from the pituitary. Side-effects include loss of libido and sweats.

Metastatic disease
May be treated with hormone manipulation, orchidectomy (removal of the testes) and palliative radiotherapy which is very effective in the management of bone metastases.

CANCER OF THE TESTES

This is the most common malignancy in men aged 20–40 years. There are about 1400 new cases annually in the UK and the incidence is rising.

Testicular germ cell tumours are classified as seminomas, teratomas or yolk sac tumours.

Clinical features
- Unilateral testicular swelling – all men should self-examine for this. It is sometimes associated with pain.
- As the disease progresses there may be weight loss, lethargy and respiratory symptoms if associated with lung metastases.
- Headache from cerebral metastases may occur.
- Back pain from glandular involvement retroperitoneally.

Investigations
- Testicular ultrasound.
- Various blood tests for hormone levels.

- Chest X-ray, CT scan of thorax, abdomen and pelvis and brain scan if cerebral secondaries are suspected.

Treatment
- Surgery – orchidectomy.
- May be followed by radiotherapy to lymph nodes.
- Chemotherapy may be used in stage II as an alternative using either the combination drug cisplatin or the single agent carboplatin.
- Postorchidectomy surveillance is monthly for the first year and approximately 20–25% relapse, usually within the first year.
- In over 96% of cases, a stage I seminoma may be disease free following orchidectomy and low-dose radiotherapy.
- In metastatic teratoma all patients receive chemotherapy. There is a 75–85% 5-year survival.

CANCER OF THE OVARY

This is the fifth most common carcinoma in women. Most patients do not present until the disease is advanced.

It is most common between 60 and 85 years of age and in nulliparous women. It is less common in users of the oral contraceptive pill.

Clinical features
- Early disease is normally asymptomatic.
- More advanced disease presents with abdominal pain, distension of the abdomen, ascites

(common), occasionally vaginal bleeding.

Investigations
- Abdominal ultrasound, laparoscopy, aspiration of ascites for cytology, CT scan.
- Most cases are diagnosed at laparotomy.

Treatment
Staging is done and treatment is based on this. Stage I is limited to the ovaries, stage II has extended to the pelvis, stage III has peritoneal implants of the tumour outside the pelvis and stage IV has distant metastases.

Surgery is the mainstay of treatment and the aim is to remove as much of the tumour as possible.

Chemotherapy with platinum-based drugs such as cisplatin is given monthly for 6 months. Response can be measured by CT scan.

Most women (70%) do not present until stage III or IV and the survival rates at 5 years are 17% and 5%.

CANCER OF THE CERVIX

The incidence in the UK is 24 per 100 000, affecting 3% of all women. It represents 20% of female cancers. The average age for detection of a precancerous lesions is 33–38 years and for invasive disease is between 50 and 60 years.

Invasive carcinoma has decreased over the years but abnormal cervical smears have increased, especially in those under 25 years of age.

Risk factors

- Associated with human papilloma virus (type 16) which is a sexually transmitted virus.
- Often associated with chronic cervicitis and cervical dysplasia.
- More common in lower socioeconomic groups.

Pathogenesis

It is a progressive disease and premalignant lesions occur 10–12 years before the development of invasive carcinoma.

Progressive changes

Cervical intraepithelial neoplasia (CIN). Also called cervical dysplasia. Some of the cervical cells are replaced by abnormal neoplastic ones. Does not always progress to cancer and many will spontaneously return to normal. Carefully followed by smears.

Cervical carcinoma in situ. Almost all the cervical epithelium shows the features of cancer but the underlying tissue is not affected.

Invasive carcinoma. There is invasion into adjacent tissues and spread to distant organs such as the lungs via the lymphatics.

Cervical cancer is staged from 0 to IV.

Clinical features

- Regular screening by cervical (Papanicolaou) smear is needed as the early disease is asymptomatic.
- Vaginal bleeding and discharge are common symptoms.
- Bleeding may follow intercourse or occur between menstrual periods. Postmenopausal bleeding may also occur.
- Colposcopy is examination of the cervix by the use of a light and a small microscope. This is done as an outpatient.

Treatment

- This depends on the stage of the disease.
- Premalignant and early cancer is treated with cryosurgery or laser therapy. Cone biopsies also remove a small amount of tissue and may be all that is needed to treat an early cancer. These procedures do not affect child-bearing ability.
- For invasive carcinoma the treatment depends upon the stage and may include hysterectomy, pelvic lymphadenectomy and more extensive pelvic surgery.
- Radiotherapy and chemotherapy are also used in some cases.

RADIOTHERAPY

Radiotherapy uses high-energy rays, usually X-rays, to kill cancer cells. It is a highly potent cytotoxic agent and reacts with both normal and malignant cells to induce the production of free radicals, which damage the intracellular DNA. The cell can function as usual but is unable to complete cell division. Normal cells are better able to repair the damage caused by sublethal doses of radiation than cancer cells. This difference in repair capacity is exploited in radiotherapy.

The total dose of radiation to be administered is divided into fractions and the time interval between fractions is calculated to allow maximum repair of normal tissue but only limited repair of malignant tissue.

Administration of radiotherapy

External beam therapy (*teletherapy*) may be produced at a lower voltage from an X-ray source. This could be used to treat superficial skin lesions such as basal cell carcinomas. It may be produced at a higher voltage by a gamma-emitting source or by a linear accelerator. This is suitable for deep-seated tumours.

Brachytherapy is ionizing radiation emitted from a sealed source placed close to the tumour, e.g. caesium needles or iridium wires.

Determining dosage

The maximum dose is given when the intention is curative. It is influenced by:

- the radiosensitivity of the tumour. Lymphomas are more sensitive than carcinomas, for instance
- the radiosensitivity of the normal tissue within the radiation field
- the volume of the normal tissue unavoidably irradiated.

In palliative radiotherapy the aim is symptom relief with the minimum side-effects possible.

Radiotherapy is usually given as an outpatient and most patients attend Monday to Friday although some may only attend once or twice a week.

Side-effects

Most side-effects are temporary and their extent depends on the area

being treated and the dose of radiation given. Many people have no problems at all.

Skin reactions
These occur less often these days the machines are more sophisticated and the maximum effect of the radiation is below the skin.

The extent of damage will depend on:

- the total dose of radiation administered
- the dose in each fraction
- the area of skin in the treatment field
- how fair-skinned the patient is.

This skin is specially sensitive where two skin surfaces come into contact, where there has been recent trauma and where the epidermis is thin and smooth.
There are four types of skin reaction.

- Inflammation – skin colour turns pink to red and may be slightly oedematous. Rather like sunburn.
- Dry desquamation – the skin becomes dry and scaly as the sebaceous glands are destroyed but this is not permanent.
- Moist desquamation – there is blistering and peeling of the epithelial layers. This is reversible but treatment should stop for a while.
- Long-term effects will result if the sweat or sebaceous glands are destroyed. Side-effects may occur up to 5 years later with atrophy of the skin.

The skin may be gently washed using a mild unperfumed soap and patted dry. No deodorants, perfumes or lotions should be applied to the area except those provided.

Tiredness and fatigue
This is quite common, especially towards the end of the treatment and it may last for some time after the treatment has stopped.

Scalp and brain
- Alopecia (hair loss). The hair follicles are especially sensitive to radiotherapy.
- The hair loss is usually temporary.

Head and neck
- Soreness of the mouth and throat due to drying of the mucous membranes, which they consist of epithelial cells that are sensitive to radiotherapy.
- Taste may change as some taste buds will be destroyed. Ability to eat may be affected and small, frequent meals should be taken.
- Extra fluids should be drunk and Complan or Build-up may help.
- Alcohol and tobacco may irritate the mouth and it is best to avoid them during treatment.
- Oral hygiene is very important and the teeth may be brushed but a very soft toothbrush should be used. A mouthwash may help to keep the mouth clean and moist but only one prescribed should be used.
- Soluble paracetamol may help.

Abdomen and pelvis
- Nausea and vomiting. Antiemetics will be prescribed.

- Diarrhoea as the lining of the intestine is affected – antidiarrhoeal tablets may be prescribed.
- Cystitis and sexual dysfunction may occur.

Cancer BACUP (www.cancerbacup.org.uk) provides helpful leaflets for the patient and their families on radiotherapy. There is a freephone helpline (telephone number available on the website) where information and support are provided by specialist nurses. All information provided aims to be high quality and up to date.

CHEMOTHERAPY

This is the treatment of cancer with cytotoxic drugs that destroy dividing cells. The aim of chemotherapy is to destroy the abnormal cancer cell, shrinking the primary tumour and also killing metastasized cells, while the normal body cells are spared.

The difference between the cancer cell and other body cells is the rate at which it reproduces and divides. Chemotherapy drugs attack the cell at different stages in the cell cycle when it is preparing for division or actually dividing.

The duration of the cell cycle varies from tissue to tissue. Some tissues are subject to much wear and tear, e.g. skin and cells lining the gastrointestinal tract. Others such as liver cells lie dormant unless damaged. The cell cycle can be as short as a few hours and as long as a number of years! Healthy cells that need to divide frequently, such as blood cells, can also be damaged by cytotoxic drugs but these cells are better able to repair themselves than cancer cells.

Often two or more drugs are used at the same time and this is called *combination therapy*.

Chemotherapy may be used to:

- cure cancer
- control cancer and prevent it from spreading
- relieve symptoms.

It may be used in addition to surgery or radiotherapy.

There are three distinct groups of cytotoxic drugs.

- Cell cycle non-specific drugs that bind to DNA and disable cell division, attacking the tumour cells whether they are dividing or dormant.
- Cycle-specific drugs that must be administered when cells are proliferating.
- Tissue-specific agents that deprive tissue of a substance needed for division.

Cell cycle non-specific drugs

Alkylating agents
These are amongst the most widely used of cancer chemotherapy agents. They act by inserting an alkyl group into the DNA and damaging it, thus interfering with cell replication.

Cyclophosphamide
- Used in chronic lymphatic leukaemia, lymphomas and some solid tumours.
- May be given orally or intravenously.

- A urinary metabolite may cause haemorrhagic cystitis: 3–4 l of extra fluids a day should be given to prevent this.

Chlorambucil
- Chronic lymphatic leukaemia, non-Hodgkin's lymphoma, ovarian cancer and Hodgkin's.
- Extra side-effects are rashes and marrow suppression.

Melphalan
- Myeloma, lymphomas, solid tumours.
- Given at intervals of 3–4 weeks.

Busulfan
- Chronic myeloid leukaemia.
- Frequent blood counts are needed as irreversible bone marrow aplasia may occur.

Lomustine (nitrosurea)
- Hodgkin's and solid tumours.
- Can cross the blood–brain barrier due to lipid solubility.

Cytotoxic antibiotics
These are derived from soil fungi, a variety of streptomyces species that are too toxic to be used as anti-microbials. All bind to DNA and they are widely used. They may act as radiomimetics so should not be given alongside radiotherapy.

Doxorubicin
- One of the most successful, well-used antitumour drugs.
- Acute leukaemias, lymphomas and solid tumours.
- Given by fast running infusion at 2-day intervals.

- May have toxic effects on the heart.
- Acts by intercalating the DNA.

Bleomycin
- Lymphomas and solid tumours.
- Causes no marrow suppression.
- By injection only.

Cell cycle specific
These are mostly antimetabolites. They mimic a normal metabolite and become incorporated into new nuclear material but do not function. Often combine irreversibly with vital cellular enzymes.

Folate antagonists
Folate is needed for the synthesis of DNA.

Methotrexate
- Causes myelosuppression.
- Damages the epithelium of the GI tract.
- In high doses can be toxic to the kidney – not given in renal disease.
- Used in combination regimes.
- May be given orally, intravenously, intramuscularly or intrathecally.
- Used as maintenance in childhood acute lymphatic leukaemia, choriocarcinoma, lymphomas, some solid tumours.
- Resistance may develop in tumour cells.
- High-dose therapy may be used for periods up to 12–36 hours. This could be lethal if doses of folate were not given to rescue the normal body cells, which recover better than the tumour cells.

Pyrimidine antagonists
- Cytarabine – mostly used to induce remission in myeloid leukaemia.
- Fluorouracil –used to treat solid tumours of the breast and colon. Can be used topically for malignancies of the skin.

Purine antagonists
- Mercaptopurine – maintenance for acute leukaemias.
- Thioguanine – acute leukaemias.

Mitotic poisons

Vinca alkaloids
From the periwinkle plant.

- Interfere with microtubule assembly and cause metaphase arrest.
- Given by injection.
- Relatively non-toxic but vincristine can cause peripheral neuropathy.
- Vincristine, vindesine, etoposide – can be given orally.
- Vinblastine – not neurotoxic but more myelosuppressive.

Taxanes
Derived from the yew tree.

- Taxol and taxotere act by spindle promotion.
- They are active against breast and ovarian cancer and are also used in small cell lung cancers.

Cisplatin
- Has a platinum atom in it and is extremely toxic. Blocks DNA replication.
- Causes very severe nausea and vomiting.

- Needs hydration therapy before administration.
- Useful in ovarian and testicular cancer.

Tissue-specific agents

A number of tumours of the endocrine system require hormones for their growth. Oestrogens and progestins are essential for some breast and endometrial tumours and prostatic tumours may need androgens.

Both hormones and hormone antagonists can be useful in the treatment of cancers of the reproductive system and their metastases.

Hormones

Medroxyprogesterone acetate is a progestogen that is used as second- or third-line management of breast cancer. It is also used for endometrial cancer.

Diethylstilbestrol is an oestrogen that used to be widely employed in the treatment of prostate cancer but its role is declining due to its side-effects.

Androgens are occasionally used as second- or third-line treatment in breast cancers. They are testosterone esters and examples are primoteston and virormone.

Hormonal antagonists

Tamoxifen

- An antioestrogen that is effective against oestrogen-dependent breast cancers.
- It is an oestrogen receptor antagonist and is the drug of choice in postmenopausal women with metastatic disease.

- Overall 30% of patients with metastatic disease respond to hormonal manipulation.
- Oestrogen receptor-positive tumours respond in 60% of cases.
- Tumours that are non-oestrogen dependent only respond in 10% of cases.
- Not all breast cancers are oestrogen dependent and some may be progesterone dependent.

Cyproterone acetate (Cyprostat).

An antiandrogen used in cancer of the prostate.

Disruption of pituitary function

The pituitary controls the secretion of sex hormones. Antiluteinizing hormone analogues act on the pituitary to reduce secretion of gonadotrophic hormones. They reduce secretion of androgens in males and are as good as orchidectomy in cancer of the prostate. Examples are buserelin, goserelin, leuprorelin or triptorelin.

Combination chemotherapy

Courses are known by the first letters of the drugs they contain. For example, an ICE course used in the treatment of acute myeloid leukaemia is a combination of the anticancer drugs idarubicin, cytarabine and etoposide.

- Different drugs exert their influence at different points in the cell cycle and so may be synergistic, e.g. cisplatin and 5-fluorouracil.
- Decreases the chances of drug resistance developing in the tumour.

Adverse effects of chemotherapy

These depend very much on the drug given. Some effects are immediate and some are delayed. As the drugs attack dividing cells, some of the side-effects are similar to those of radiotherapy.

Immediate effects may include nausea and vomiting, mouth ulcers and anorexia.

Delayed effects may include alopecia and suppression of bone marrow cells.

Thrombocytopenia, agranulocytosis, anaemia and leucopenia can occur. The reduced white cell count means lowered immunity and this itself may make it more difficult for the body to fight the cancer.

Regular blood counts are done and if the white cell count falls too low the treatment may have to be delayed.

Drug administration

Extreme care has to be taken when these drugs are administered parenterally. Should extravasation occur, the accidental leakage of the irritant drug into the tissues can lead to severe local necrosis (death) and permanent tissue damage. The drugs are usually given via a Hickman line to avoid this risk.

Those giving the drugs have to take precautions to avoid contact with the drug and gown and gloves are worn when preparing and giving these drugs. Direct contact with the skin can lead to dermatitis, inflammation, blistering and other allergic responses.

Written guidelines are provided to cover the preparation, administration and disposal of these drugs. Should any spillage or contamination of yourself or others occur, the guidelines must be followed and help sought immediately.

Chemotherapy is given in cycles and toxicity is monitored carefully. The World Health Organization has produced a grading for toxicity

4.11 SURGERY

Operations are classified according to a scale of magnitude, which relates broadly to the risks involved and the physiological disturbance.

- *Minor surgery* – this may sometimes be done in the community and may only involve a local anaesthetic, e.g. skin lesions. It may also be carried out in a day surgery unit, e.g. needle biopsy.
- *Intermediate surgery* – this is usually done in a day surgery unit and would include such operations as a hernia repair.
- *Major surgery* – much abdominal surgery falls into this category, e.g. cholecystectomy.
- *Complex major surgery* would include another aspect, e.g. cholecystectomy with anastomosis.
- *Complex major plus* includes heart surgery.

COMPLICATIONS OF SURGERY

- Early – within 24 hours
- Intermediate – up to 3 weeks postoperative
- Late – any time after, maybe up to years on occasions.

Complications may be:

- local – at the operation site
- general – affecting other systems, e.g. respiratory system.

According to Lafferty and Rennie (1998), this classification can be used for any operation, e.g. appendicectomy.

Abnormal bleeding
Causes include the following:

- Inherited deficiencies of coagulation factors such as haemophilia.

- Acquired coagulation deficiencies that may occur in liver disease and when vitamin K absorption is reduced.
- Drugs such as anticoagulants, e.g. heparin and warfarin. Anticoagulant therapy needs continuous monitoring. Aspirin also increases bleeding time.
- Thrombocytopenia may cause bleeding, especially when the platelet count is below $40 \times 10^9/l$. Causes include such blood disorders as leukaemia (see p. 184).
- Abnormalities of the vessel wall such as vasculitis and scurvy.

Abnormal clotting
Causes of thrombosis fall into one of the following categories.

- abnormalities in the vessel wall
- alterations in the state of blood flow
- alterations in the blood

	Local	General
Early	Bleeding	Anaesthetic Cardiac
Intermediate	Wound infection	Chest infection Deep venous thrombosis Pulmonary embolus
Late	Incisional hernia Ugly scar	Faecal fistula

PHARMACOLOGY

5.1 Drugs and the law 308

5.2 Administration of drugs 309

5.3 Nurse prescribing 310

5.4 Pharmacology in practice 311

5.5 Classification of drugs 315

5.6 Poisoning 325

5.1 DRUGS AND THE LAW

There are two main Acts of Parliament that control the prescription and administration of many drugs. These are The Medicines Act 1968 and The Misuse of Drugs Act 1971.

THE MISUSE OF DRUGS ACT 1971

This relates to drugs which are liable to cause dependence if misused. Certain drugs are referred to as 'Controlled Drugs' and known as CDs. Accurate records of all purchases, amounts of drug issued and dosages given have to be kept. There must be special labels on the containers of these drugs to make them clearly recognizable.

In hospitals there are regulations controlling these drugs.

- They are stored in a double-locked cupboard of their own.
- The key must be carried by the nurse in charge.
- There is a special Controlled Drugs Order Book for those drugs in frequent use which can be kept as stock. The sister in charge must sign each order.
- Each administration of these drugs has to be recorded in the Controlled Drug Book with the patient's name, the dose of the drug, the time it was given and the signature of the nurse who administers the drug and another who has checked all these details.

The content of the CD cupboard is checked regularly by the pharmacist against the contents of the CD Book and any discrepancies are fully investigated.

There are also prescription rules applying to these drugs, including that the prescription must always be in the prescriber's own handwriting and a computerized prescription form cannot be used.

The Misuse of Drugs Regulations 1985 divides drugs into five schedules, each with its own requirements governing supply, prescribing and record keeping.

Schedule 1 are drugs that are not used medicinally and possession and supply are prohibited. An example would be lysergic acid diethylamide (LSD).

Schedule 2 includes drugs subject to full controlled drug requirements. Examples include:

diamorphine (heroin)	morphine
pethidine	glutethimide
amfetamine	cocaine
fentanyl	methadone
dihydrocodeine injection	codeine phosphate injection

Schedule 3 are subject to the same special prescription requirements (except phenobarbital) but not to the safe custody requirements (except buprenorphine and diethylpropion). They do not need a special register but invoices must be retained for 2 years. Examples include:

buprenorphine	meprobamate
pentazocine	phentermine

Schedule 4 drugs are subject to minimal control and include 34 benzodiazepines, examples being diazepam and temazepam.

Schedule 5 includes those drugs which, because of their strength, are exempt from virtually all CD regulations other than retention of invoices for 2 years.

5.2 ADMINISTRATION OF DRUGS

As a registered nurse, the administration of medicines is an important aspect of your professional practice and the UKCC produced an advisory paper in 1992, in the form of a small booklet entitled 'Standards for the Administration of Medicines'. This is obtainable free of charge from the UKCC (now the NMC).

In this booklet there is emphasis on the trained nurse using thought and professional judgement when administering medication and so going beyond the mechanistic delivery of the prescribed dose on the treatment sheet. This would involve ensuring the correctness of the prescription and explaining the medication to the client if he did not already understand.

The effects of the medication should be assessed and evaluated and any side-effects reported to the medical team.
Drugs are very necessary in the treatment of some clients but the wrong drug could on occasions be lethal and safety is of prime importance in the administration of medicines.

The 'five rights' are a reminder of some of the essential points of care:

- right client
- right drug
- right dose
- right time
- right route.

POINTS TO NOTE

- The nurse should never administer a medication without knowing its action and there should always be a copy of the British National Formulary (BNF) available when medicines are given so that any new drugs can be found and their action clarified.
- The nurse must be certain of the identity of the patient to whom the medication is to be administered and should also have knowledge of his planned care.
- The prescription must be very clear and legible. Doctors are asked to print the drug name and in hospital must always use the generic name of the medication and not the trade name.
- If there is any ambiguity or query regarding the drug, the dose or the route of administration, which should all be very clear on the prescription sheet, the nurse must refuse to administer the medication and should contact the prescriber.
- When a medication has been administered, this must be recorded at the time in a clear and accurate manner and with a signature which is legible. If the patient refuses his medication this should also be recorded and the nurse in charge should assess the situation and contact the prescriber.

- A medicine must never be charted before it is given. When you sign for that drug you are saying that the client has actually taken it.
- Always check that the client understands the medication that he is receiving and is aware of any important side-effects. Emphasize the importance of the treatment and explain its mode of action in simple terms.
- If an error is made in the administration of a medicine, this should immediately be reported to the nurse in charge, who will inform the prescriber.
- Evaluate the action of the prescribed medication and record any positive or negative effects, informing the prescriber of these.

WHO CAN ADMINISTER MEDICINES IN A HOSPITAL SETTING?

The UKCC (1992b) states that 'prescribed medications should only be administered by registered practitioners who are competent for the purpose and aware of their personal accountability'. It also states that a first- or second-level nurse 'should be able to administer medicines without involving a second person' but do note that there may be exceptions to this dependent on local circumstances. Examples are paediatrics, where there may be insufficient specialist nurses, or areas that may be dependent on temporary agency staff.

5.3 NURSE PRESCRIBING

The medicinal Products: Prescription by Nurses Act 1992 permitted some nurses with a health visiting and district nursing qualification to prescribe certain drugs and dressings from a nurse prescribers' formulary.

The original list included:

- simple analgesics such as aspirin and paracetamol
- laxatives such as senna and lactulose
- antacids such as magnesium hydroxide mixture
- nystatin oral suspension for the treatment of thrush
- catheter maintenance solutions such as chlorhexidine
- mouthwash solutions
- parasiticidal preparations such as permethrin for scabies and head lice.

Following a 3-month consultation with nursing, medical and pharmacy professionals, ministers announced in May 2001 that nurse prescribing would be extended to more nurses with a wider range of medicines to cover four broad bands of practice:

- minor ailments
- minor injuries
- health promotion
- palliative care.

The nurse prescribers no longer have to be district nurses or health visitors but must be first-level registered nurses or midwives. They must be on the UKCC register as having completed the ENB approved course for nurse prescribing. This extended prescribing commenced in April 2002.

There is a nurse prescribers' extended formulary (NPEF) detailing those items that may be prescribed. This is incorporated every 6 months into the British National Formulary (BNF).

Those preparing for extended nurse prescribing undertake a specific programme of preparation at degree level with 25 taught days in a university and 12 days learning in practice. The programme is part time over a period of 3 months and includes assessment of theory and practice.

5.4 PHARMACOLOGY IN PRACTICE

Pharmacology is the study of drugs and their actions. It includes absorption, metabolism and elimination of the drug as well as the mode of action of the drug. Drug absorption will vary depending on the route of administration.

DRUG ADMINISTRATION

The aims of administration are:

- to establish optimal drug concentration at the target site
- to maintain optimal concentration for the required period of time
- to minimize adverse drug reactions due to general distribution.

Routes of administration

Oral
This is usually the most convenient route. Medication for oral administration may come in several forms.

Tablets. The drug has been diluted, powdered and compressed by a tabletting machine into a shape that will be easy to swallow. Tablets are often coated with sugar or some colouring material.

Some tablets have an *enteric coating (EC)*, which is usually shiny in nature and is an acid-resistant layer to prevent dissolution in the stomach. This is used for drugs that may be irritant to the stomach lining.

Some oral medications may be specially formulated for *slow release* and will have SR after their name.

Capsules. These usually contain oily or nauseous preparations in an envelope made of gelatine or a similar substance. Examples are ampicillin and cod liver oil. The medication is liberated when the outer capsule is digested in the stomach or intestine.

Mixtures. These are liquid preparations in a water or other solvent base which usually contain a number of ingredients. An example is magnesium trisilicate mixture, which is used as an antacid. Bottles containing mixtures should be shaken before administration as ingredients may separate out during storage.

Linctus. Used as a cough suppressant and made with a strong syrup base and flavouring agents. An example is linctus codeine.

Oral drug absorption. This is the passage of the drug from the gut lumen, through the gut mucosa and into the bloodstream. Although some absorption takes place in the stomach, the surface area here is much less than the small intestine, where most of the absorption takes place.

The absorption of oral medication is influenced by many factors.

Food in the stomach. Drugs are usually absorbed more quickly if the stomach is empty and in the case of most antibiotics, the client is instructed to take the medication 1 hour before food for this reason.

Drugs which may irritate the stomach should be given with or after food and this instruction will usually be on the container. An example is aspirin.

Interactions with other drugs. Drugs that inhibit gastric emptying, e.g. atropine, amfetamine, morphine, may reduce the rate of absorption of other drugs.

Diseases of the gastrointestinal tract, e.g. ulcerative colitis, may lead to poor absorption of the medication.

Transit time. The time taken for passage through the small intestine. The longer the medication is in the gut, the more of it will usually be absorbed.

Gastrointestinal movement aids the absorption of a drug and as the drug passes through the intestine, it is fragmented and dissolved. If there is excessive peristalsis, as in diarrhoea, the drug will not have time to be absorbed.

Laxatives also decrease absorption.

Acid in the stomach. This will destroy some drugs, e.g. acid-sensitive penicillins, so they have to be given by injection.

Enzymes. These will break down proteins and amino acids such as insulin, which therefore has to be given by injection.

Metal ions and tetracycline. Tetracycline forms a complex with either calcium or iron and if either of these is given with tetracycline a large molecule is formed that cannot be absorbed and the patient will not get the benefit of either drug.

As there is calcium in milk, tetracycline should not be taken with a drink of milk. Magnesium and aluminium also complex and may be found in antacids.

A drug concentration in the intestine depends on the:

- amount ingested
- rate with which it is released from the formulation
- volume of gastrointestinal contents with which it is mixed.

Sublingual

The drug is administered under the tongue. This route is used when drugs are metabolized very quickly by the liver and if swallowed, would pass into the circulation and reach the liver before their target organ, thus being destroyed before they have any action. An example is glyceryl trinitrate given for angina.

This route is also useful if the patient is not allowed fluids or feels sick, e.g. postoperatively the analgesic buprenorhine is given sublingually.

Rectal

Drugs may be given rectally for local or systemic action. For local action a suppository or an enema may be given when the patient is constipated to promote a bowel action. Glycerin suppositories are the most common. Glycerol is a mild irritant to the rectal mucosa and thus stimulates the defaecation reflex.

Steroid enemas are administered for local action on an inflamed bowel in ulcerative colitis.

Normally the rectum is empty and a suppository will melt and be absorbed via the rectal mucosa into the bloodstream, making this a good route for systemic drug administration.

The rectal route is especially useful when:

- a drug is irritant to the stomach mucosa, e.g. indomethacin for inflammatory pain
- the patient is vomiting or nauseated, e.g. prochlorperazine, an antiemetic
- there is difficulty in swallowing
- the patient is drowsy or unconscious.

Examples of drugs given rectally are:

- paracetamol – especially in fever
- diazepam – for convulsions
- prochlorperazine (Stemetil) as an antiemetic
- diclofenac (Voltarol) – a NSAID.

Transdermal (via the skin)
Drugs are usually given in the form of a patch that releases the drug through a rate-controlling membrane. It is absorbed through the skin and into the blood supply. Hormone replacement therapy and glyceryl trinitrate may be given this way.

Topical application
This is for local effect on the skin and mucous membranes.

- Creams – these are emulsions of oil and-water that are well absorbed into the skin and may be used for dry and scaly skin or as the base for other drugs, such as steroids in eczema.
- Eye drops – sterile preparations for instillation into the eye. This could be for an infection, e.g. chloramphenicol drops, or to have an effect on the pupil or the drainage system.
- Ear drops – these are for application to the external auditory meatus, e.g. cerumol which helps to dissolve wax in the ear.
- Vaginal pessaries or cream – for local action.

An advantage of topical application is that a high local concentration can be achieved, usually without a systemic effect. A disadvantage is that absorption can sometimes occur with serious effects.

Inhalation
This route is used for drugs that are absorbed via the respiratory mucosa for systemic action, e.g. volatile anaesthetics, and for drugs acting on the respiratory system.

The drug may be administered as:

- a gas, as in anaesthetics
- an aerosol, as in salbutamol inhalers used to treat asthma. Aerosols are particles dispersed in a gas and small enough to remain suspended for a long time

- a powder dispensed from a rotary inhaler as in sodium cromoglycate (Intal) for the treatment of asthma
- a nebulizer – the machine converts a solution of the drug into an aerosol. These are used in respiratory conditions, e.g. salbutamol for asthma.

Injection
Injections may be given:

- intradermally – into the skin. Used for allergy testing and diagnostic tests, e.g. Mantoux. Less than 0.1 ml may be given
- subcutaneously – under the skin. Used for insulin and heparin administration. Up to 2 ml may be administered. Sites for subcutaneous injection are shown in Figure 5.2. Absorption of the

drug does depend on local blood supply and may be more rapid with exercise
- intramuscularly – into a muscle. Up to 5 ml may be given into one site. The sites used are shown in Figure 5.1. Again, absorption is variable dependent on the site and the state of the circulatory system
- intravenously – into the venous circulation. This route may only be used by doctors and qualified nursing staff who have done a course in intravenous drug administration
- intrathecally – into the spinal theca. This route may be used in meningitis
- into various body cavities, e.g. the peritoneum, the pleura.

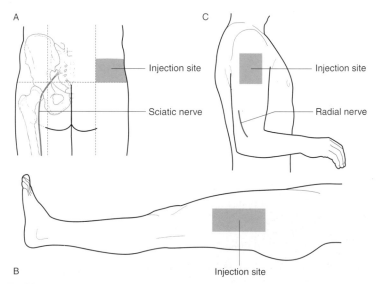

Fig. 5.1 Sites used for intramuscular injection. A. Upper outer quadrant of the buttock. B. Anterior lateral aspect of the thigh. C. Deltoid region of the arm. From Jamieson/Clinical Nursing Practice, reproduced with permission.

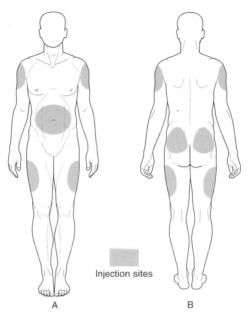

Fig. 5.2 Sites used for subcutaneous injection. A. Anterior aspect. B. Posterior aspect. From Jamieson/Clinical Nursing Practice, reproduced with permission.

The administration of any injection is an aseptic procedure and must involve good hand-washing and drying techniques.

Some advantages of intravenous administration

- The drug is delivered into the bloodstream and so is able to act immediately.
- There is no reliance on absorption and the whole dose of the drug reaches the bloodstream, enabling better calculation of the amount the patient actually receives.
- A continuous infusion allows the rate of administration to be controlled and the action of the drug thus modified.

Some disadvantages of intravenous administration

- Once the drug is given it cannot be removed from the body.
- Any allergic response is likely to be more severe.
- There is danger of infection if rigorous asepsis is not applied.
- Only those with special training can administer the drug.

5.5 CLASSIFICATION OF DRUGS

ANAESTHETICS

- Drugs that produce a loss of sensation.
- In local anaesthesia sensory nerve impulses are blocked and the

- patient remains alert. An example of a local anaesthetic is lidocaine (lignocaine) hydrochloride.
- In general anaesthesia there is loss of consciousness and the patient is unaware of, and unresponsive to, painful stimulation.
- Examples of general anaesthetics given intravenously are thiopentone sodium and propofol.
- General anaesthesia may also be maintained by the inhalation of anaesthetic gases and examples are nitrous oxide and halothane.

ANALGESICS

- Drugs that relieve pain.
- Paracetamol is a non-opioid drug that is not irritant to the stomach and of similar efficacy to aspirin but has no antiinflammatory action. When simple analgesia is needed it is usually tried first. The dose is 1 g every 4–6 hours. In overdosage it can cause liver failure.
- Codeine and dihydrocodeine are stronger than paracetamol but also cause more side-effects, such as constipation. Dihydrocodeine also may cause nausea and vomiting.
- Compound analgesic preparations usually contain paracetamol with a low dose of an opioid analgesic. Examples are co-codamol (paracetamol 500 mg plus codeine phosphate 8 mg), co-dydramol (paracetamol 500 mg and dihydrocodeine 10 mg) and co-proxamol. Co-proxamol is widely prescribed and is paracetamol 325 mg with dextropropoxyphene 32.5 mg. The latter produces some

euphoria. It may cause side-effects of dizziness and nausea in some patients and is very dangerous in overdosage when the dextropropoxyphene may cause respiratory depression.

- Non-steroidal anti-inflammatory drugs (NSAIDs) such as aspirin and ibuprofen are used for chronic pain of an inflammatory nature but are also useful in the treatment of mild to moderate pain, especially if it is musculoskeletal in origin.
- They are irritant to the stomach mucosa.
- Ibuprofen is the mildest; diclofenac and naproxen are of moderate strength and indomethacin is stronger.
- The side-effects of dyspepsia and stomach ulceration increase in severity with the strength of the drugs.

Opioid analgesics are the strongest and are reserved for severe visceral pain or analgesia in palliative care. Examples are morphine sulphate, diamorphine and pethidine. These drugs produce dependence if used over a period of time.

Morphine given for acute pain over a short period does not produce serious problems with dependency. MST Continuous, which is a modified-release formulation of morphine, is not suitable for acute pain.
Side-effects of morphine include:

- drowsiness
- nausea
- dizziness
- constipation.

Diamorphine is the drug of choice for severe chest pain as in myocardial infarction. It is more soluble and has a faster action than morphine. It may produce nausea and an antiemetic such as metoclopramide (10 mg) or prochlorperazine (12.5 mg) is often given as well.

In cases of chronic pain the doctor may prescribe mild analgesia to start with but if this does not control the pain, a stronger drug should be prescribed from further along the 'analgesic ladder'.

Analgesia in palliative care

- The aim in terminal illness is to keep the patient as comfortable, pain free and alert as possible.
- The number of drugs given should be as few as necessary to obtain symptom control and oral medication is usually satisfactory.
- Analgesics are always more effective in preventing the development of pain than in the relief of established pain.
- Non-opioid analgesics may well be sufficient in some cases if administered regularly. These would include paracetamol, aspirin and other NSAIDs.
- NSAIDs are especially useful in the control of bone secondaries and some occur in suppository form, e.g. naproxen, flurbiprofen and indomethacin.

Morphine is the most useful of the opioid analgesics as it not only relieves pain but also promotes a state of euphoria and mental detachment. Morphine may be given by mouth as an oral solution, 4 hourly, and the doctor should increase the dose if pain is occurring between doses.

Modified-release tablets of morphine (MST Continuous or Oramorph SR) are an alternative and have the advantage that they only need to be taken every 12 hours.

The starting dose if the patient is not already taking a strong analgesic is usually 10–20 mg every 12 hours but the dose would need to be higher if the patient has already been taking an opioid analgesic.

The BNF gives detailed dose regimens that the doctor may use for prescribing.

> ⚠ Modified-release morphine should never be given more frequently than every 12 hours.

Box 5.1	The analgesic ladder
Step 1	Non-opioids – paracetamol, aspirin and other NSAIDs
Step 2	Mild opioids and combinations – codeine, dihydrocodeine, co-proxamol, co-codamol, co-dydramol, etc.
Step 3	Strong opioids – morphine, diamorphine, etc.

Other routes of administration include rectally as a suppository while fentanyl is now available to be given transdermally as a patch. Morphine is not usually given by repeated administration of IM injections as this is both inconvenient and uncomfortable for the terminally ill patient.

- If morphine cannot be taken orally, a syringe driver may be used to administer the drug by slow continuous subcutaneous infusion.
- Diamorphine rather than morphine is used as this has a higher solubility, enabling larger doses to be given in a small volume.
- Symptoms can be controlled with the minimum of discomfort to the patient.

> ⚠ **Always remember that all opioid analgesics can cause constipation and this may be the source of much distress for the patient. If the patient is not able to tolerate a high-fibre diet, laxatives may have to be used.**

- Larger doses of opioids may cause respiratory depression and hypotension. Other side-effects include nausea, vomiting and drowsiness.
- Repeated administration does cause dependence and tolerance but this should not be a deterrent to pain control in the terminally ill.

ANTACIDS

- Drugs that neutralize the acidity of the gastric juice.
- They may be given in dyspepsia, gastritis, peptic ulcers and oesophageal reflux.

- Examples are magnesium trisilicate and aluminium hydroxide.

ANTHELMINTICS

- Drugs which destroy or eliminate intestinal worms.
- Examples are mebendazole and piperazine for threadworm and roundworm and niclosamide for tapeworm infections.

ANTIARRHYTHMICS

- Drugs given to prevent or reduce irregularities of cardiac rhythm.
- Examples are digoxin, adenosine, amiodarone and lidocaine.

Digoxin was originally derived from the foxglove. It is used in the treatment of heart failure, atrial fibrillation and atrial flutter. Digoxin slows the heart rate and increases the force of contraction.

It is toxic in doses only just above therapeutic and the patient may suffer from digoxin toxicity. Signs are:

- disturbed vision
- pulsus bigemus (coupling)
- abdominal pain
- confusion

Adenosine is a naturally occurring compound within the body. It can be used in the treatment of supraventricular arrhythmias (see p. 146). It is given by rapid intravenous injection as the body destroys it very quickly.

Side-effects may include severe bradycardia, flushing, dyspnoea and bronchospasm but are usually short-lived.

Amiodarone is a valuable antiarrhythmic drug used in both ventricular and atrial tachyarrhythmias. It is used in the treatment of rapid atrial fibrillation. The drug has a very long half-life and stays in the body for months after it has been discontinued.

Side-effects are common and include hypotension, microdeposits in the cornea, pulmonary fibrosis and discoloration of the skin in sunlight (*photosensitivity*).

Lidocaine (lignocaine) is a local anaesthetic but is also an antiarrhythmic drug. It is used in ventricular arrhythmias and is usually given by intravenous infusion in this case.

Side-effects can include anxiety, restlessness, dizziness and tremors as well as nausea and occasionally seizures.

ANTIBIOTICS

- Antibacterial substances originally derived from other living organisms such as fungi.
- Antibiotics are given for bacterial infections. They do not kill viruses and viral infections should not be treated with these drugs.
- Duration of therapy depends on the nature of the infection and the response to treatment. It is most important that a course of treatment is completed even if the patient feels better and it is also important that the drugs are taken at the correct time to maintain the necessary level of drug in the blood.
- Examples of antibiotics are penicillin, ampicillin, erythromycin, cephalosporins, gentamicin, metronidazole, trimethoprim and vancomycin.

Penicillin was one of the first antibiotics. It is bactericidal (kills bacteria) and interferes with the synthesis of the bacterial cell wall. It is used in a wide variety of bacterial diseases such as:

- throat infections
- pneumonia
- meningitis
- syphilis.

It is effective against many Gram-positive cocci such as *streptococci*, *meningococci* and *gonococci* and also most anaerobic (can live in the absence of oxygen) bacteria such as Clostridia (gas gangrene).

Penicillin G (benzylpenicillin) has to be given by injection as the acid in the stomach destroys it, but penicillin V is a derivative that can be given orally.

Side-effects are rare but some people are dangerously allergic to penicillin and anaphylaxis (see p. 15) may result. The nurse should always check if the patient is allergic to penicillin before starting a course of the drug.

Ampicillin is derived from penicillin but is a broad-spectrum antibiotic (kills both Gram-negative and Gram-positive bacteria). It may be given orally or intravenously.

Erythromycin is effective against a wide range of organisms and is often used if the patient is allergic to penicillin. It may be given orally or intravenously but is always well diluted, as it is irritant to the veins. It is also irritant to the GI tract and may cause nausea and diarrhoea.

Cephalosporins include first-generation drugs such as cefalexin, second-generation such as cefuroxime and cefaclor, third-generation such as cefotaxime and the fourth-generation drug cefepime. The spectrum of activity of the drugs is different and the third- and fourth-generation drugs are more active against Gram-negative bacteria. They are less susceptible to bacterial destruction than penicillin. Cefotaxime can penetrate the CNS and so is very useful in meningitis.

Gentamicin is a bactericidal antibiotic used in the treatment of septicaemia, meningitis and other CNS infections, biliary tract infections and many other instances. It can only be given by injection, as it is not absorbed in the GI tract. Plasma concentration monitoring is needed to ensure neither excessive nor subtherapeutic levels of the drug. The level should be checked after 3–4 doses of gentamicin, before administration to ensure the trough dose is sufficient and approximately 1 hour after intravenous or intramuscular administration to ensure the peak concentration is not too high. This is because gentamicin is toxic to the kidneys and the auditory nerve at high concentration.

Metronidazole is effective against anaerobic bacteria and protozoa. Surgical sepsis, leg ulcers, pressure sores and pseudomembranous colitis can all be treated. The drug is used prophylactically in gut and dental surgery. It can be used to treat trichomoniasis, an infection due to the protozoan *Trichomonas vaginalis* that often infects the vagina and causes inflammation of the genitalia with vaginal discharge. The drug may be given orally, rectally or intravenously and has a half-life of about 8 hours.

Side-effects include gastrointestinal disturbances, headache, dizziness, ataxia and occasionally seizures. Alcohol should be avoided whilst taking metronidazole.

Trimethoprim is a bacteriostatic drug (prevents bacteria multiplying). It is usually used in infections of the respiratory and urinary tract. It may be administered with a sulphonamide drug as co-trimoxazole but only in certain circumstances advised by the Committee on Safety of Medicines. Adverse effects include nausea and other GI disturbances.

Vancomycin is valuable in multiresistant staphylococcal infections and in those allergic to penicillin and cephalosporins. It can be given orally or intravenously and side-effects include ototoxicity (damage to hearing) and nephrotoxicity (damage to the kidney). It is contraindicated in renal failure as dangerously high levels of the drug can be reached.

ANTICOAGULANTS

- These are drugs that prevent or reduce clotting of the blood in the blood vessels.
- They may be given prophylactically to prevent a deep vein thrombosis occurring postoperatively for example, or may be given when a thrombosis has already occurred, as in pulmonary embolism.

- Heparin has to be given by injection but acts immediately.
- Warfarin is an oral anticoagulant for long-term therapy.

Heparin is discussed in more detail on p. 143.

ANTIDEPRESSANTS

- Drugs that help to relieve depression.
- These may be tricyclics such as amitriptyline and imipramine or monoamine oxidase inhibitors (MAOIs) such as phenalzine or isocarboxid. The latter interact with several types of food such as cheese, yeast extracts and food that is 'going off'. The patient is given a card with instructions. Failure to adhere to these may lead to a dangerous rise in blood pressure.
- Selective serotonin reuptake inhibitors (SSRIs) are newer drugs and are less dangerous in overdose situations and less sedative in action. Examples are fluoxetine (Prozac) and paroxetine (Seroxat).

ANTIEPILEPTICS (ANTICONVULSANTS)

- Drugs which control epilepsy.
- The aim of treatment with these drugs is to prevent the occurrence of seizures. Ideally this should be with only one drug and the combination of antiepileptic drugs is to be avoided where possible because of the complex interactions that may occur.

- Abrupt withdrawal of the drug may precipitate rebound seizures and individual doses should not be missed.
- Examples of antiepileptic drugs are carbamazepine, phenytoin, sodium valproate and vigabatrin.

ANTIEMETICS

- Drugs that reduce nausea and vomiting.
- They should only be used when the cause of the vomiting is known as they may cause symptom relief that could delay diagnosis.
- Examples are prochlorperazine (Stemetil), metoclopramide (Maxalon), domperidone and ondansetron.

ANTIFUNGALS

- Drugs given for fungal infections. Sometimes fungal infections are associated with a defect in host resistance.
- Nystatin is used for *Candida albicans* infections of the skin and mucous membranes (thrush) but is too toxic to be taken orally.
- Amphotericin is active against most types of fungi and may be taken orally to treat intestinal candidiasis as well as systemic fungal infections.

ANTIHISTAMINES

- Drugs which reduce some of the effects of released histamines.
- Histamine is released by the mast cells in an allergic reaction and antihistamines are given for

allergies such as hay fever where they reduce the rhinitis, sneezing and rashes due to allergies.

- They are also used for insect bites and stings to reduce the irritation and inflammation.
- Often make the patient drowsy as a side-effect.
- Examples are chlorpheniramine (Piriton) and promethazine hydrochloride (Phenergan).
- The non-sedative antihistamine terfenadine (Triludan) has occasionally caused fatal arrhythmias, especially when taken with erythromycin, and should not be taken with grapefruit juice.

ANTIHYPERTENSIVE DRUGS

- Drugs that reduce blood pressure.
- Examples are beta-adrenergic antagonists (beta-blockers) such as atenolol, ACE inhibitors such as captopril, calcium channel blockers such as nifedipine and diuretics such as bendrofluazide. These are discussed on p. 139.

ANTIPLATELET DRUGS

- Decrease platelet aggregation.
- Examples are aspirin, dipyridamole and clopidogrel.
- Aspirin is given to try and prevent cerebrovascular disease and myocardial infarction in those at risk. Only a small dose is needed daily (75 mg).

ANTIPSYCHOTICS

- Also known as neuroleptics and used in the treatment of

psychoses such as schizophrenia or acute behavioural disturbance.

- They may also be used to alleviate acute anxiety.
- Sometimes they are given in the form of depot injections.
- Over a period of time they may give parkinsonian side-effects such as a tremor and movement disorders.
- Examples are chlorpromazine (Largactil), haloperidol, clozapine, thioridazine (Melleril) and risperidone.

ANTIPYRETICS

- Drugs that reduce the body temperature.
- Examples are aspirin and paracetamol.
- Aspirin is not given to children under the age of 12 because of an association with Reye's syndrome.

ANTISPASMODICS

- Drugs that relax smooth muscle as found in the gut.
- They are useful in abdominal colic or distension as in irritable bowel disorder.
- Examples are mebeverine hydrochloride (Colofac), hyoscine butylbromide (Buscopan) and peppermint oil.

ANTIVIRALS

- Combat viral infections.
- There are very few drugs in this category and it is fortunate that spontaneous recovery occurs from most viral infections.

- Acyclovir (Zovirax) is active against the herpes virus and may be used as a topical application for cold sores (herpes simplex) or shingles (herpes zoster).
- Acyclovir may be given intravenously in herpes encephalitis and may be given by mouth to the immunocompromised in chicken pox. It does not eradicate the virus, which lies dormant in the body but may flare up again when conditions are suitable.
- Zidovudine (Azidothymidine, AZT) is given for human immunodeficiency virus (HIV) disease.

ANXIOLYTICS

- Drugs given to reduce anxiety.
- An example is diazepam (Valium).
- These drugs are used for alleviating definite acute and severe anxiety states and the lowest possible dose is given for the shortest possible time as they produce dependency.
- Diazepam does have other uses and may be given rectally or intravenously to halt status epilepticus or febrile convulsions.

BETA-BLOCKERS

- Block the beta-adrenergic receptor and so reduce the effect of noradrenaline and adrenaline on the body.
- They are used as treatment for hypertension and angina.
- Some of them are cardioselective, e.g. atenolol, which reduces side-effects.

- Are also used in migraine, anxiety, hyperthyroidism and certain arrhythmias but should not be given to those with asthma as they may induce an asthma attack.
- Propranolol is a non-selective beta-blocker, which will block the beta receptors in the lungs and so is more likely to cause an asthma attack than atenolol.

BRONCHODILATORS

- Relax bronchial smooth muscle and thus cause dilatation of the air passages.
- Examples are salbutamol (Ventolin), a beta-2 receptor agonist, ipratropium bromide (Atrovent), an anticholinergic drug, and aminophylline.
- Salbutamol and ipratropium can both be given by inhaler or by nebulizer. Aminophylline may be given intravenously, diluted in dextrose, or as slow-release tablets.

CORTICOSTEROIDS

- Steroid hormones are synthesized by the adrenal cortex and cortisol is the naturally occurring hormone.
- Corticosteroids are anti-inflammatory and suppress the immune system. They have many uses in inflammatory conditions, allergic responses and autoimmune diseases but also have many side-effects, especially with long-term use.
- They are usually given in the form of an inhaler in asthma –

beclometasone (Becotide) and budesonide (Pulmicort) are examples. Steroids may also be given orally, usually as prednisolone, and intravenously as hydrocortisone.

CYTOTOXICS (CHEMOTHERAPEUTIC AGENTS)

- Toxic to dividing cells and used in the treatment of cancer.
- Examples are methotrexate and vincristine.
- The drugs are toxic to all dividing cells and thus have side-effects such as a fall in the white cell count and hair loss.They are discussed in more detail on p. 301.

DIURETICS

- Make the patient pass more urine. They are best given in the morning if possible. Examples are furosemide (frusemide) and benoroflumethiazide (bendrofluazide).
- Diuretics are given to reduce the circulating blood volume in heart failure and in hypertension. Salts such as potassium are also lost in the urine and to prevent this, a potassium-sparing diuretic such as amiloride may need to be given with the diuretic.

FIBRINOLYTICS

- Drugs that digest fibrin in blood clots.
- These drugs are used to dissolve the blood clot and restore the

circulation to the heart following a myocardial infarction.
- An example is streptokinase. Their use is described on p. 143.

HYPNOTICS

- Induce sleep. An example is triazolam.
- These drugs produce dependency and are becoming less frequently prescribed.

IMMUNOSUPPRESSIVES

- Suppress the immune system and are used in autoimmune disorders or following organ transplantation to reduce rejection of the donor organ.
- An example is azathioprine.

INOTROPES

- Affect the contraction of the heart muscle.
- Drugs such as digoxin have a positive inotropic action and increase the force of the heart beat.
- Some drugs such as beta-blockers have a negative inotropic effect and decrease the force of the heart beat.

LAXATIVES

- Drugs used to promote a softer or bulkier stool or to encourage a bowel action.
- Given for constipation.
- Examples are lactulose and senna.

MIOTICS

- Drugs which constrict the pupil of the eye.

- They are used in glaucoma to open up the drainage channels in the trabecular meshwork resulting from spasm of the ciliary muscle and constriction of the pupil is a side-effect.
- An example is pilocarpine.

MUSCLE RELAXANTS

- Used in conjunction with general anaesthesia to produce complete muscle relaxation, especially in abdominal surgery.
- As they prevent muscles contracting, they also stop respiration and the patient has to be ventilated.
- They are used in intensive care units when a patient needs long-term ventilation to stop the patient 'fighting the ventilator'.
- Examples are atracurium and vecuronium.

MYDRIATICS

- Dilate the pupil of the eye.
- An example is homatropine.
- They may be used when the doctor needs to have a clear view of the retina as in examination of the eye in diabetes.

NON-STEROIDAL ANTIINFLAMMATORY DRUGS – SEE ANALGESICS.

VACCINES

These are preparations of antigenic material that can be given to stimulate the production of antibodies and thus confer immunity to a disease. They consist of:

- a live attenuated form of the infective agent, as in rubella vaccine
- an inactivated preparation of the virus, as in influenza vaccine, or the bacteria, as in typhoid vaccine
- detoxified exotoxins produced by the microorganism, as in tetanus vaccine (see p. 111).

5.6 POISONING

A poison is any substance which, when introduced into a living organism, destroys life or injures health.

ACCIDENTAL POISONING

May be encountered at any age, but the causes differ.

Neonatal poisoning
Usually as a result of therapeutic doses of drugs or self-poisoning in the late stages of labour. Could be due to the miscalculation of doses.

Children
Accidental poisoning is commonest between the ages of 1 and 5 years when children like to explore the environment with their mouths as well as their eyes and fingers!

Older children and adults
Usually as a result of a mishap at school or at work, e.g. inhalation of gases or fumes from organic solvents or ingestion whilst pipetting.

The elderly
Especially if confused, may forget they have taken a dose of their drug or make mistakes with doses.

DELIBERATE SELF-POISONING

This is the commonest form of poisoning in adults. It accounts for at least 95% of all poisoning admissions to hospital The peak age is between 20 and 35 years but it is not uncommon below the age of 15.

Symptoms and signs

Usually poisoned adults are able to tell us what they have taken but the presence of signs and symptoms may help us to see how severe the poisoning is.

Coma

This is one of the common signs of poisoning and is usually due to depression of the central nervous system by:

- hypnotics
- antidepressants
- anticonvulsants
- tranquillizers
- opioid analgesics
- alcohol.

It is uncommon in acute salicylate poisoning (aspirin) and does not occur with paracetamol poisoning unless another drug has been taken as well, e.g. co-proxamol which is paracetamol combined with dextropropoxyphene. The latter is a morphine derivative and will depress the CNS and the respiratory centre.

Convulsions

Caused by CNS stimulation by anticholinergics, sympathomimetics, tricyclic antidepressants and monoamine oxidase inhibitors.

Respiratory features

- Cough, wheeze and breathlessness often occur after inhalation of irritant gases such as ammonia, chlorine and smoke from fires.
- Cyanosis may be due to a combination of factors in the unconscious patient. Can also be due to methaemoglobinaemia caused by poisons such as chlorates, nitrates, nitrites, phenol and urea herbicides.
- Hypoventilation is common with any CNS depressant.
- Usually respiration gets shallower rather than slower.
- Marked reduction in rate is likely to be due to opioids.
- Hyperventilation is most commonly due to salicylate poisoning and occasionally to CNS stimulant drugs and cyanide.
- Pulmonary oedema may follow inhaled poisons and paraquat poisoning (contained in some weed-killers).

Cardiovascular features

- Tachycardia may be due to anticholinergics, sympathomimetics and salicylates.
- Bradycardia may be caused by cardiac glycosides, e.g. digoxin and beta-blockers.
- Dysrhythmias may be caused by a variety of drugs and any antiarrhythmic drugs cause dysrhythmias if taken in excess.
- Hypotension may occur in any severe poisoning.

- CNS depressants may lower the systolic blood pressure to 70–80 mmHg. The BP falls lower as the coma gets deeper.
- Diuretics lower the blood pressure by depleting the blood volume.
- Hypertension is uncommon in overdosage.

Pupil changes

- Very small and pinpoint pupils, especially if the respiratory rate is slowed, suggest opioid analgesics.
- Dilated pupils suggest tricyclic antidepressants or other anticholinergics or antihistamines.

Tinnitus is a very common feature of salicylate poisoning.

ANTIDOTES

Most important here is naloxone (Narcan) which is the antidote to all narcotic drugs. It may completely reverse a coma within 1–2 minutes and will increase the respiratory rate.

Flumenazil is the antidote for severe benzodiazepine poisoning but is not always used in less severe cases.

Acetylcysteine (Parvolex) is given in paracetamol poisoning and can prevent liver failure if given soon enough after the overdose.

SCREENING FOR POISONS

The purpose of screening is to identify and quantify poisons amenable to treatment. There is no point in doing an emergency screening if the result has no bearing on the treatment that will be given.

Paracetamol is the drug that is most likely to be screened for.

MANAGEMENT OF THE PATIENT

About 90% of adults and children have minimal symptoms and require little medical care. Half the remainder are seriously ill and recovery depends upon good care. Management of coma is a vital part of this care.

- Ensure the airway, breathing and blood pressure are adequate (ABC) (see p. 12).
- Assess the level of consciousness (see p. 31).
- Contact the poisons information services if there is any uncertainty about the toxicity of the substance or the management of the poison.
- Consider whether an antidote is available or necessary.
- Consider the need to prevent absorption of the poison.
- Consider whether it is necessary to attempt to increase elimination of the poison.

POISONS INFORMATION SERVICE

No one can expect to know all the constituents of the drugs, household products, agricultural and industrial preparations that may be taken. Toxic effects and appropriate treatment may not be known either. Poisons information services were set up to supply such information. They give a UK-wide toxicology service for healthcare professionals within the NHS and provide information on the diagnosis, treatment and management of poisoning. There are six UK centres but the move now is away from telephone contact and poisons information is supplied online by a database – TOXBASE (www.spib.axl.co.uk).

MINIMIZING THE ABSORPTION OF INGESTED POISONS

- Emptying the stomach
- Administering activated charcoal
- Whole-bowel irrigation

Emptying the stomach

There is an ongoing debate as to the usefulness of emptying the stomach.

There are always dangers involved and sometimes it may lead to more rapid absorption of the drug.

Gastric lavage is sometimes used but be aware of the following points.

- Should never be attempted without intubation and an anaesthetist present if the patient is very drowsy or comatose.
- Should never be attempted when a corrosive material has been ingested.
- Gastric lavage is of doubtful value if it is conducted more than 1–2 hours after ingestion.
- Worthwhile recovery of salicylates may be achieved up to 4 hours after ingestion.
- Danger of inhalation of stomach contents.
- Petrol is more dangerous in the lungs than in the stomach and so gastric lavage should not be attempted.

Syrup of ipecacuanna is the best agent for inducing emesis but is very rarely recommended as it can be dangerous and cannot be used alongside the administration of active charcoal.

- Emesis induced in this manner is of limited value and there is no evidence that it prevents clinically significant absorption even if used within 1–2 hours.
- The adverse effects may complicate diagnosis.
- It causes excessive vomiting and if absorbed may have cardiac effects.

Activated charcoal

- There is a trend towards abandoning the above methods in mild or moderate poisoning and replacing them with repeated doses of activated charcoal.
- The charcoal is not absorbed and combines with some drugs in the stomach and intestine (adsorbs them) to prevent their absorption too.
- Ten times as much charcoal is needed as the drug you wish it to combine with.
- The sooner it is given, the more effective it will be.
- It is best given within the first hour of ingestion but may be effective up to 2 hours after ingestion and longer if modified-release preparations are taken.
- It is a tasteless, black, gritty slurry and patients do not like to take it.
- It should not be given before ipecacuanha as it stops absorption of the latter.

It does not adsorb all toxins but is good for:

- paracetamol
- benzodiazepines
- digoxin
- paraquat
- phenytoin
- salicylates
- quinine.

It is useful for poisons that are toxic in small amounts such as tricyclic antidepressants. It can enhance the elimination of some drugs when they have been absorbed.

Repeated doses are given for:

- aspirin
- carbamazepine
- phenobarbital

- theophylline
- quinine.

INCREASING THE ELIMINATION OF POISONS

Methods include:

- forced diuresis (aspirin) – no longer recommended
- haemodialysis – salicylates, phenobarbital.
- repeat-dose oral charcoal (gut dialysis).

All patients who have taken an intentional overdose should be admitted to hospital and given a psychiatric referral as the overdose is often a 'cry for help'.

References

Barr L, Cowan R, Nicholson M 1997 Churchill's pocketbook of oncology. Churchill Livingstone, Edinburgh

CASCADE Investigators 1993 Randomized antiarrhythmic drug therapy in survivors of cardiac arrest. The CASCADE study. American Journal of Cardiology 72: 280–287

Diabetes UK 2002 (www.diabetes.org.uk)

Edwards SL 1998 Critical thinking and analysis: a model for written assignments. British Journal of Nursing 7(3): 159–166

Edwards SL 2002 Myocardial infarction: nursing responsibilities in the first hour. British Journal of Nursing 11(7): 454–468

Fritsch D 1995 hypothermia in the trauma patient. AACN Clinical Issues 6(2): 196–211

Gibbs G 1988 Learning by doing: a guide to teaching and learning methods. Oxford Polytechnic FEU, Oxford

Hincliffe S, Norman S, Schober J 1998 Nursing practice & health care: a foundation text, 3rd edn. Arnold, London

Holtzclaw B 1993 Monitoring body temperature. Clinical Issues in Advanced Practice 25(4): 751–759

Johns C 1994 Guided reflection. In: Palmer A, Burns S, Bulman C (eds) Reflective practice in nursing. Blackwell Science, London

Kinghorn S, Gamlin R 2001 Palliative nursing: bringing comfort and hope. Baillière Tindall, London

Kumar P, Clark M 1998 Clinical medicine. Baillière Tindall, London

Lafferty K, Rennie J (eds) 1998 Concise surgery. Arnold, London

Mallett J, Dougherty L (eds) 2000 Manual of clinical nursing procedures, 5th edn. Blackwell Sciences, London

Morgan S 1990 Comparison of three methods of managing fever in the neurologic patient. Journal of Neuroscience Nursing 22(1): 19–24

Nolan J, Nolan M 1993 Can nurses take an accurate blood pressure? British Journal of Nursing 2(14): 724–729

O'Brien E, Beevers D, Marshall H 1995 ABC of hypertension, 8th edn. BMJ Books, London

UKCC 1989 Exercising accountability. UKCC, London

UKCC 1992a Code of professional conduct. UKCC, London

UKCC 1992b Standards for the administration of medicines. UKCC, London

Further reading

Crawford Adams J, Hamblen DL 1999 Outline of fractures, 11th edn. Churchill Livingstone, Edinburgh

Department of Health 1989 Report of the Advisory Group on Nurse Prescribing. DoH, London

Department of Health 2002 Extending independent nurse prescribing within the NHS in England – a guide for implementation. DoH, London

Edwards SL 1997 Measuring temperature. Professional Nurse Study Supplement 13(12): S5–S7

Edwards SL 1997 Recording blood pressure. Professional Nurse Study Supplement 13(2): S8–S11

Edwards SL 1998 High temperatures. Professional Nurse 13(8): 521–526

Edwards SL 1998 Malnutrition in hospital patients: where does it come from? British Journal of Nursing 7(16): 954–974

Edwards SL 1998 Hypovolaemia: pathophysiology and management options. Nursing in Critical Care 3(2): 73–82

Edwards SL 1999 Hypothermia. Professional Nurse 14(4): 253–258

Edwards SL 2000 Fluid overload and monitoring indices. Professional Nurse 15(9): 568–572

Edwards SL 2001 Regulation of water, sodium and potassium: implications for practice. Nursing Standard 15(22): 36–42

Edwards SL 2001 Shock: types, classifications and explorations of their physiological effects. Emergency Nurse 9(2): 29–38

Edwards SL 2001 Using the Glasgow Coma Scale: analysis and limitations. British Journal of Nursing 10(2): 92–101

Edwards SL 2002 Physiological insult/injury: pathophysiology and consequences. British Journal of Nursing 11(4): 263–274

Ellis H 2002 Lecture notes on general surgery. Blackwell Science, Oxford

Galbraith A, Bullock S, Manias E, Hunt B, Richards A 1999 Fundamentals of pharmacology. Addison Wesley, London

Hinchliff S, Montague S, Watson R 1996 Physiology for nursing practice, 2nd edn. Baillière Tindall, London

Hinchliff S, Norman S, Schober J (eds) 1998 Nursing practice and health care: a foundation text, 3rd edn. Arnold, London

Horton R 1995 Handwashing: the fundamental infection control principle. British Journal of Nursing 4(16): 926–933

Laurence D, Bennett P, Brown M 1997 Clinical pharmacology. Churchill Livingstone, Edinburgh

Manley K, Bellman L (eds) 2000 Surgical nursing: advancing practice. Churchill Livingstone, Edinburgh

Marieb E 1999 Human anatomy and physiology. Addison Wesley Longman, London

McCance K, Huether S 2002 Pathophysiology. Mosby, St Louis

Neal M 1997 Medical pharmacology at a glance. Blackwell Science, Oxford

Oh T (ed) 1998 Intensive care manual, 4th edn. Butterworth Heinemann, Oxford

Souhami R, Moxham J 2002 Textbook of medicine. Churchill Livingstone, London

Trounce J 1998 Clinical pharmacology for nurses. Churchill Livingstone, London

Wilson J 1995 Infection control in clinical practice. Baillière Tindall, London

Units of measurement

UNITS OF MEASUREMENT – INTERNATIONAL SYSTEM OF UNITS (SI), THE METRIC SYSTEM AND CONVERSIONS

The International System of Units (SI) or Système International d'Unités is the measurement system used for scientific, medical and technical purposes in most countries. In the United Kingdom SI units have replaced those of the Imperial System, e.g. the kilogram is used for mass instead of the pound (in everyday situations, both mass and weight are measured in kilograms although weight, which varies with gravity, is really a measure of force).

The SI comprises seven base units with several derived units. Each unit has its own symbol and is expressed as a decimal multiple or submultiple of the base unit by using the appropriate prefix, e.g. millimetre is one thousandth of a metre.

Base units

Quantity	Base unit and symbol
length	metre (m)
mass	kilogram (kg)
time	second (s)
amount of substance	mole (mol)
electric current	ampere (A)
thermodynamic temperature	kelvin (∞K)
luminous intensity	candela (cd)

Derived units

Derived units for measuring different quantities are reached by multiplying or dividing two or more base units.

Quantity	Derived unit and symbol
work, energy, quantity of heat	joule (J)
pressure	pascal (Pa)
force	newton (N)
frequency	hertz (Hz)
power	watt (W)
electrical potential, electromotive force, potential difference	volt (v)
absorbed dose of radiation	gray (Gy)
radioactivity	becquerel (Bq)
dose equivalent	sievert (Sv)

Factor, decimal multiples and submultiples of SI units

Multiplication factor	Prefix	Symbol
10^{12}	tera	T
10^{9}	giga	G
10^{6}	mega	M
10^{3}	kilo	k
10^{2}	hecto	h
10^{1}	deca	da
10^{-1}	deci	d
10^{-2}	centi	c
10^{-3}	milli	m
10^{-6}	micro	μ
10^{-9}	nano	n
10^{-12}	pico	p
10^{-15}	femto	f
10^{-18}	atto	a

Rules for using units and writing large numbers and decimals

- The symbol for a unit is unaltered in the plural and should not be followed by a full stop except at the end of a sentence: 5 cm not 5 cm. or 5 cms.
- Large numbers are written in three-digit groups (working from right to left) with spaces not commas (in some countries the comma is used to indicate a decimal point): fifty thousand is written as 50 000; five hundred thousand is written as 500 000.
- Numbers with four digits are written without the space, e.g. four thousand is written as 4000.
- The decimal sign between digits is indicated by a full stop positioned near the line, e.g. 50.25. If the numerical value of the decimal is less than 1, a zero should appear before the decimal sign: 0.125 not .125.
  Decimals with more than four digits are also written in three-digit groups but this time working from left to right, e.g. 0.000 25.
- 'Squared' and 'cubed' are expressed as numerical powers and not by abbreviation: square centimetre is cm^2 not sq. cm.

Commonly used measurements requiring further explanation

- Temperature – although the SI base unit for temperature is the kelvin, by international convention temperature is measured in degrees Celsius (°C).
- Energy – the energy of food or individual requirements for energy are measured in kilojoules (kJ); the SI unit is the joule (J). In practice many people still use the kilocalorie (kcal), a non-SI unit, for these purposes.

  1 calorie = 4.2 J
  1 kilocalorie (large calorie) = 4.2 kJ

- Volume – volume is calculated by multiplying length, width and depth. Using the SI unit for length, the metre (m), means ending up with a cubic metre (m^3), which is a huge volume and is certainly not appropriate for most purposes. In clinical practice the litre (L or l) is used. A litre is based on the volume of a cube measuring 10 cm × 10 cm × 10 cm. Smaller units still, e.g. millilitre (ml) or one thousandth of a litre, are commonly used in clinical practice.

- Time – the SI base unit for time is the second (s), but it is acceptable to use minute (min), hour (h) or day (d). In clinical practice it is preferable to use 'per 24 hours' for the excretion of substances in urine and faeces: g/24 h.
- Amount of substance – the SI base unit for amount of substance is the mole (mol). The concentration of many substances is expressed in moles per litre (mol/l) or millimoles per litre (mmol/l) which replaces milliequivalents per litre (mEq/l). Some exceptions exist and include haemoglobin and plasma proteins in grams per litre (g/l); and enzyme activity in International Units (IU, U or iu).
- Pressure – the SI unit of pressure is the pascal (Pa) and the kilopascal (kPa) replaces the old non-SI unit of millimetres of mercury pressure (mmHg) for blood pressure and blood gases. However, mmHg is still widely used for measuring blood pressure. Other anomalies include cerebrospinal fluid, which is measured in millimetres of water (mmH$_2$O), and central venous pressure, which is measured in centimetres of water (cmH$_2$O).

MEASUREMENTS, EQUIVALENTS AND CONVERSIONS (SI OR METRIC AND IMPERIAL)

Length

1 kilometre (km)	= 1000 metres (m)
1 metre (m)	= 100 centimetres (cm) or 1000 millimetres (mm)
1 centimetre (cm)	= 10 millimetres (mm)
1 millimetre (mm)	= 1000 micrometres (μm)
1 micrometre (μm)	= 1000 nanometres (nm)

Conversions

1 metre (m)	= 39.370 inches (in)
1 centimetre (cm)	= 0.3937 inches (in)
30.48 centimetres (cm)	= 1 foot (ft)
2.54 centimetres (cm)	= 1 inch (in)

Volume

1 litre (L)	= 1000 millilitres (mL)
1 millilitre (mL)	= 1000 microlitres (μL)

NB The millilitre (mL) and the cubic centimetre (cm^3) are usually treated as being the same.

Conversions

1 litre (L)	= 1.76 pints (pt)
568.25 millilitres (mL)	= 1 pint (pt)
28.4 millilitres (mL)	= 1 fluid ounce (fl oz)

Weight or mass

1 kilogram (kg)	= 1000 grams (g)
1 gram (g)	= 1000 milligrams (mg)
1 milligram (mg)	= 1000 micrograms (µg)
1 microgram (µg)	= 1000 nanograms (ng)

NB To avoid any confusion with milligram (mg) the word microgram (µg) should be written in full on prescriptions.

Conversions

1 kilogram (kg)	= 2.204 pounds (lb)
1 gram (g)	= 0.0353 ounce (oz)
453.59 grams (g)	= 1 pound (lb)
28.34 grams (g)	= 1 ounce (oz)

Temperature conversions

To convert Celsius to Fahrenheit:
multiply by 9, divide by 5, and add 32 to the result:
e.g. 36°C to Fahrenheit:
$36 \times 9 = 324 \div 5 = 64.8 + 32 = 96.8°F$
therefore 36°C = 96.8°F

To convert Fahrenheit to Celsius:
subtract 32, multiply by 5, and divide by 9:
e.g. 104°F to Celsius:
$104 - 32 = 72 \times 5 = 360 \div 9 = 40°C$
therefore 104°F = 40°C

Temperature comparison

°Celsius	°Fahrenheit	°Celsius	°Fahrenheit
100	212	37.5	99.5
95	203	37	98.6
90	194	36.5	97.7
85	185	36	96.8
80	176	35.5	95.9
75	167	35	95
70	158	34	93.2
65	149	33	91.4
60	140	32	89.6
55	131	31	87.8
50	122	30	86
45	113	25	77
44	112.2	20	68
43	109.4	15	59
42	107.6	10	50
41	105.8	5	41
40	104	0	32
39.5	103.1	−5	23
39	102.2	−10	14
38.5	101.3	NB Boiling point = 100°C = 212°F	
38	100.4	Freezing point = 0°C = 32°F	

Normal values

The values below represent an 'average' reference range, in adults, for blood, cerebrospinal fluid, urine and faeces. These ranges should be used as a guide only. Reference ranges vary between individual laboratories and readers should consult their own laboratory for those used locally. This is especially important where reference values depend upon the analytical equipment and temperatures used.

BLOOD (HAEMATOLOGY)

Test	Reference range
Activated partial thromboplastin time (APTT)	30–40 s
Bleeding time (Ivy)	2–8 min
Erythrocyte sedimentation rate (ESR)	
Adult women	3–15 mm/h
Adult men	1–10 mm/h
Fibrinogen	1.5–4.0 g/l
Folate (serum)	4–18 µg/l
Haemoglobin	
Women	115–165 g/l (11.5–16.5 g/dl)
Men	130–180 g/l (13–18 g/dl)
Haptoglobins	0.3–2.0 g/l
Mean cell haemoglobin (MCH)	27–32 pg
Mean cell haemoglobin concentration (MCHC)	30–35 g/dl
Mean cell volume (MCV)	78–95 fl
Packed cell volume (PCV or haematocrit)	
Women	0.35–0.47 (35–47%)
Men	0.4–0.54 (40–54%)
Platelets (thrombocytes)	$150–400\times10^9$/l
Prothrombin time	12–16 s
Red cells (erythrocytes)	
Women	$3.8–5.3\times10^{12}$/l
Men	$4.5–6.5\times10^{12}$/l
Reticulocytes (newly formed red cells in adults)	$25–85\times10^9$/l
White cells total (leucocytes)	$4.0–11.0\times10^9$/l

BLOOD-VENOUS PLASMA (BIOCHEMISTRY)

Test	Reference range
Alanine aminotransferase (ALT)	10–40 U/l
Albumin	36–47 g/l
Alkaline phosphatase	40–125 U/l
Amylase	90–300 U/l
Aspartate aminotransferase (AST)	10–35 U/l
Bicarbonate (arterial)	22–28 mmol/l
Bilirubin (total)	2–17 μmol/l
Caeruloplasmin	150–600 mg/l
Calcium	2.1–2.6 mmol/l
Chloride	95–105 mmol/l
Cholesterol (total)	ideally below 5.2 mmol/l
HDL–cholesterol	
Women	0.6–1.9 mmol/l
Men	0.5–1.6 mmol/l
$PaCO_2$ (arterial)	4.4–6.1 kPa
Copper	13–24 μmol/l
Cortisol (at 08.00 h)	160–565 nmol/l
Creatine kinase (total)	
Women	30–150 U/l
Men	30–200 U/l
Creatinine	55–150 μmol/l
Gamma-glutamy transferase (γGT)	
Women	5–35 U/l
Men	10–55 U/l
Globulins	24–37 g/l
Glucose (venous blood, fasting)	3.6–5.8 mmol/l
Glycosylated haemoglobin (HbA_1)	4–6%
Hydrogen ion concentration (arterial)	35–44 nmol/l
Iron	
Women	10–28 μmol/l
Men	14–32 μmol/l
Iron-binding capacity total (TIBC)	45–70 μmol/l
Lactate (arterial)	0.3–1.4 mmol/l
Lactate dehydrogenase (total)	230–460 U/l
Lead (adults, whole blood)	<1.7 μmol/l
Magnesium	0.7–1.0 mmol/l
Osmolality	275–290 mmol/kg
PaO_2 (arterial)	12–15 kPa
Oxygen saturation (arterial)	>97%
pH	7.36–7.42
Phosphate (fasting)	0.8–1.4 mmol/l
Potassium (serum)	3.6–5.0 mmol/l
Protein (total)	60–80 g/l
Sodium	136–145 mmol/l
Transferrin	2–4 g/l
Triglycerides (fasting)	0.6–1.8 mmol/l
Urate	
Women	0.12–0.36 mmol/l
Men	0.12–0.42 mmol/l
Urea	2.5–6.5 mmol/l

Test	Reference range
Uric acid	
Women	0.09–0.36 mmol/l
Men	0.1–0.45 mmol/l
Vitamin A	0.7–3.5 μmol/l
Vitamin C	23–57 μmol/l
Zinc	11–22 μmol/l

CEREBROSPINAL FLUID

Test	Reference range
Cells	0–5 mm^3
Chloride	120–170 mmol/l
Glucose	2.5–4.0 mmol/l
Pressure (adult)	50–180 mm/H$_2$O
Protein	100–400 mg/l

URINE

Test	Reference range
Albumin/creatinine ratio	<3.5 mg albumin/mmol creatinine
Calcium (diet dependent)	<12 mmol/24 h (normal diet)
Copper	0.2–0.6 μmol/24 h
Cortisol	9–50 μmol/24 h
Creatinine	9–17 mmol/24 h
5-Hydroxyindole-3-acetic acid (5HIAA)	10–45 μmol/24 h
Magnesium	3.3–5.0 mmol/24 h
Oxalate	
Women	40–320 mmol/24 h
Men	80–490 mmol/24 h
pH	4–8
Phosphate	15–50 mmol/24 h
Porphyrins (total)	90–370 nmol/24 h
Potassium (depends on intake)	25–100 mmol/24 h
Protein (total)	no more than 0.3 g/l
Sodium (depends on intake)	100–200 mmol/24 h
Urea	170–500 mmol/24 h

FAECES

Test	Reference range
Fat content (daily output on normal diet)	<7 g/24 h
Fat (as stearic acid)	11–18 mmol/24 h

Drug measurement and calculations

The International System of Units (SI) is used for drug doses and concentrations and patient data (including weight and body surface area), drug levels in the body and other measurements (see Appendix 1 for more information)

Weight

Grams (g) and milligrams (mg) are the units most often encountered in drug dosages. Doses of less than 1 g should be expressed in milligrams, e.g. 250 mg rather than 0.25 g. Similarly, doses less than 1 mg should be expressed in micrograms, e.g. 200 micrograms rather than 0.2 mg. Whenever drugs are prescribed in microgram dosages, the units should be written in full, e.g. digoxin 250 micrograms, as the use of the contracted terms μg or mcg may in practice be mistaken for mg and, as this dose is one thousand times greater, disastrous consequences may follow.

Drug dosages are often described in terms of unit dose per kg of body weight, i.e. mg/kg, μg/kg, etc. This method of dosage is frequently used for children and allows dosages to be tailored to the individual patient's size.

Volume

Litres (L or l) and millilitres (mL or ml) account for almost all measurements expressed in unit volume for the prescription and administration of drugs.

Concentration

When expressing concentration of dosages of a medicine in liquid form, several methods are available.

- Unit weight per unit volume – describes the unit of weight of a drug contained in unit volume, e.g. 1 mg in 1 ml, 40 mg in 2 ml. Examples of drugs in common use expressed in these terms: pethidine injection 100 mg in 2 ml; chloral hydrate mixture 1 g in 10 ml; phenoxymethylpenicillin oral solution 250 mg in 5 ml.

- Percentage (weight in volume) – describes the weight of a drug expressed in grams (g) which is contained in 100 ml of solution, e.g. calcium gluconate injection 10% which contains 10 g in each 100 ml of solution, or 1 g in each 10 ml or 100 mg (0.1 g) in each 1 ml.
- Percentage (weight in weight) – describes the weight of a drug expressed in grams (g) which is contained in 100 g of a solid or semi-solid medicament, such as ointments and creams, e.g. fusidic acid ointment 2% which contains 2 g of fusidic acid in each 100 g of ointment.
- Volume containing '1 part' – a few liquids and to a lesser extent gases, particularly those containing drugs in very low concentrations, are often described as containing 1 part per 'x' units of volume. For liquids, 'parts' are equivalent to grams and volume to millimetres, e.g. adrenaline injection 1 in 1000 which contains 1 g in 1000 ml or expressed as a percentage (w/v) – 0.1%.
- Molar concentration – only very occasionally are drugs in liquid form expressed in molar concentration. The mole is the molecular weight of a drug expressed in grams and a one molar (1 M) solution contains this weight dissolved in each litre. More often the millimole (mmol) is used to describe a medicinal product, e.g. potassium chloride solution 15 mmol in 10 ml indicates a solution containing the molecular weight of potassium chloride in milligrams × 15 dissolved in 10 ml of solution.

Body height and surface area

Drug doses may be expressed in terms of microgram, milligram or gram per unit of body surface area. This is frequently the case where precise dosages tailored to individual patients' needs are required. Typical examples may be seen in cytotoxic chemotherapy or in drugs given to children. Body surface area is expressed as square metres or m^2 and drug dosages as units per square metre or units/m^2, e.g. cytarabine injection 100 mg/m^2.

Formulae for calculation of drug doses and drip rates

Oral drugs (solids, liquids)

$$\text{Amount required} = \frac{\text{Strength required} \times \text{Volume of stock strength}}{\text{Stock strength}}$$

Parenteral drugs
(a) Solutions (IM, IV injections)

$$\text{Volume required} = \frac{\text{Strength required} \times \text{Volume of stock strength}}{\text{Stock strength}}$$

(b) Powders
It is essential to follow the manufacturer's directions for dilution, then use the appropriate formula.

(c) IV infusions

$$\text{Rate (drops/min)} = \frac{\text{Volume of solution (ml)} \times \text{Number of drops/ml}}{\text{Time (min)}}$$

Macrodrip (20 drops/ml) – clear fluids

1. $$\text{Rate (drops/min)} = \frac{\text{Volume of solution (ml)} \times 20}{\text{Time (min)}}$$

2. Macrodrip (15 drops/ml) – blood

$$\text{Rate (drops/min)} = \frac{\text{Volume of solution (ml)} \times 15}{\text{Time (min)}}$$

(d) Infusion pumps
Rate (ml/h) = Volume (ml) ÷ Time (h)
(e) IV infusions with drugs

$$\text{Rate (ml/h)} = \frac{\text{Amount of drug required (mg/h)} \times \text{Volume of solution (ml)}}{\text{Total amount of drug (mg)}}$$

NB After selecting the appropriate formula, ensure that all strengths are in the same units, otherwise convert.
1% solution contains 1 g of solute dissolved in 100 ml of solution.
1:1000 means 1 g in 1000 ml of solution, therefore 1 g in 1000 ml is equivalent to 1 mg in 1 ml.

Other useful formulae
Children's dose (Clarke's Body Weight Rule)

$$\text{Child's dose} = \frac{\text{Adult dose} \times \text{Weight of child (kg)}}{\text{Average adult weight (70 kg)}}$$

Children's dose (Clarke's Body Surface Area Rule)

$$\text{Child's dose} = \frac{\text{Adult dose} \times \text{Surface area of child (m}^2)}{\text{Surface area of adult (1.7 m}^2)}$$

Acknowledgements
The measurement section was adapted from Henney C R et al 1995 Drugs in Nursing Practice, 5th edn. Churchill Livingstone, Edinburgh, with permission; and the formulae from Havard M 1994 A Nursing Guide to Drugs, 4th edn. Churchill Livingstone, Edinburgh, with permission.

Glossary

Acidosis	Abnormally high acidity of body fluids and tissues
Albumin	A protein found in the blood plasma and important in maintaining plasma volume
Allogenic	Pertaining to grafted tissue derived from a donor of the same species
Anaemia	Reduction in the quantity of oxygen-carrying haemoglobin in the blood
Anastomosis	Artificial connection or join between two tubular body parts, usually small intestine
Angiography	Demonstration of blood vessels after an injection of contrast medium
Angiopathy	Disorder of the blood vessels
Anion	Negatively charged ion e.g. bicarbonate
Anthopometry	Measurement of parts of the body
Anuria	Failure of the kidneys to produce urine
Aplasia	Total or partial failure of development of an organ or tissue
Arthropathy	Joint disease
Ascites	Fluid in the peritoneal cavity
Atelectasis	Failure of part of the lung to expand
Atheroma	Deposition of lipid material in the intimal layer of arteries
Blast cells	Formative, immature cells
Catecholamines	A group of chemicals secreted by the body that includes adrenaline, noradrenaline, dopamine and some other neurotransmitters
Cation	A positively charged ion e.g. sodium and potassium
Cholecystitis	Inflammation of the gallbladder
Coagulopathy	Disorder of blood clotting
Colloid	Substances, which are unable to pass through the cell membrane; diffusible but not soluble in water Used to describe some intravenous fluids e.g. haemocel

Crystalloid	Organic salts that will pass through the cell membrane. Used to describe intravenous fluids such as saline 0.9%
Cytokine	Secretions of the lymphoid system that act as signals to other lymphoid cells
Dysphagia	Difficulty in swallowing
Dysphasia	Disorder of language following brain damage e.g. a stroke
Dysplasia	Abnormal development or formation of tissue
Empyema	Pus in the pleural cavity
Enteritis	Inflammation of the small intestine often resulting in diarrhoea
Epigastrium	Upper central region of the abdomen
Erythema	Flushing of the skin due to dilatation of the blood capillaries
Erythropoietin	Hormone released by the kidney that stimulates the formation of red blood cells
Euthyroid	Having a thyroid gland that functions normally
Exacerbation	Increased severity of symptoms
FEV_1	Forced expiratory volume in the first second of exhalation in a respiratory function test. Is usually 80% of the total FEV
Gastrin	Hormone released into the bloodstream by the stomach and stimulating the production of gastric juice
Gluconeogenesis	Synthesis of glucose by the body from non-carbohydrate sources e.g. protein
Glucocorticoids	Any steroid hormone that promotes gluconeogenesis e.g. cortisol
Gynaecomastica	Breast enlargement in the male
Haematocrit	Volume of red cells in the blood expressed as a percentage of the total blood volume
Haematemesis	Vomiting blood
Haematuria	Blood in the urine
Haemodilution	Decrease in the proportion of red cells relative to plasma, brought about by an increase in total volume of the plasma
Haemoptysis	Coughing up blood
Haemothorax	Blood in the pleural cavity
Halitosis	Bad breath
Hepatocyte	Liver cell
Hepatomegaly	Enlargement of the liver that is palpable
Hirschprung's disease	Congenital intestinal disease of nervous tissue leading to intractable constipation
Hypercalcaemia	Excessive calcium in the blood

Hypercarbia	Raised carbon dioxide in arterial blood
Hypersplenism	Depression of blood cell counts by an enlarged spleen in the presence of an active bone marrow
Hyperuricaemia	Excessive uric acid in the blood; characteristic of gout
Hypokalaemia	Abnormally low potassium level in the blood
Hyponatraemia	Abnormally low sodium level in the blood
Hypovolaemia	Diminished quantity of total blood
Hypoxaemia	Diminished amount of oxygen in arterial blood
Hypoxia	Diminished amount of oxygen in the tissues
Idiopathic	Condition of unknown or spontaneous origin e.g. some forms of epilepsy
Ileus	Intestinal obstruction – term usually restricted to paralytic rather than mechanical obstruction
Ischaemia	Deficient blood supply to any part of the body
Ketoacidosis	Acidosis due to accumulation of ketone bodies
Leucocytosis	Increase in the number of white blood cells in the blood
Leukaemia	Malignant disease in which increased numbers of any type of white blood cell are produced
Lipolysis	Fat breakdown into fatty acids by the enzyme lipase
Lymphoid	Tissue responsible for the production of lymphocytes and antibodies
Macrocytic	Describing an abnormally large red blood cell
Mallory-Weiss syndrome	Tearing of the tissues around the junction of the oesophagus and stomach as a result of violent vomiting
Methaemoglobin	Form of oxidized haemoglobin that cannot carry oxygen
Microcytic	Describing abnormally small red blood cells
Mineralocorticoids	Hormonal secretion of the adrenal cortex – aldosterone mainly
Myopathy	Disease of the muscles
Nephroureterectomy	Removal of the kidney along with part or the whole of the ureter
Neoplasm	New growth that may be cancerous or non-cancerous
Neutropenia	Reduced number of neutrophils (type of white blood cell) in the blood
NSAID	Non-seroidal anti-inflammatory drug e.g. aspirin
Oliguria	Production of an abnormally small volume of urine May be due to sweating, dehydration, blood loss or kidney disease
Pancreatitis	Inflammation of the pancreas
Papilloedema	Swelling of the optic disc
Petechiae	Small haemorrhagic round flat dark red spots caused by bleeding into the skin or beneath the mucous membrane

Pneumothorax	Air in the pleural cavity
Polycythaemia	Increase in the number of circulating red blood cells
Polydipsia	Excessive thirst leading to the drinking of large quantities of fluids
Polyuria	Passing excessive amounts of urine
Proteolysis	Protein breakdown
Queckenstedt's test	Performed during a lumbar puncture. Compression of the internal jugular vein produces a rise in CSF pressure if there is no obstruction to circulation of fluid in the spinal region
Remission	Period of abatement of a disease
Resection	Surgical excision
Salpingitis	Inflammation of the fallopian tubes
SCIDS	Severe combined immune deficiency – genetic disorder affecting one baby in 25 000. The baby has no resistance to infection and has to be enclosed in a protective plastic bubble from birth
Septicaemia	The persistence and multiplication of living bacteria in the blood stream
Splenomegaly	Enlargement of the spleen
Steatosis (hepatic)	Infiltration of hepatocytes with fat
Subphrenic abscess	A collection of pus in the space below the diaphragm
Supine	Lying on the back with the face upwards
Thrombocyropenia	Reduction in the number of platelets in the blood
Tinnitus	Any noise, often buzzing, thumping or ringing in the ears
Toxaemia	Blood poisoning caused by the products of bacteria
Toxoplasmosis	Disease due to the protozoan *toxoplasma gondii*. Often spread from cats
Transferrin	Protein that acts as a carrier for iron in the bloodstream
Uraemia	Excessive amounts of urea and nitrogenous waste in the bloodstream

Index

Entries in *italics* refer to figures, tables and information boxes.
Abbreviations used in this index include:

AIDS – Acquired Immunodeficiency Syndrome
CDC – Centers for Disease Control
COAD – Chronic Obstructive Airways Disease
DVT – Deep Vein Thrombosis
HIV – Human Immunodeficiency Virus

AABC of resuscitation 12
abacterial cystitis 223
abdomen
   bowel obstruction 203
   radiotherapy side-effects 301
   rigid 198, 201
abdominal ascites *see* ascites
abdominal discomfort
   care/management 152
   right heart failure 152
abdominal guarding 201
abdominal pain, acute 200
   appendicitis 211
   common causes in adults 200
   gall stones 213
   pancreatitis 219, 220
   perforate peptic ulcers 198
abdominal paracentesis 87–88
   special care considerations 87–88
abscess
   cerebral 247, *247*
   lung 168
accelerated idioventricular tachycardia 148
accidental hypothermia 98
accidental poisoning 325
accountability 7
ACE inhibitors *see* angiotensin-converting
      enzyme (ACE) inhibitors
Acetest, ketones in urine 61
acetylcholine (ACh) 238
acetylcysteine 327
achalasia 192

aciclovir 323
acid–base balance 58, 67
   bicarbonate level 124
   changes in stored blood *127*
acidosis 67, 123
   acute renal failure 225–226
   respiratory 68
   see also metabolic acidosis
acquired haemolytic anaemias 179
acquired immunity 284
acquired immunodeficiency disease
      (AIDS) *see* AIDS
acromegaly 251
ACTH 258, 259
   tumours producing 260
activated charcoal, poisoning 328–329
activated partial thromboplastin time
      (APPT) 143
active external/internal rewarming
      99–100
acute abdomen 200
acute renal failure (ARF) *see* renal failure
acute tubular necrosis (ATN) 224
adaptation, stress response 35–36
Addison's disease 259
adenosine 318
   cardiac arrhythmias 144
admissions (hospital)
   coronary care unit 142–143
   general principles/procedures 102–103
adrenal glands 258–260
   hormones secreted 258

autoantibodies 287
autoimmune diseases 272, 287–288
    organ-specific *288*
    rheumatoid arthritis 271, 272
    systemic 287
    thyroid 253, 256
    treatment 288
autoimmunity 287–288
autonomic nervous system (ANS) 31
autonomy 8–9
    ethical principles 8
autoregulation, intracranial pressure 55
autotransfusion 126
avascular necrosis 282
    fractures 282
axillary temperature 50

bacteria
    pneumonia causing 166
    septic shock due to 15
bactericidal alcoholic solution, hand
        washing 113
balloon tamponade, bleeding oesophageal
        varices 195, 216
barium studies
    achalasia diagnosis 192
    enemas 76
    preparation for 76
barium sulphate 77
barrier nursing
    infection control 112
    informing patients/visitors 112–113
basal cell carcinomas
base units 335
basic life support
    cardiac arrest 12–13
    sequence of actions 13
Bence-Jones protein, multiple myeloma 188
benign tumours 291
benzylpenicillin 319
bereavement 110–111
berry aneurysm 236
beta–2 agonists, COAD 163
beta-blockers 323
    cardioselective 141, 323
    hypertension 139
    hyperthyroidism 254
    stable angina 141
bicarbonate level 124
    blood 68

bile 212
bile duct stones 214–215, 217
biliary colic 214
    gall stones 213
    nursing care/management 214
biliary contrast radiology 77
biliary obstruction 217
biliary surgery, complications 215
biliary system *212*, 212–215
bilirubin
    serum levels 64
    in urine 60
biochemical measurements
    normal values *340–341*
        blood *65, 340–341*
    nutritional assessment 42
biopsy 80
bladder cancer 230
bladder lavage 90
bleeding
    abnormal after surgery 306
    oesophageal 194
    see also blood loss; haemorrhage
bleeding disorders 181–183
    fluid loss 125
bleomycin 303
blood 172–189
    breast cancer spread 296
    chronic renal failure 226
    culture 62
    normal values *65, 173, 339, 340–341*
    pH 67, 123
    in urine 59, 221
    viscosity 63, 64
        anomalous 64
    volume reduction 125
blood flow 63
    cerebral 55, 56, 97
blood gases, arterial 67–68
blood loss
    fluid loss due to 125
    hypotension due to 139
    see also bleeding; haemorrhage
blood pressure 46–47
    definition 46
    Glasgow Coma Scale 34
    measurement 46, *48, 49*
    potential sources of error *48*
    taking an accurate reading *49*
    types of shock 14

see also hypertension; hypotension
blood products, synthetic, transfusion 126, 128
blood tests 62–68
  drug analysis 64–65
blood transfusion 126–128
  autotransfusion 126
  changes in stored products 126, *127*
  fluid overload 18
blood-venous plasma, normal values *340–341*
blood vessel injuries, fractures 282–283
blue bloaters 162
B lymphocytes 284
body mass index (BMI)
  normal 42
  nutritional assessment 41–42
body temperature *see* temperature
body water, total 117
body weight, nutritional assessment 41
bolus feeding, enteral 135
bone 266
  chronic renal failure 226
  fractures *see* fractures
  grafts 282
  shortening due to fracture malunion 282
  tumours 269–271
bone diseases 266–283
  Paget's disease 268–269
Bourbonnais pain assessment tool 37
bowel
  inflammatory disorders 203–206
  strangulation 202
    causes 202
  washout 208
  see also large bowel
bowel obstruction
  causes 202
  clinical features 202–203
  Crohn's disease 205
  investigations 203
  management 202
  treatment 203
bowel sounds, abnormal 203
bowel surgery
  complications 209
  preparation 208–209
  psychological preparation 208
brachytherapy 300

Braden Scale, pressure sore risk assessment 39
bradycardia 146
  causes 70
  junctional 146
  poisoning causing 326
  pulse rate 43
  sinus 144
bradykinesia, Parkinson's disease 239–240
bradypnoea 45
brain 230–232
  electrical discharges 20
  radiotherapy side-effects 301
  tumours *see* intracranial tumours
brainstem, functional abnormalities 34
breast cancer 294–296
  carcinoma *in situ* 295
  diagnosis 294–295
  localized spread 295–296
  pathogenesis 295
  presentation 295
  risk factors 294
  routes of spread 295–296
  screening 294
  staging 296
  treatment 295, 304
breathing
  pursed lips 162
  right-sided heart failure 153
  stroke patients
    continued care 156
    initial care 155
  see also respiration
breathlessness 45
  COAD 162
  left heart failure 149, 151
  nursing care/management 151
  palliative care 108
  respiration depth 45
  right heart failure 151
British Guidelines on Asthma Management 160, *161*
British National Formulary (BNF) 309, 311
British Thoracic Society (BTS) guidelines, asthma medication 160, *161*
bronchiectasis 164–165
  causes 164
  clinical features 164
  nursing care/management 164–165

bronchitis, chronic 162
bronchodilators 323
  asthma 160
  COAD treatment 163–164
bronchopneumonia 166
bronchoscopy 80
bulbar palsy, progressive 244
bulk-forming agents 204
busulfan 302

calcium antagonists
  hypertension 139
  stable angina 141
calcium balance 121–122
calculating drug doses 345–348
cancer 291–305
  see also tumours; individual organs/types
cancer BACUP 301
  website 301
capsules 311
carbimazole 254
  side-effect 254
carbohydrates, malnutrition 131
carbon dioxide
  acid–base balance and 123
  end-tidal, monitoring 69
  partial pressure (PCO$_2$), blood test 67, 68
carbonic acid 123
carboxyhaemoglobin 73
carcinogenesis 293
  age-related incidence 293
carcinoma in situ 292
  bladder 230
  breast 295
  cervical 299
carcinomas see individual carcinomas
cardiac arrest 11–13
  primary 11–12
  rhythms association 12
  secondary 12
cardiac arrhythmias 144–149
  cardiac arrest associated 12
  causes 70–71, 145
  consequences 145
  diagnosis 71
  drug therapy 144
  ECG diagnosis 70–71
  management aims 145–146
  poisoning causing 326
cardiac enzymes 143

in blood 65–67, 66–67
  myocardial infarction 143
cardiac failure 149–153
  see also left heart failure; right-sided
    heart failure
cardiac involvement, rheumatoid arthritis
    273
cardiac output
  cardiogenic shock 16
  decreased, acute renal failure 224
  hypotensive shock 14
cardiac pacemaker 69
cardiogenic shock 16
  compensatory mechanisms 16
  fluid overload 18
cardiopulmonary resuscitation (CPR) 11
cardiovascular accident (CVA)
  see stroke
cardiovascular features, deliberate self-
    poisoning 326–327
cardiovascular system 138–159
  chronic renal failure 226
  pump failure, hypotension due to 140
  thyrotoxicosis 253
caring, cost to the nurses 111
carpal tunnel syndrome, rheumatoid
    arthritis 273
cast bracing, uncomplicated fractures 280
catecholamine release
  stress response 37
  trauma 19
catheterization, urinary see urinary
    catheterization
catheters
  central venous pressure (CVP) 54
  parenteral nutrition delivery 133
  urinary 89–90
CD4 cell, AIDS 290
cell cycle non-specific drugs 302–303
cell cycle specific drugs 303–304
Centers for Disease Control (CDC), AIDS
    classification 290
central catheter, parenteral nutrition
    delivery 133
central nervous system (CNS) 230, 231
central painful stimulus, Glasgow Coma
    Scale 32
central venous line
  complications 54
  parenteral nutrition delivery 133

complications 134
central venous pressure (CVP)
    catheter 54
        common complications 54
    increased 52
    monitoring 52–54, 53
    normal 54
    reduced 54
cephalosporins 320
cerebellum 232
cerebral abscess 247, 247
cerebral autoregulation 55
cerebral blood flow (CBF) 55, 97
cerebral oedema 34, 219
cerebral perfusion pressure (CPP) 56
cerebral underperfusion, signs 47
cerebrospinal fluid (CSF) 55
    examination 74
    excess 248
    flow obstructed 74
    normal values 341
    pressure 74
cervical cancer 298–299
cervical carcinoma in situ 299
cervical intraepithelial neoplasia (CIN) 299
chemotherapeutic agents 324
chemotherapy 301–305
    adverse effects 305
    combination 302, 304
    drug administration 305
    see also cytotoxic drugs
chest pain 140, 142
chest tubes 88
Cheyne-Stokes breathing 45, 109
childhood rickets 268
children
    dermatitis 287
    poisoning 325
chill stage, pyrexia 94–95
chlorambucil 302
chlorhexidine gluconate 86
chloride balance 123–124
chloride shift 123
cholangiography
    intravenous 77
    percutaneous 213
cholangitis, ascending 215
cholecystectomy, gall bladder disease 213, 214
cholecystitis

acute 214
    nursing care/management 214
    gall stones 213
cholecystography 77
    oral 213
cholelithiasis 212
    see also gall stones
Christmas disease 181
chronic obstructive airways disease (COAD) 91, 162–164
    clinical features 162–163
    drug therapy 163–164
    nursing care/management 163
    oxygen therapy 91
    predisposing factors 162
chronic renal failure (CRF) see renal failure
circulating volume
    maintenance 125–130
    pulmonary artery wedge pressure 55
cirrhosis of liver 215, 216
    causes 216
cisplatin 303–304
clean asepsis 115
cleaners, infection control 115
clinical complaints 4
clinical supervision 10–11
Clinitest 61
closed fractures see simple fractures
clothing, protective, infection control 114
clotting, abnormal after surgery 306
coagulation defects 181–182
    abnormal bleeding after surgery 306
    investigations 182
    treatment 182
codeine 316
Code of Professional Conduct (UKCC) 10
codes of practice 10
'cogwheel' effect 239
colectomy 204, 210
colloid therapy
    versus crystalloid therapy 128
    hypovolaemia 125
colon see large bowel
colonoscopy 80
colorectal cancer 209–210
colorectal polyps 209
colostomy 206–207
    indications 207
    permanent (sigmoid) 206, 207
    temporary (transverse loop) 206, 207

coma 32–34
  deliberate self-poisoning 326
combination chemotherapy 302, 304
comfort eating 28
comminuted fracture 276, 277
communication 2, 27–28
  barriers/problems 28, 30
  non-verbal 27
  Parkinson's disease 240
  potential problems 30, 30
  process and elements 27
  right heart failure management 153
  stress reduction 27
  stroke patients 155, 156
  tracheostomy patients 83
  use of aids 28, 29
compartment syndrome, fractures 283
compensated shock 14
compensatory mechanisms
  cardiogenic shock 16
  hypovolaemic shock 17
  intracranial pressure 55
complaints
  clinical 4
  formal 3
  procedure 4
complementary therapies, dying patients
      109
complete fracture 277
complex major plus surgery 305
complex major surgery 305
complicated fracture 278
compound fractures 276, 276
  treatment 280–281
compression fracture 277, 278
computed tomography (CT scanning) 79
confidentiality 9
  principles of judgement 9
congestive cardiac failure 149, 150
consent, informed 4, 8
constipation 189, 191
  bowel obstruction 203
  causes 191
  gastrointestinal disease 189
  palliative care 108
  Parkinson's disease 240
  treatment 191
continuing hypoperfusion 14
continuous ambulatory peritoneal dialysis
      (CAPD) 228

contrast media
  care and precautions for use 77
  X-rays 76–77
Controlled Drugs (CDs) 308
Controlled Drugs Order Book 308
convulsions
  deliberate self-poisoning 326
  febrile 237
  see also seizures
cooling patients
  hyperpyrexia due to hypothalamus
      damage 97
  hyperthermia 96–97
COPD see chronic obstructive airways
      disease (COAD)
co-proxamol 316
coronary angioplasty, angina pectoris 142
coronary artery bypass grafting, angina
      pectoris 141
coronary care unit (CCU), admissions
      142–143
coronary thrombosis see myocardial
      infarction (MI)
coroners 110
corticosteroids 323–324
  COAD treatment 164
  multiple sclerosis 242
cortisol 258
  release, trauma 19
cortisol release factor (CRF) 258
cranial nerves 232
  lesions 233
creams, topical 313
creatinine, in blood 64
creatinine kinase (CK) 66, 67
  MB isoform 66
  myocardial infarction 66, 143
crepitus 275
crisis stage, pyrexia 95
Crohn's disease 205–206
  clinical features 205
  complications 205
  investigations 205
  nursing care/management 205–206
crush fracture 278
crystalloid therapy
  versus colloid therapy 128
  hypovolaemia 125–126
cultural diversity 108
cultural issues 28

Cushing disease 251
  hypertension 138
Cushing's syndrome 120, 259–260
  aetiology 259–260
  clinical features 260
  hyperglycaemia 60
  investigations 260
  treatment 260
cyanosis 62, 63
  COAD 162
  poisoning causing 326
cyclophosphamide 302
cyproterone acetate (cyprostat) 304
cystic fibrosis (CF) 220–221
cystitis 222
  abacterial 223
cystoscopy 80
cystourethroscopy 80
cytarabine 303
cytology 80 81
cytotoxic antibiotics 302–303
cytotoxic drugs 302–304, 324
  cell cycle non-specific drugs 302–303
  cell cycle specific drugs 303–304
  tissue-specific agents 304

dead space ventilation (VD) 72
death 109
  actions after 109
  general principles/procedures 108–111
  last offices 110
  see also dying patients
death certificate 110
decimals, rules for writing 336
deep vein thrombosis (DVT) 158–159
  clinical features 158
  fatigued patients, risk 152
  management 158–159
  postoperative risk 106
  prevention 159
  pulmonary embolism 169
  risk factors 158
defervescence stage, pyrexia 95
dehydration
  fluid loss 125
  hypernatraemia 120
  hypotension due to 139
  pyrexia causing 96
  urine specific gravity 58
  see also hypovolaemia

delayed hypersensitivity 285
delayed union, fractures 281
deliberate self-poisoning 326–327
  symptoms 326–327
delirium 244
delirium tremens 216
dementia 244–245
demyelinating diseases 241–243
depressed fracture 278
depression
  Parkinson's disease 240–241
  rheumatoid arthritis 273
derived units 335
dermatitis 286, 287
  types 287
desquamation, skin reaction to
    radiotherapy 300
dexamethasone suppression test 260
dextrose (5%), fluid overload 18
Diabetes Control and Complications Trial
    (DCCT), type 1 diabetes 264
diabetes insipidus 249–250
  clinical presentation 250
  treatment 250
diabetes mellitus 260–266
  classification *261*
  clinical trials 264
  diagnosis 261
  diet 264
  emergencies 264–266
  glycosuria 60–61
  hyperglycaemia 60
  hypoglycaemia 265–266
  long-term complications 266
  type 1 261–263, 272
    clinical features 261–262
    glucose monitoring 263
    insulin therapy 262–263
  type 2 263–264
diabetic ketoacidosis 58–59, 265–266
  causes 265
  treatment 265–266
  urine odour 61
diabetic nephropathy 266
diabetic neuropathy 266
diabetic retinopathy 266
diagnostic strips *see* reagent test strips
dialysis
  acute renal failure 226
  end-stage renal failure 227–228

dialysis (cont'd)
  peritoneal, end-stage renal failure 228
diamorphine 317, 318
diarrhoea 189, 190–191
  causes 190
  gastrointestinal disease 189
  nursing care/management 190–191
  ulcerative colitis 203
diastolic blood pressure 46
diazepam 323
diet
  cultural restrictions 28
  diabetes mellitus 264
  elemental 206
  gall stone disease management 214
  gall stones due to 213
  nutritional assessment 41
dietary intake, improvement 131–132
dietary reference values (DRVs), nutrition
    130
diet history, nutritional assessment 41
digoxin 318, 324
  administration 152
  blood analysis 65
  cardiac arrhythmias 144
  right heart failure 152
dihydrocodeine 316
dipsticks see reagent test strips
direct laryngoscope 14
direct monitoring, blood pressure 46
discharge 5
  planning 103–104
  self-discharge 5
dislocation 278
displacement fracture 278
disseminated intravascular coagulation
    (DIC) 182–183
  blood transfusion therapy 126
  causes 183
  diagnosis 183
  inflammatory/immune response 20
  treatment 126, 183
diuresis, acute renal failure 225
diuretics 324
  administration 152
  COAD treatment 164
  hypertension 139
  left heart failure 150
  oedema 151, 152
  right heart failure 152

domestic staff, infection control 115
donors, dying patients 109
dopamine 237, 241
Doppler-shift ultrasound 78
dosage calculations 345–348
doxorubicin 302–303
drainage
  intrapleural see intrapleural drainage
  wounds 84–85
drains
  chest 88, 89
  wounds 85
dressing
  right-sided heart failure 153
  stroke patients 155
    continued care 156
    initial care 155
dressings (wound) 85–86
  classification of types 85–86
  ideal 85
drinking
  right heart failure 153
  stroke patients 155, 156
drugs
  absorption 311–312
  administration 309–310, 311–315
    errors 310
    'five rights' 309
    in hospital setting 310
    points to note 309–310
  administration routes 311–315
    inhalation 313–314
    injection 314, 314–315, 315
    oral 311–312
    rectal 312–313
    sublingual 312
    topical 313
    transdermal 313
  analysis, blood 64–65
  classification 315–325
  dosage calculations 345–348
  interactions 312
  law and 308–309, 343–345
  prescribing by nurses 310–311
  schedules 308–309
  therapy of specific diseases see
      individual diseases/drugs
  transit time 312
dry desquamation, skin reaction to
    radiotherapy 300

dry pleurisy 171
duodenal ulcer 197
  see also peptic ulcers
duodenoscopy 80
duodenum 195–200
  haemorrhage 199
dying patients
  emotional distress 111
  general principles/procedures 108–111
  organ donation potential 109
  palliative care 107–108
  stroke patients
    continued care 157
    initial 155
  see also death
dysarthria 232
dyspepsia, gastrointestinal disease 189
dysphagia 189, 192
dysphasia 232
dysplasia 203, 292
dyspnoea 45
  see also breathlessness
dysrhythmias, cardiac see cardiac
    arrhythmias

ear drops 313
ear temperature 50
eating
  Parkinson's disease 240
  psychological issues 28
  right-sided heart failure 153
  stroke patients 155, 156
economic status, effect on patient
    recovery 29–30
ectopic beats 44
  atrial 147
  pulse rate 44
  ventricular 97, 148
eczema 286–287
  disease patterns 287
  exacerbating factors 287
elderly patients
  poisoning 325
  temperature control 51
  understanding 30
electrocardiogram (ECG)
  12-lead 71
  cardiac arrhythmias 146, 147, 148
  hyperkalaemia 120
  PQRST waveform 70, 70

electrocardiogram (ECG) rhythm strip
    69–71
electrolytes
  balance 117–130
    body fluid compartments 118–124
    intercompartment movement 118
    measurement 119–124
    units of measurement 118
  in blood 64
  changes in stored blood 127
  imbalances 119–124
    parenteral nutrition complication
      134
    treatment 124
electronic thermometers 51
elemental diet 206
eliminating substances see excretion
embolism
  fat 283
  pulmonary 169
embryonic cancers 293
emergency situations 11–22
  endotracheal intubation 13–14
  fitting/seizures/epilepsy 20–22
  fluid overload 17–18
  shock see shock
  trauma 18–20
  see also cardiac arrest
emotional care 108
emotional distress, dying patients 111
empathy, COAD patients 163
emphysema 162
empyema 171
  gall bladder 213, 214
encephalitis 246–247
  acute viral 246
  clinical features 246–247
  investigations 247
  treatment 247
encephalitis lethargica 238
encephalopathy, portosystemic 216
endocrine system 249–266
  thyrotoxicosis 252
endoscopic retrograde
    cholangiopancreatography (ERCP)
    213
endoscopy 80
endotracheal intubation 13–14
  complications 14
  indications 14

end-stage renal failure (ESRF) 227–228
  renal replacement therapy 227–228
end-tidal carbon dioxide ($P_{ET}CO_2$) 69
enemas 312–313
energy requirements, unwell patients 136
enteral feeding (EF) 134–136
  administration methods 135
  complications 135–136
  tube types 134–135
enteric coating (EC) 311
epidural bolt/screw/sensor, intracranial
      pressure monitoring 56
epilepsy 20–22, 236–237
  causes 20, 237
  nursing care/management 237
  see also seizures
epithelium, tumours of 291–292
equipment, infection control 116
erythrocyte sedimentation rate
      (ESR) 65
erythromycin 319
essential hypertension 139
essential thrombocythaemia 181
ethical principles, autonomy 8
European Resuscitation Council (ECR),
      advanced life support guidelines 13
euthyroidism 252
evaluation, nursing process 25
Ewing's sarcoma 270–271
excreta, infection control 115
excretion
  poisons 329
  right-sided heart failure 153
  stroke patients 155, 156
exhaustion, stress response 36
exophthalmos 252, 253
expiratory reserve volume (ERV) 71
external fixation, uncomplicated fractures
      280
external rewarming, active 99–100
extracellular fluid (ECF) 117
extracellular fluid (ECF) compartment
      117, 118
extradural haematoma 234–235, 235
extrinsic asthma 159
extubation, tracheostomy 82
eye drops 313
eyes
  protection, infection control 114
  rheumatoid arthritis 273

thyrotoxicosis 253

faecal incontinence 203
faeces
  infection control 115
  normal values 341
familial polyposis coli 208
fanning, hyperthermia management 96–97
fasting, physiological effects 131
fat embolism, fractures 283
fatigue
  care/management 152
  DVT risk 152
  radiotherapy side-effects 301
  rheumatoid arthritis 273
  right heart failure 152
fat stores, utilization 131
febrile convulsions 237
females, urinary catheterization
      procedure 90
fibrinolytics 324
  myocardial infarction 143
fibrinous pleurisy, rheumatoid arthritis 273
fibrosis, lung, rheumatoid arthritis 273
film membrane wound dressings 85
fingerprick glucose monitoring, diabetes
      263
first aid, fracture treatment 278
fistula
  Crohn's disease 205
  gastrocolic 205
  tracheo-oesophageal 191
fitting 20–22
  see also epilepsy; seizures
fixation, fractures 280
flatulence 189
flexural dermatitis 287
fluid balance 117–130
  acute renal failure 225
  intake/output 117–118, 118
  maintenance 125–130
  recording 118
  see also electrolytes, balance
fluid loss
  causes 125
  hypovolaemic shock 16–17
  see also dehydration; hypovolaemia
fluid overload 17–18
  precipitating factors 17–18
flumenazil 327

fluorouracil 303
foam wound dressings 85
focal seizures 237
folate antagonists 303
folate deficiency anaemia 174, 175
food plan, personal 131–132
forced expiratory volume in 1 second
     (FEV₁) 72
formal complaints 3
fractures 275–283
     causes 275–276
     classification 276, 276
     clinical features 275
     complete/incomplete 277–278
     complications 281–283
     diagnosis 275
     displacement 278
     healing 281
     non-union and malunion 282
     pathological 276
     patterns 277, 277–278
     restoration of function 281
     skull 235
     stress 276
     treatment 278–281
          open (compound) fractures 280–281
          uncomplicated fractures 278–280
     types 276–278
     vertebral 267
fresh frozen plasma (FFP), transfusion
     therapy 126
fulminant hepatic failure (FHF) 218–219
     paracetamol overdose 218
functional residual capacity (FRC) 72
fungating wounds, palliative care 108

gait
     festinating 239
     shuffling 238, 239
gall bladder 212
     empyema 213, 214
gall stone disease 212
gall stones 212–214
     clinical features 213
     investigations 213
     nursing care/management 213–214
     types 212–213
gamma-glutamyl transpeptidase, serum
     levels 64
gastrectomy 198

Bilroth I partial 198
     side-effects 198
gastric carcinoma see under stomach
gastric emptying, poisonings 328
gastric lavage, poisoning 328
gastric ulcer see peptic ulcers
gastritis 196
     clinical features 196
gastrocolic fistula 205
gastrointestinal diseases
     diarrhoea 189
     oral drug absorption and 312
     symptoms 189
gastrointestinal haemorrhage 199
gastrointestinal system 189–221
     chronic renal failure 226
     thyrotoxicosis 253
gastro-oesophageal reflux 192–193
gastroscopy 80
gastrostomy tube, enteral feeding
     134–135
general anaesthesia 316
generalized lymphadenopathy 188
generalized peritonitis 201
generalized seizures 21, 237
gentamicin 320
     blood analysis 65
germ cell tumours, testicular 297
Gibbs reflective cycle (1988) 11, 11
gigantism 251
Glasgow Coma Scale (GCS) 31–34, 33
     modes of behaviour 33
glass thermometers 51
gliomas 292
glomerular filtration rate (GFR) 56, 226
glomerulonephritis 228–229
     acute (poststreptococcal) 229
     acute renal failure 224
     causes 228
     clinical features 228–229
gloves, disposable 114
glucagon, in hypoglycaemia 265
glucocorticoids 258–259
     release 258
          increased in Cushing's syndrome
          259–260
          reduced 259
          stress response 37
          trauma 19
gluconeogenesis 131

glucose
  control of blood levels 263, 264
  fingerprick monitoring 263
  insulin action 260
  tolerance test, oral 261
  in urine 60–61
glucose-6-phosphate dehydrogenase
    (G6PD) deficiency 179
glucose tolerance test, oral 261
glycerin suppositories 313
glyceryl trinitrate (GTN) 140, 141
glycogen 95, 131
glycogenolysis 131
glycolysis 131
glycosuria 60–61, 221
goal setting 25
goitre 252
  endemic 252
gowns, infection control 114
graft rejection, prevention 288–289
graphic anxiety scale 35
Graves' disease 253
gravity controllers 129
gravity drip, enteral feeding 135
gravity flow infusion devices 128
gravity infusion devices 128–129
greenstick fracture 277, 277
grief 110–111
  abnormal 110
    recognition 111
growth hormone hypersecretion, pituitary
    tumour 251
guarding 201
Guidelines for Professional Practice (1996) 10

haemarthrosis 182
haematemesis 189
  bleeding varices 195, 215
  peptic ulcers 198
haematocrit levels 63–64
haematological disorders, splenomegaly 180
haematology, normal values 65, 339
haematoma
  extradural 234–235, 235
  subdural 235, 235
haematuria 59, 221
haemodialysis, end-stage renal failure
    227–228
haemodilution 125–126
haemofiltration 228

haemoglobin
  abnormalities 177–179
  levels 62–63
    normal 62, 65
    oxygen saturation measurement 50
    slow reduction 62
  measurement, nutritional assessment
    42
haemolytic anaemia 176
  acquired 179
  causes 176
  clinical features 176
haemolytic jaundice 217
haemophilia 181
haemorrhage
  bleeding varices 195, 215
  intraabdominal 201
  stomach/duodenum 199
  subarachnoid 236
  thyroid surgery complication 255
  see also bleeding
haemorrhagic disease of newborn 182
haemostasis 181
haemothorax 171
hairline fracture 277
hair loss, radiotherapy 301
handling see moving and handling
hand washing
  infection control 113–114
  procedure 113–114
Hartmann's procedure 207
Hashimoto's disease 256
head/neck, radiotherapy side-effects 301
healing process
  fractures 281
  phases 84
  wound care 84
health and safety 5–7
  moving and handling see moving and
    handling
health assessment 31–43
healthy living advice, COAD treatment
    164
heart
  contractility 43, 69
  in rheumatoid arthritis 273
  see also entries beginning cardiac
heart attack see myocardial infarction (MI)
heartbeat 43, 69, 70
heartburn 189

heart failure *see* cardiac failure
heart rate 43
  Glasgow Coma Scale 34
heat cramps 96
heat exhaustion 96
heat stroke 96
height, nutritional assessment 41
Helicobacter pylori 195–196
  diagnosis/treatment 196
hemiplegia 231
heparin 321
  low molecular weight (LMWH) 144
  myocardial infarction 143–144
hepatic failure, fulminant 218–219
hepatitis, acute viral 217–218
hepatitis A (HAV) 217
hepatitis B (HBV) 217–218
hepatitis C (HCV) 218
hepatitis D (HDV) 218
hepatitis E 218
hepatocellular jaundice 217
hepatorenal syndrome 216
hereditary spherocytosis 176
hernia
  bowel strangulation due to 202
  hiatus *193*, 193–194
  para-oesophageal 193–194
hiatus hernia *193*, 193–194
high blood pressure *see* hypertension
history taking, nutritional assessment
      40–41
HIV-1 289–291
  diagnosis 290
  genetic variation 289–290
  symptomatic infection 290
  transmission 289
  see also AIDS
Hodgkin's disease 186–187
  clinical features 186–187
  staging *187*
  treatment 187
holistic care 24
  principles 24
hormonal antagonists, chemotherapy 304
hormonal therapy, tumours 304
hormone replacement therapy
      (HRT) 267
  breast cancer risk 294
Hospital Anxiety and Depression scale
      (HAD) 35

hospitalization, anxiety 34
hospitals
  admissions *see* admissions (hospital)
  discharge planning 103–104
      see also discharge
human immunodeficiency virus (HIV-1)
      see HIV-1
humidification, oxygen therapy 92
humidity, tracheostomy care 81
hydrocephalus 248
hydrocolloid wound dressings 86
hydrocortisone, Addison's disease 259
hydrogel wound dressings 86
hygiene, infection control 116–117
hypercalcaemia 121–122
hypercarbia 165
hyperchloraemia 124
hyperglycaemia 60
hyperkalaemia 120
  acute renal failure 225
hypermagnesaemia 123
hypernatraemia 119–120
  causes 119, 120
hyperparathyroidism 257–258
  causes 257
  clinical features 257–258
  investigations 258
  treatment 258
hyperphosphataemia 122
hyperpyrexia 94–96
  due to hypothalamus damage 97
hypersecretion, growth hormone in
      pituitary tumour 251
  diagnosis 251
hypersensitivity 285–286
  delayed 285
  general predisposition 286
  immediate 285
  localized anaphylaxis (atopy) 286
  type 1 285
      common antigens *285*
hypertension 138–139
  causes 138–139
  classification 138
  control in stroke prevention 154
  essential 139
  medication 139
  phaeochromocytoma 260
  treatment 139
hypertensive shock 14

hyperthermia 96–97
  causes 96
  malignant 96
  tepid sponging/fanning 96–97
hyperthyroidism 252
  treatment 254–256
  see also thyrotoxicosis
hyperventilation
  poisoning causing 326
  respiration pattern 45
hypervolaemia
  central venous pressure 54
  fluid overload 18
  plasma osmolality 63
  pulmonary artery wedge pressure
      (PAWP) 55
  urine output changes 56
hypnotics 324
hypoadrenalism, primary 259
hypocalcaemia 121
hypocaloric feeding 136
hypochloraemia 124
hypoglycaemia 264–265
  causes 264
  clinical features 264
  treatment 264–265
hypokalaemia 120–121, 249
  causes 121
hypomagnesaemia 123
hyponatraemia 119
hypoparathyroidism 256, 258
hypophosphataemia 122
hypotension 139–140
  acute renal failure 224
  causes 139–140
  management/care 140
  poisoning causing 326
hypotensive shock 14
hypothalamus damage, hyperthermia,
      fanning/tepid sponging 97
hypothermia 97–100
  accidental 98
  inadvertent/intraoperative 98–99
  mild 97
  moderate 97–98
  postanaesthetic/postoperative 99
  rewarming methods 99–100
  severe/profound 98
  special care considerations 100
  temperature measurement 51

therapeutic 98–99
hypothyroidism 256–257
  aetiology 256–257
  clinical features 257
  investigations 257
  thyroid surgery complication 256
  treatment 257
hypovolaemia
  acute renal failure 224
  central venous pressure 54
  colloid therapy 125
  crystalloid therapy 125–126
  plasma osmolality 63
  pulmonary artery wedge pressure
      (PAWP) 55
  respiration patterns 45
  septic shock 15
  urine output changes 56
hypovolaemic shock 16–17
  causes 16
  compensatory mechanisms 17
hypoxaemia 165
  correction in COAD 163
hypoxia
  causes 47, 91
  determination 47, 50
  oxygen therapy 91

ibuprofen 316
ileitis, terminal 205
ileostomy 207–208
  uses/reasons for 208
immediate hypersensitivity 285
immobilization, uncomplicated fracture
      treatment 279–280
immune system 283–291
  ageing 285
  barriers to infections 284
immunity
  acquired 284
  innate 284
immunizations 111
immunocompromised patients,
      pneumonia 166
immunodeficiency diseases 289–291
immunosuppressives 324
  ulcerative colitis 204
impacted fracture 277–278
imperial measurements, conversions
      (SI/metric) 337–338

implementation, nursing process 24–25
implied consent 4
inadvertent therapeutic hypothermia, causes 99
incomplete fracture 277–278
incontinence, faecal 203
indirect monitoring, blood pressure 46–47
    potential errors 47
induced therapeutic hypothermia 98
infantile eczema 207
infants, temperature control 51
infection(s) 281
    fractures 281
    host barriers 284
    hyperthermia 96–97
    nervous system 245–247
    splenomegaly 180
infection control 111–117
    immunizations 111
    practices 112–117
    universal precautions 6–7
infiltrating carcinoma, pathogenesis 295
inflammation
    skin reaction to radiotherapy 300
    splenomegaly 180
inflammatory barriers, innate immunity 284
inflammatory bowel disorders 203–206
    see also Crohn's disease; ulcerative colitis
inflammatory disease
    joints 271–275
    nervous system 245–247
inflammatory immune response (IIR) 19–20
    systemic immune response syndrome 20
inflammatory joint disease 271–275
inflammatory phase, healing process 84
inflammatory response 284
informed consent 4, 8
infusion devices 128–130
    ambulatory 129–130
infusion pumps 129
inhalation, of drugs 313–314
inhalers 313–314
    asthma 160–161, 324
injections 314–315
    sites 314, 315
innate immunity 284
inotropes 324

inspiratory capacity (IC) 72
inspiratory reserve volume (IRV) 71
insulin
    administration 263
    analogues 262
    biphasic 263
    deficiency see diabetes mellitus
    diabetes mellitus, type I 262–263
    normal actions 260
    resistance 263
    soluble fast-acting 262
    types 262, 262–263
insulin-dependent diabetes mellitus (IDDM) see diabetes mellitus, type 1
interferon, multiple sclerosis 243
interferon beta-1a 243
intermediate surgery 305
intermittent continuous feeding, enteral feeding 135
internal fixation, uncomplicated fractures 280
internal rewarming, active 99–100
international system of units (SI) 335–337
    conversions (metric/imperial) 337–338
    factors/multiples of 336
interviewing patients 26–27
intestinal disorders 202–203
    see also entries beginning bowel
intraabdominal haemorrhage 201
intracellular fluid (ICF) 117
intracellular fluid (ICF) compartment 117, 118
intracranial pressure (ICP)
    elevated 34
    monitoring 55–56
    normal range 55
intracranial tumours 247–248
    clinical features 247–248
    investigations 248
    nursing care/management 248
    primary/secondary 247
intradermal injections 314
intramuscular injections 314, 315
intrapleural drainage 88–89
    complications 88
    important considerations 89
    uses 88
intrathecal injections 315
intravenous cholangiography 77

intravenous injections 314
  advantages/disadvantages 315
intrinsic asthma 159–160
intubation, endotracheal *see* endotracheal
      intubation
invasive carcinoma, cervical 299
investigations 56–81
iodine-containing contrast media 77
iodine therapy, radioactive 254
ionizing radiation, protection from
      75–76
ipecacuanna, syrup 328
ipratropium 323
iron deficiency anaemia 173–174
  causes 173
  treatment 173–174
ischaemia 140
  acute, legs 157
ischaemic heart disease (IHD) 138
isolation, infection control 112
isoniazid 168

jaundice 217
  pancreatic cancer 220
  types 217
jejunostomy tube, enteral feeding 134
Johns' model of structured reflection
      (1994) 11, *12*
joint diseases 266–283
  inflammatory 271–275
joint injuries
  dislocation 278
  fractures 283
joint stiffness 272, 283
junctional bradycardia 146
juvenile chronic arthritis 274

ketoacidosis, diabetic *see* diabetic
      ketoacidosis
ketone bodies 131, 262
ketones 262
  in urine 61, 262
ketosis, malnutrition-induced 131
Ketostix, ketones in urine 61
kidney
  functions 221–222
  stones 59, 223–224
  see also entries beginning renal
knowledge of clientele 28–30
Korotkoff sounds 46, *47*

lactic dehydrogenase (LDH) *66*, 67
  myocardial infarction 143
laparoscopy 80
large bowel
  endoscopy 80
  surgery, complications 209
large vessel disease, diabetes mellitus 266
laryngeal nerves, damage 256
laryngeal oedema 255, 285
laryngoscopy, direct 14
last offices, after death 110
lateral sclerosis, amyotrophic 243
late ventricular fibrillation 149
latex catheter, urinary catheterization 89
laxatives 191, 324
left heart failure 149–151
  acute, clinical features 149
  causes 149
  central venous pressure 54
  congestion in *150*
  nursing care/management 149–151
left ventricular failure (LVF) *see* left heart
      failure
legal issues 3–5
legs, acute ischaemia 157
leucocytosis 201
leukaemia 184–186
  acute lymphatic/lymphoblastic (ALL)
      184, 185
  acute myelogenous (AML) 184–185
  causal factors 184
  chronic lymphatic (CLL) 185, 186
  chronic myeloid/granulocytic (CML)
      185, 186
  classification 184–185
  diagnosis 184
  pathophysiology 185–186
  treatment 185–186
levodopa, Parkinson's disease 241
lichenification 286
lidocaine (lignocaine) 316, 319
  cardiac arrhythmias 144
life support
  advanced 13
  basic 12–13
light, pupil reactions 32–34
lignocaine *see* lidocaine (lignocaine)
linctus 311
linear analogue scale (LAS), anxiety 35
linen, infection control 115

liver, cirrhosis *see* cirrhosis of liver
liver disease 215–219
  clinical features 215
  complications 215–216
liver function tests (LFTs) 64
liver transplantation 219
liver tumours 216
  metastatic 216, 219
lobar pneumonia 166
localized anaphylaxis (atopy) 286
localized lymphadenopathy 188
localized peritonitis 200–201
log role 93
  procedure 93–94
lomustine 302
London Pain Chart 38
low blood pressure *see* hypotension
lower motor neurone lesions 234
low grade treatment, non-Hodgkin's
  lymphoma (NHL) 188
low molecular weight heparins (LMWHs)
  144
lumbar puncture 73–75
  contraindications 73–74
  patient positioning 74
  uses 73
lung
  abscess 168
  fibrosis, rheumatoid arthritis 273
  interstitial diseases 165
  pressure collapse 172
lung cancer 170–171
  clinical features 170
  investigations 170
  metastatic complications 170
  nursing care/management 170–171
lymphadenopathy 188
  generalized 188
  localized 188
  persistent generalized,
    AIDS/HIV-1 290
lymphatic system, breast cancer spread
  296
lymphomas 186–188
  Hodgkin's *see* Hodgkin's disease
  non-Hodgkin's *see* non-Hodgkin's
    lymphoma (NHL)

macrocytic anaemia 174
macronutrients 130

macrovascular disease, diabetes mellitus
  266
magnesium balance 122–123
magnetic resonance imaging (MRI) 79–80
major surgery 305
malaise, rheumatoid arthritis 273
malignant tumours 291
Mallory–Weiss tears, oesophageal
  bleeding 194
malnutrition 130–131
  physiological effects 131
  undernutrition 42–43
malunion, fractures 282
mammography 294
manipulative reduction, uncomplicated
  fractures 278
masks, infection control 114
maturation phase, healing process 84
measurement units 335–338
  conversions (SI/metric/imperial)
    337–338
  equivalents 337–338
  rules for writing 336
mechanical traction, fractures 278
medical asepsis 115
medication, administration 152–153
Medicinal Products: Prescription by
  Nurses Act (1992) 310, 345
Medicines Act (1968) 344–345
megacolon, toxic 204
melaena 189
melphalan 302
meningioma 248
meningitis 245–246
  bacterial causes 245–246
  clinical features 246
  diagnosis 246
  nursing care/management 246
  viral 246
meningococcal meningitis 245
meningococcal prophylaxis 246
mercaptopurine 303
mesenchyme, tumours 292
metabolic acidosis 58–59, 68
  ketones in urine 61
  malnutrition-induced 131
metabolic alkalosis 68
metabolic complications, parenteral
  nutrition delivery 134
metabolic defects 179

metal ions, oral drug interactions 312
metastases 291
 liver 216, 219
 prostate gland cancer 297
 tumours with 293
metastatic complications, lung cancer 170
methaemoglobinaemia 326
methotrexate 303
metric measurements, conversions
  (SI/imperial) 337–338
metronidazole 320
metyrapone 260
micronutrients 130
microvascular disease, diabetes mellitus
  266
mid-arm muscle circumference (MAMC)
  42
mid upper arm circumference (MUAC)
  42
mineralocorticoid release, stress response
  37
minor surgery 305
minute volume (MV), total 72
miotics 324–325
Misuse of Drugs Act (1971) 308–309,
  343–344
Misuse of Drugs Regulations (1985) 308
mitotic poisons 303
mixed tissue tumours 292
mixture drugs 311
mobilization 94
 right-sided heart failure 153
 stroke patients 155, 156
moderate hypothermia 97–98
moist desquamation, skin reaction to
  radiotherapy 300
monoamine oxidase inhibitors (MAOIs)
  321
monomorphic ventricular tachycardia 148
morphine 316, 317–318
 side-effects 316
motor disorders, stroke 154
motor neuron 232
motor neuron disease 232, 234, 243–244
 course 244
 progressive muscular atrophy 243
 treatment 244
mouth care 86–87
 nursing management 153
 palliative 108

moving and handling 5–6
 log role 93–94
 principles of safety 5–6
 risk assessment 5
 safety factors 5
MPTP, Parkinson's disease due to 239
MST Continuous 316, 317
mucous plug formation, tracheostomy
  82–83
multidisciplinary communication 2
multiple myeloma 188–189
 clinical features 188–189
 treatment 189
multiple sclerosis (MS) 241–243
 aetiology 241
 clinical features 242
 investigations 242
 prognosis 242
 treatment 242–243
multiple system organ failure (MSOF)
 inflammatory/immune response 20
 neuroendocrine response 19
muscle, Volkmann's ischaemic contracture
  282
muscle diseases 248–249
muscle mass index 42
muscle relaxants 325
muscular atrophy, progressive 243
myasthenia gravis 249
Mycobacterium tuberculosis 168–169
 drug-resistant 169
mydriatics 325
myelodysplastic syndromes 186
 leukaemia 186
myelofibrosis 180
myocardial infarction (MI) 142–149
 cardiac arrhythmias 144–149
  see also cardiac arrhythmias
 cardiac enzymes 65, *66*, 143
 clinical features 142
 inferior 146
 mortality rate 142
 nursing care/management 142–144
 'silent' 142
myopathies 248–249

naloxone 327
napkin dermatitis 287
nasal cannulae 91
nasoduodenal tube, enteral feeding 134

nasogastric tube, enteral feeding 134
National Institute for Clinical Excellence
    (NICE) 243
nebulized drugs 314
  asthma 161
needlestick injuries 289
neonatal poisoning 325
neoplasia 291
  cervical intraepithelial 299
neoplasms 291
nephropathy, diabetes mellitus 266
nephrotic syndrome 229
nerve injury, fractures 283
nervous system 230–249
  chronic renal failure 226–227
  thyrotoxicosis 253
  tumours 292
nervous tissue damage, clinical signs 232
neuroendocrine response
  multiple system organ failure 19
  trauma 18–19
neurogenic shock 16
neuroleptic drugs 322
neurological observations, Glasgow Coma
    Scale 34
neuromuscular disease, dysphagia 192
neuropathy
  diabetes mellitus 266
  rheumatoid arthritis 273
nipple, Paget's disease 295
nitrates, urine testing 60
nitrites, urine testing 60
nitrosurea 302
non-Hodgkin's lymphoma (NHL) 187–188
  clinical features 187–188
  treatment 188
non-insulin-dependent diabetes mellitus
    (NIDDM) 263–264
  see also diabetes mellitus
non-rapid eye movement sleep (NREM)
    102
non-steroidal antiinflammatory drugs
    (NSAIDs) 316
non-union, fractures 282
non-verbal communication 27
noradrenaline 19
normal saline, fluid overload 18
normal values 65, 339–341
  blood 65, 173, 339, 340–341
  cerebrospinal fluid 341

  faeces 341
  plasma 340–341
  urine 341
normotensive shock 14
nosocomial infection, prevention 113
notification, infection control 116
no-touch technique, infection control 114
numbers, rules for writing 336
numerical rating scales, pain assessment 37
nurse prescribers' extended formulary
    (NPEF) 311
nurse prescribers' formulary 310
nurses
  prescribing 310–311
  stress of caring for dying patients 111
nursing, barrier see barrier nursing
nursing care issues 81–100
nursing care/management, systems
    approach 137–306
nursing process 24–25
  steps 24–25
nutrition 130
  dietary reference values 130
  improving dietary intake 131–132
  Recommended Daily Amounts 130
nutritional assessment 40–43
  history taking 40–41
nutritional support 130–136
nystatin 321

observation
  non-verbal communication 27
  patient 26
observations and measurements
    43–56
obstructive jaundice, causes 217
odour, urine testing 61
oedema
  care/management 151–152
  cerebral 34, 219
  laryngeal 255, 285
  pulmonary see pulmonary oedema
  right heart failure 151
oesophageal varices 195, 215
  treatment 195
oesophagitis, reflux see reflux oesophagitis
oesophagogastroduodenoscopy (OGD) 80
oesophagus 191–195
  atresia 191
  bleeding 194

oesophagus (*cont'd*)
  obstruction, dysphagia 192
  tumours 194
oestrogen receptors 304
oliguria 222
  acute renal failure 225
oncology 291
open fractures *see* compound fractures
operative reduction, uncomplicated
        fractures 278–279
opioid analgesics 316–317
  side-effects 316, 318
oral complications, of treatments 86
oral glucose tolerance test 261
oral hygiene 86–87
  palliative care 108
organ donation, dying patients 109
  suitable/unsuitable donors 109
organization 1–22
  self 2–11
organ-specific autoimmune diseases *288*
orientation, nursing care/management
        152
osmolality, plasma 63
osteitis deformans 268–269
osteoarthritis (OA) 274–275, 283
  clinical features 275
  nursing care/management 275
  primary/secondary 274
osteomalacia, adults 268
osteomyelitis 269, *269*
osteoporosis 267–268
  aetiology 267
  clinical features 267
  investigations 267
  treatment/prevention 267–268
osteosarcomas 270
ovarian cancer 298
overdose, paracetamol, fulminant hepatic
        failure 218
overfeeding, enteral feeding 135–136
oxygen
  partial pressure (PO_2) 50, 67
  preoxygenation before suctioning of
        tracheostomy 81–82
  saturation measurement 47, 50
    pulse oximetry 72–73
  toxicity 91
oxygen dissociation curve 50
oxygen mask 91

oxygen therapy 91–92
  in COAD 162
  humidification 92

packed cell volume (PCV) 173
packed red cells, blood transfusion
        therapy 126
Paget's disease of bone 268–269
Paget's disease of nipple 295
pain 37–38
  assessment tools 37–38
  relief *see* analgesics
  undertreatment, effects 38
painful stimulus, Glasgow Coma Scale 32
palliative care
  analgesics 317–318
  general principles/procedures 107–108
pancreas 219–222
pancreatic cancer 220
pancreatitis 219–220
  acute 219–220
    clinical features 219
    hyperglycaemia 60
    nursing care/management 219–220
  chronic 220
papilloedema 232
paracentesis, abdominal 87–88
paracetamol 316
  overdose, fulminant hepatic failure 218,
        219
para-oesophageal hernia 193–194
parasympathetic nervous system 31
parathormone (PTH) 257
parathyroid glands 257–258
parenteral nutrition (PN) 132–134
  administration routes 133
  complications 133–134
  delivery 133
  indications 132
  management 133
  regimes 133
  septic shock risk 15
  solution 133
Parkinson's disease 237–241
  aetiology 238–239
  clinical features *238*, 239–240
  common problems 240–241
  drug treatment 241
Park's pouch 208
partial gastrectomy, side-effects 198

partial seizures *21*, 237
partial thyroidectomy 255
passive external rewarming 99
pathological fractures 276
patient-controlled analgesia (PCA) 129
patients
  anxiety 34
  assessment/investigation 23–100
  communication with *see*
    communication
  complaints 3–4
  explanations on barrier nursing
    112–113
  goal setting involvement 25
  hygiene, infection control 116–117
  identification of problems 24–30
  interviewing 26–27
  lumbar puncture positioning 74
  moving and handling 5–6
  moving/handling *see* moving and
    handling
  observation 26
  personal hygiene *see* personal hygiene
  preoperative care participation 104
  property 3
  refusal of treatment 4–5
peak expiratory flow (PEF) rate 72, 160
peau d'orange 295
pelvis, radiotherapy side-effects 301
penicillin 319
penicillin G 319
peptic ulcers 195, 197–199
  aetiology 197
  chronic 198–199
  clinical features 197
  complications 198–199
  investigations 197
  perforation 198
  surgery 198
  treatment 197, 198–199
  Zollinger–Ellison syndrome 197
percutaneous cholangiography 213
percutaneous endoscopically guided
    gastrostomy (PEG) 134
percutaneous transhepatic
    cholangiography (PTC) 77
pericarditis, rheumatoid arthritis 273
perioperative care, general
    principles/procedures 105
peripheral nerves, lesions 232

peripheral painful stimulus, Glasgow
    Coma Scale 32
peripheral pulses 44–45
peripheral resistance, reduced,
    hypotension due to 140
peripheral vascular disease 157
peritoneal dialysis 228
peritonitis 200–201
  appendicitis leading to 210, 211
  common causes 200–201
  generalized 201, 211
  localized 200–201, 211
  treatment 201
pernicious anaemia 174–175
  clinical features 174–175
  investigations 175
  treatment 175
persistent generalized lymphadenopathy,
    AIDS/HIV-1 290
personal food plan 131–132
personal hygiene
  infection control 116–117
  right-sided heart failure 153
  stroke patients 155, 156
pH blood 67, 123
  urine 58–59
phaeochromocytoma 260
phagocytic barriers, innate immunity
    284
pharmacology 307–329
  practical aspects 311–315
phenothiazines, parkinsonism 239
phenytoin, blood analysis 65
phosphorus balance 122
photophobia 236
photosensitivity 319
physical examination, nutritional
    assessment 41
physiological barriers, innate immunity
    284
'pill-rolling' movement *238*, 239
pink puffers 162
pituitary function disruption,
    chemotherapy 304
pituitary gland 249–251
  posterior, diseases 249–251
pituitary hormones 249, *250*
pituitary tumours 250–251
  diagnosis 251
  growth hormone hypersecretion 251

pituitary tumours (*cont'd*)
  local effects 251
  overproduction type 250–251
  treatment 251
  underproduction type 251
planned assessment, patients 31
planning, nursing process 24
plasma
  loss 125
  normal values *340–341*
  osmolality 63
plaster of Paris
  restricted circulation 279–280
  uncomplicated fractures 279–280
    observation 279–280
plateau stage, pyrexia 94–95
platelets 181–183
  normal count 181
  overproduction/excess 181
  reduced number 181
playing, stroke patients continued care
    156
pleura, conditions affecting 171
pleural cavity, drainage *see* intrapleural
    drainage
pleural effusion 151, 171
  causes 171
  clinical features 171
pleurisy
  dry 169
  fibrinous, rheumatoid arthritis 273
pneumonia 165–168
  aspiration 166
  bacteria causing 166
  characteristics 165–166
  immunocompromised patients 166
  nursing care/management 166–168
  primary/secondary *167*
pneumothorax 171–172
  causes 171–172
  clinical features 172
  nursing care/management 172
  tension 172
poisoning 325–329
  accidental 325
  adult 325
  antidotes 327
  deliberate self 326–327
  elimination increase after 329
  information services 327–328

minimizing absorption 328–329
  patient management 327
  screening 327
  TOXBASE website 328
polycythaemia 179–180
polycythaemia rubra vera 179–180
polymorphic ventricular tachycardia 148
polyps, colorectal 209
porphyria 221
portal hypertension 180–181, 195
  splenectomy 180–181
portosystemic encephalopathy 216
positioning of patients 93–94
  lumbar puncture 74
postanaesthesia therapeutic hypothermia
    99
posterior pituitary gland, diseases
    249–250
postoperative care 106–107
  special nursing considerations 106–107
postoperative complications 106
postoperative therapeutic hypothermia
    99
postural instability, Parkinson's disease
    240
posture, for handling patients 5–6
potassium balance 120–121
Pott's fracture 278
precautions, universal 6–7
prednisolone, COAD 164
pregnancy, X-ray contact avoidance 76
preoperative care
  general principles/procedures 104–105
  patient participation 104
  screening 104–105
  subtotal thyroidectomy 255
preoxygenation, suctioning 81
pressure collapse, lung *172*
pressure sores
  pathogenesis 38
  predisposing factors 39
  risk assessment 38–39
primary biliary cirrhosis 216
primary hypoadrenalism 259
primary intention, healing process 84
primary pneumonia *167*
primary polycythaemia 179–180
primary ventricular fibrillation 149
procedures 56–81, 101–136
  fluid/electrolyte balance 117–130

general principles 102–111
infection control 111–117
nutritional support 130–136
proctitis 204
professional issues 7–11
accountability 7
advocacy 9–10
autonomy 8–9
clinical supervision 10–11
code of practice 10
confidentiality 9
reflective practice 11
responsibility 7–8
see also individual issues
progressive bulbar palsy 244
progressive muscular atrophy 243
property (patient's) 3
propranolol 323
prostate gland cancer 296–297
clinical features 296–297
investigations 297
metastatic disease 297
risk factors 296
treatment 297
protection, ionizing radiation 75–76
protective clothing, infection control 114
protective isolation, infection control 112
proteinuria 59, 221
pseudoseizures 237
psychological disturbances 28–29
psychological preparation
bowel surgery 208–209
stomas 208
psychological status, nutritional
assessment 40–41
pulmonary artery wedge pressure
(PAWP) 54–55
measurements 55
normal 55
pulmonary disorders, chronic 72, *165*
obstructive 72, *165*
restrictive 72, *165*
pulmonary embolism (PE) 169
clinical features 169
DVT as cause 169
end-tidal CO_2 69
nursing care/management 149–150,
169
pulmonary hygiene, tracheostomy care 81
pulmonary oedema *165*

clinical features 149
left heart failure as cause 149
poisonings 326
pulmonary tuberculosis 168–169
clinical features 168
drug therapy 168–169
nursing care/management 168
pulse deficit 44
pulse oximetry 72–73
pulse pressure 44
pulse rate 43–45
irregular 44
normal 43
pulses 43, 44–45
pump-assisted feeding, enteral feeding
135
pupils
changes, deliberate self-poisoning 327
size and reaction to light, Glasgow
Coma Scale 32–34, *34*
purine antagonists 303
Purkinje fibres 43, 69
pyelonephritis 222
pyloric stenosis 199
pyrexia 94–96
beneficial effects 95
detrimental effects 95–96
management 96–97
stages 94–95
pyrimidine antagonists 303

Queckenstedt's test 74–75

radial pulse rate 43
radiation therapy 75
radioactive iodine therapy 254
radiography (X-rays) 75–80
angiography 77–78
avoidance in pregnancy 76
biliary contrast 77
contrast media 76–77
protection from ionizing radiation
75–76
radioisotope scanning 79
radiolucent materials 75
radioopaque materials 75
radiotherapy 299–301
administration 300
dosage determination 300
side-effects 300–301

rapid eye movement sleep (REM) 102
reagent test strips
  glycosuria 61
  haematuria 59
  ketones in urine 61
  proteinuria 59
  urine specific gravity 58
Recommended Daily Amounts (RDA),
      nutrition 130
rectally administered drugs *see*
      suppositories
rectal temperature 50
recurrent laryngeal nerve, damage 256
red blood cells (RBCs) 172–180
  membrane defects 176–177
      treatment 177
  transfusion 126
red cell count (RCC) 173
reduction, fracture treatment 278–279
reflective practice 11
  Gibbs reflective cycle (1988) 11, *11*
  Johns' model of structured reflection
      (1994) 11, *12*
reflux oesophagitis 192–193
  clinical features 193
  drugs 193
  treatment 193
refractory shock 14
refusal of treatment 4–5, 28
regenerative phase, healing process 84
rehabilitation, fractures 281
religious issues 28
renal calculi *see* renal stones
renal cell carcinoma 230
renal colic 223–224
  clinical features 223
  nursing care/management 223–224
renal failure
  acute 224–226
    causes 224–225
    clinical features 225
    nursing care/management 225–226
  chronic 226–227
    causes 226
    clinical features 226–227
    nursing care/management 227
  end-stage 227–228
renal function 221–222
renal osteodystrophy 226
renal pelvis, transitional cell carcinoma 230

renal replacement therapy 227–228
renal stones 59, 223–224
  clinical features 223
  nursing care/management 223–224
renal system 221–230
renal transplantation 228
renal vasoconstriction, acute renal failure
      224
reperfusional ventricular fibrillation 149
residual volume (RV) 71
resistance, stress response 35–36
respiration 45
  depth 45
  Glasgow Coma Scale 34
  pattern 45
  rate 45
  see also breathing
respiratory acidosis 68
respiratory alkalosis 68
respiratory failure 165
  classification of causes *165*
respiratory features, deliberate self-
      poisoning 326
respiratory investigations 71–72
respiratory system 159–172
  thyrotoxicosis 253
responsibility 7–8
  to others 7
  professional 7–8
  for self 7
rest, promotion 102
restricted circulation, clinical features
      279–280
resuscitation, AABC 12
retention catheter 89–90
reticuloendothelial system, tumours 292
retinopathy, diabetes mellitus 266
rewarming methods 99–100
  active external 99–100
  active internal 100
  passive 99
Reye's syndrome 322
rheumatoid arthritis 271–274
  aetiology 272
  clinical features 272–273
  drug treatment 274
  incidence 271–272
  investigations 273–274
  joints affected *271*
  nursing care/management 274

rheumatoid factor 272
rickets, childhood 268
rifampicin 168
right-sided heart failure 151–153
  care/management 151–153
  clinical features 151
  congestion in *150*
  nursing principles 153
rigidity, Parkinson's disease 239
rimeterol 160
risk assessment
  moving and handling 5
  pressure sores 38–39
rolling hernia 193–194
Royal Marsden Manual of Clinical Nursing
    Procedures (2000) 116
rt-PA (alteplase), myocardial infarction 143

safety issues 3–5
  nursing management 154–155, *155*
salbutamol 160, 323
  nebulized 161
saline, normal, fluid overload 18
sarcoma 292
  Ewing's 270–271
scalp, radiotherapy side-effects 301
schedule 1 drugs 308
schedule 2 drugs 308
schedule 3 drugs 308
schedule 4 drugs 308
schedule 5 drugs 309
screening
  breast cancer 294
  poisoning 327
  preoperative 104–105
seborrhoeic dermatitis 287
secondary hypertension 138
secondary intention, healing process 84
secondary pneumonia *167*
secondary ventricular fibrillation 149
secretions, mobilization, tracheostomy
    care 81
seizures 20–22, 236
  causes 237
  generalized *21*, 237
  partial *21*, 237
  precipitating factors 22
  treatment 22
  types 20, *21*, 237
  see also convulsions; epilepsy

selective serotonin reuptake inhibitors
    (SSRIs) 321
selegeline, Parkinson's disease 241
self-discharge 5
self-organization 2–11
self-poisoning, deliberate 326–327
self-responsibility 7
Sengstaken–Blakemore tube 195, 216
sensory disorders, stroke 154
septic shock 15–16
  causes 15
  clinical features 15–16
seroconversion illness, AIDS/
    HIV-1 290
serum biochemistry *65*
serum proteins, levels 64
severe hypothermia 98
shock 14–17
  anaphylactic 15
  cardiogenic 16
  causes 14
  hypovolaemic 16–17
  multiple forms 17
  neurogenic 16
  septic 15–16
  stages 14
shortening, fractures 282
sickle cell crisis
  clinical features 178
  treatment 178–179
sickle cell disease, clinical features 178
sickle cell syndromes 178–179
sickle cell trait, clinical features 178
sigmoid colostomy 206, *207*
Silastic, urinary catheterization 89
silicone, urinary catheterization 89
simple fractures 276, *276*
  treatment 278–280
single-use chemical thermometers 51
sinoatrial node 43, 69, 70
  bradycardia 146
sinus arrhythmia, pulse rate 43
sinus bradycardia 146
  causes 146
sinus rhythm 146, *147*
sinus tachycardia 147
skin
  care, in right heart failure 152
  chronic renal failure 226
  functions 83–84

skin (cont'd)
  lichenification 286
  microflora 113
  reactions to radiotherapy 300–301
  structure 83
  temperature 52
  testing 286
  thyrotoxicosis 253
  xeroderma 287
skinfold thickness measurements,
    nutritional assessment 42
skin-tunnelled catheter, parenteral
    nutrition delivery 133
skip lesions 206
skull fractures 234, 235
sleep
  minimizing interruptions 103
  paradoxical 102
  promotion 102
  right-sided heart failure 153
  stroke patients, continued care 157
sleep cycles 102
sleep deprivation 102
sliding hiatus hernia 193
  management 194
slow release (SR) drugs 311
small vessel disease, diabetes mellitus 266
soap and water, hand washing 113
social needs 108
social status
  effect on patient recovery 29–30
  nutritional assessment 40–41
sodium balance 119–120
specialist infusion pumps 129–130
specific gravity (SG), urine 58
specimen, collection/sending 56–57
spherocytosis, hereditary 176
sphygmomanometers, blood pressure
    measurement 46
spider naevi 215
spinal cord, lesions 232, 234
spiritual care 108
spleen 180–181
splenectomy, portal hypertension
    180–181
splenomegaly 180
  causes 180
  rheumatoid arthritis 273
spongiosis 286
sputum, bronchiectasis 164

squamous cell carcinoma, oesophageal
    194
stable angina, management 141
staff allocation, infection control 116
staging
  breast cancer 296
  Hodgkin's disease 187
Standards for the Administration of
    Drugs (UKCC, 1992) 309
Staphylococcus aureus 287
starvation, physiological effects 131
status epilepticus 237
steatorrhoea 189, 212
sterile asepsis 115–116
steroid inhalers, asthma 160
Still's disease 274
stoma(s) 206–210
  early complications 208
  psychological preparation 208
  types 206–208
stomach 195–200
  carcinoma 199–200
    clinical features 199–200
    treatment 200
  emptying, poisoning 328
  haemorrhage 199
stored blood products, changes 126, 127
strangulation of bowel 202
streptokinase, myocardial infarction 143
stress 35–37
  hyperglycaemia 60
  management 27
  to nurses, of caring for dying patients
    111
  physiological responses 36–37
stress fractures 276
stressors 35, 36
stroke 153–157
  clinical features 154
  continuing care/rehabilitation 155–157
  initial management 154–155
  predisposing factors 154
stroke volume 44
subarachnoid bleeding, traumatic 236
subarachnoid haemorrhage (SAH) 236
subcutaneous injections 314, 314
subcutaneous nodules, rheumatoid
    arthritis 272–273
subdural bolt, intracranial pressure
    monitoring 56

subdural catheter, intracranial pressure monitoring 56
subdural haematoma 235, *235*
sublingual drugs 312
sublingual temperature 50
subtotal thyroidectomy 254–255
sucralfate 198
suctioning
 tracheostomy *see* tracheostomy care
 wound drainage 85
sulphasalazine 204
supervision, clinical 10–11
suppositories 312–313
 examples and uses 313
surgery 305–306
 angina pectoris 141–142
 complications 306, *306*
 hyperthyroidism 254–255
surgical asepsis 115–116
Swan–Ganz catheter 54
sympathetic nervous system 31
 stimulation in trauma 19
symptom control, general principles/procedures 107–108
synthetic blood products, blood transfusion therapy 126, 128
syringe infusion pumps 129
syrup of ipecacuanna, poisoning 328
systemic autoimmune diseases 287
systemic immune response syndrome (SIRS) 20
systemic lupus erythematosus (SLE) 221, 287
systems approach to nursing 137–306
systolic blood pressure 46

tablets 311
tachycardia 146–147
 accelerated idioventricular 148
 atrial 147
 causes 70
 narrow complex 147
 poisoning causing 326
 pulse rate 43
 sinus 147
 ventricular 148
tachypnoea 45
tamoxifen 304
taxanes 303
teamwork 2–3

temperature (body) 50–52
 circulatory effects 50
 elevated 34
  fluid loss 125
  see also hyperthermia; pyrexia
 Glasgow Coma Scale 34
 infants/elderly patients 51
 measurement 50–51
 reduced *see* hypothermia
 skin 52
 toe 52
tendon injuries, fractures 283
tensilon test 249
tension pneumothorax 172
tepid sponging, hyperthermia 96–97
teratomas 292
terfenadine 322
terminal ileitis 205
tertiary intention, healing process 84
testicular cancer 297–298
 clinical features 297
 investigations 297–298
 treatment 298
tetany, hypoparathyroidism 258
tetracycline 312
thalassaemia 177–178
 treatment 177–178
α-thalassaemia 177
β-thalassaemia 177
thalassaemia minor 177
thalassaemia trait 177
therapeutic drug monitoring 65
therapeutic hypothermia 98–99
thermodilution pulmonary artery catheter 54
thermometers 51
thioguanine 303
third space fluid shift 125
thrombocythaemia, essential 181
thrombocytopenia 181, 306
thrombolytic drugs 324
 myocardial infarction 143
thrombosis 183
 arterial 183
 deep vein *see* deep vein thrombosis (DVT)
 risk factors *184*
 venous 183
thrombus 142
thyroid cancer 256
 types *256*

thyroidectomy 256
  partial 255
  subtotal 254–255
thyroid function tests 253, *253*
thyroid gland 251–257
  goitre 252
thyroiditis, autoimmune 256
thyroid surgery
  complications 255–256
  see also thyroidectomy
thyrotoxic crisis 255
thyrotoxicosis 252–256
  causes 252
  clinical features *252*, 252–253
  diagnosis 253–254
  treatment 254–256
thyroxine 257
tidal volume (TV) 13, 71
tiredness, radiotherapy 301
tissue plasminogen activator (t-PA),
  recombinant 143
tissue-specific agents 304
tissue typing 288
T lymphocytes 284
  helper cells in AIDS 290
toe temperature 52
topical drugs 313
torsades de pointes 148
total body water 117
total lung capacity (TLC) 71–72
total minute volume (MV) 72
TOXBASE, website 328
toxic megacolon 204
tracheo-oesophageal fistula 191
tracheostomy care 81–83
  complication prevention 82–83
  humidity 81
  mucous plug formation 82–83
  secretions mobilization 81
  special care considerations 83
  suctioning 81–82
    preoxygenation 81
    procedure 82
traction, fractures 278, 280
transdermal drug administration 313
transferrin, serum, nutritional assessment
  42
transfers, general principles/procedures
  103–104
transient ischaemic attack (TIA) 153–154

transitional cell carcinoma
  renal pelvis 230
  ureter 230
transplantation, renal, end-stage renal
  failure 228
transverse loop colostomy 206, *207*
trapezium squeeze 32
trauma 18–20
  fractures due to 275–276
  immediate interventions 20
  nervous system 234–236
  neuroendocrine response 18–19
  subarachnoid bleeding 236
treatment refusal 4–5, 28
tremor, Parkinson's disease 239
triceps skinfold thickness (TSF) 42
tricyclic antidepressants 321
trimethoprim 320
triple therapy, one week regimen *196*
troponins (Tn) 67, *67*
Trousseau's sign 258
tuberculosis, pulmonary *see* pulmonary
  tuberculosis
tubular necrosis, acute, acute renal failure
  224
tumours
  age-related incidence 293
  benign/malignant 291
  bone 269–271
  epithelial 291–292
  intracranial 247–248
  mesenchymal 292
  mixed tissue 292
  naming 291–292
  nervous system 292
  pathogenesis 293
  reticuloendothelial system 292
  spread 293–294
  urological 230
  see also individual organs/types
tympanic membrane thermometer
  51
UKCC Code of Professional conduct 10
UKCC Standards for the Administration
  of Drugs (1992) 309
ulcerative colitis 203–204
  clinical features 203–204
  investigations 204
  treatment 204
ultrasound 78

limiting factors 78
principles and uses 78
uncomplicated fractures *see* simple fractures
unconsciousness 92 93
causes 92
special care considerations 92–93
undernutrition 42–43
understanding elderly patients 30
United Kingdom Prospective Diabetes Survey (UKPDS), type 2 diabetes 264
units of measurement 335–338
conversions (SI/metric/imperial) 337–338
equivalents 337–338
rules for writing 336
universal precautions 6–7
unstable angina 141
upper motor neurone lesions *234*
uraemia 222
urea, normal blood levels 64, 222
ureter, transitional cell carcinoma 230
ureteroscopy 80
urethral syndrome 223
urinary catheterization 89–91
procedure, females 90
urinary retention 90
urinary stasis 222
urinary tract infection (UTI) 222–223
causative organisms 222
clinical features 222–223
lower tract 222–223
nursing care/management 223
predisposing factors 222
upper tract 223
urine testing 60
urine
appearance 61, 221
bilirubin and urobilinogen 60
blood in 59, 221
discoloured 221
glucose 60–61, 221
infection control 115
ketones 61
nitrates and nitrites 60
normal values *341*
odour 61
output 56
pH 58–59

protein 59, 221
reduced output 221–222
specific gravity 58
testing 57–61
urobilinogen, in urine 60
urological tumours 230

vaccines 325
vacuum-assisted wound closure (VAC) system 86
vaginal pessaries/creams 313
vagotomy, highly selective 198
Valium 323
vancomycin 320
varices, oesophageal 195, 215
vasculitis, rheumatoid arthritis 273
vasodilatation, acute renal failure 224
venous thrombosis 183
ventilation 45
ventricular arrhythmias 148–149
advanced life support guidelines 13
ventricular ectopic beats 148
ventricular fibrillation (VF) 144, *144*, 148–149
hyperkalaemia causing 120
ventricular flutter 148
ventricular standstill 146
ventricular tachycardias 148
ventriculostomy, intracranial pressure monitoring 56
verapamil, cardiac arrhythmias 144
verbal consent 4
verbal rating scales, pain assessment 37
vertebral fractures 267
vinblastine 303
vinca alkaloids 303
vincristine 303
violence 6
management principles 6
viral encephalitis, acute 246
viral hepatitis, acute 217–218
viral meningitis 246
visceral injury, fractures 283
visitors, explanations on barrier nursing 112–113
visual analogue scale (VAS)
anxiety 35
pain assessment 37
visual problems, multiple sclerosis 242
vital capacity (VC) 72

vital signs, Glasgow Coma Scale 34
vitamin B$_{12}$ deficiency, anaemia 174
vitamin D deficiency 268
  treatment 268
vitamin K 217
vitamin K deficiency 182, 212
  causes 182
Volkmann's ischaemic contracture of
    muscle 282
volumetric infusion pumps 129
voluntary muscle, diseases 248–249
vomiting 189–190
  causes 189–190
    bowel obstruction 202
    gastrointestinal disease 189
  infection control 115
  nursing care/management 190
  projectile 199
von Willebrand's disease 182

warfarin 321
  pulmonary embolism 169
waste material, infection control 115
water, total body 117
Waterlow Scale, pressure sore risk
    assessment 39

water manometer 52, 53
weight, nutritional assessment 41
white blood cells 184–186
  acquired/innate immunity 284
whole blood loss 125
working, stroke patients, continued care
    156
wound(s)
  assessment 39, 40
  drainage 84–85
  dressings see dressings
  fungating, palliative care 108
wound care 83–86
  healing process and phases 84
  open (compound) fractures 280
  tracheostomy 82
written consent 4

xeroderma 287
X-ray machines 75, 76
X-rays 75
  see also radiography (X-rays)

zidovudine 291, 323
Zollinger–Ellison syndrome 197

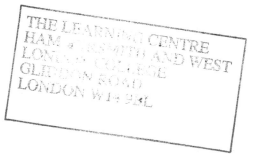